Department
of Health

Reference Guide to the Mental Health Act 1983

GRAN*G/S* UK Publishing

Adapted and Published by GRANGIS (Grand Register Library).
Online: www.grangis.com.
E-mail: contact@grangis.com.

In this version:
ISBN: 979-8-88559-079-2
Photos and paint not included in this version.

Note: Title, sub-title and version of this publication is as described. For the most recent information please visit www.gov.uk.

Introduction

Using the Act

Chapter 1

The Mental Health Act 1983 – the structure of the Act and definitions

Protecting patients' rights and autonomy

Chapter 2

The nearest relative

Assessment, transport and admission to hospital

Chapter 16
Hospital and limitation directions

Chapter 17
Committal to Crown Court for restriction order

Chapter 18
Interim hospital orders

Chapter 19
Transfer of sentenced prisoners to hospital

Chapter 20
Transfer of unsentenced prisoners to hospital

Chapter 21
Restricted patients

Chapter 22
Other legislation under which part 3 remands, orders and directions may be made

Care, support and treatment in hospital

Chapter 23
Medical treatment

Chapter 24
Medical treatment of CTO patients (part 4a)

Leaving hospital

Chapter 25

Leaving hospital (planned discharge and absence without leave)

Chapter 26

Community treatment orders

Chapter 27
Discharge

Chapter 28
Guardianship

Chapter 35
Transfer of patients to Scotland

Chapter 36
Transfer of patients to Northern Ireland

Chapter 37
Transfer to the Isle of Man or the Channel Islands

Chapter 38
Removal of foreign patients

Annexes

List of figures

Introduction

Using the Act

Chapter 1

Protecting patients' rights and autonomy

Chapter 2–6

Assessment, transport and admission to hospital

Chapter 7–11

Additional considerations for specific patients

Chapter 12–22

Care, support and treatment in hospital

Chapter 23–24

Leaving hospital

Chapter 25–29

Professional responsibilities

Chapter 30–33

Acknowledgement

'The artwork on the front cover is 'Missed' by Chris Ridge, the overall winner of our competition for artwork for the Code of Practice. 'Missed' illustrates the benefits of art therapy for people with mental health problems.'

Introduction

i. The Code of Practice and this Reference Guide should be used together to provide statutory guidance (the Code of Practice) and an explanation of the provisions of the Mental Health Act 1983 (the Act).

ii. There are a small number of clarifications to the Code of Practice and these are listed in Figure 1 at the end of this Introduction.

Presentation and content

iii. The Reference Guide is divided into 38 chapters with five annexes. Chapters have been grouped into eight clusters relating to common themes and topics. Colour coding has been used so these groups can be recognised. Comprehensive cross-referencing and annexes have been included to ensure that users can readily find related material. The eight clusters reflect the sections of the Code of Practice. The groupings are summarised below.

Using the Act: chapter 1
The chapter in this section describes the structure of the Act and provides basic definitions for the terms used in the Act.

Protecting patients' rights and autonomy: chapters 2-6
This group of chapters addresses the issues of particular importance for empowering patients, carers, nearest relatives and others with a legitimate interest in matters relating to care and treatment under the Act. It provides guidance on the nearest relatives including the identification and appointment of an acting nearest relative by the court. It also describes the role and activities of independent mental health advocates and the roles of the Care Quality Commission and the Tribunal. The limited circumstances in which correspondence to or from patients may be withheld are explained.

Assessment, transport and admission to hospital: chapters 7-11
This group of chapters is concerned with the ways in which civil (part 2) patients may be admitted to hospital, the circumstances in which patients may be transferred between hospitals if that becomes necessary as part of their care and treatment and how patients who are absent without leave may be returned.

Additional considerations for specific patients: chapters 12-22
Certain groups of patients require consideration in addition to the general guidance that applies to all patients. These chapters set out how the Act regards three specific groups of patients – those under 18 years of age, informal patients (ie those who are not detained under the Act and are receiving treatment voluntarily), and patients who have been referred to hospital after coming into contact with the criminal justice system (part 3 patients). Part 3 patients may be sent to hospital by the courts or be transferred from prison or other forms of custody, eg immigration removal centres.

Care, support and treatment in hospital: chapters 23-24
These chapters describe the provisions of the Act dealing with medical treatment for mental disorder. These provisions primarily apply to people who are liable to be detained in hospital or who are community treatment order (CTO) patients. Some provisions apply to all mental health patients, regardless of whether they are, or could be, detained under the Act.

Leaving hospital: chapters 25-29
Patients who leave hospital may be fully discharged or allowed on temporary leave under section 17 of the Act, placed under guardianship or be discharged onto a CTO. Patients on section 17 leave remain liable to be detained under the Act and patients subject to a CTO may be recalled to hospital for further medical treatment if necessary.

The Secretary of State for Justice may conditionally discharge a restricted patient at any time, by issuing a warrant to that effect and in certain circumstances restricted patients may be conditionally discharged by the Tribunal.

Where patients are placed under guardianship the guardian may be a local authority or a private individual.

The Act requires clinical commissioning groups and local authorities to arrange after-care for certain patients who have been detained for treatment under the Act to help their re-integration into the community. This after-care must meet a need arising from or related to the person's mental disorder and have the purpose of reducing the risk of a deterioration of the person's mental condition.

Professional responsibilities: chapters 30-33
The responsibilities and obligations of mental health professionals and hospital managers under the Act are set out in relation to:

- patients
- the nearest relative, and (on occasion)
- victims.

The provisions in the Act relating to the approval of approved mental health professionals (AMHP), doctors approved under the Act as having special experience in the diagnosis or treatment of mental disorder, and approved clinicians are included.

The chapter on hospital managers and the Act covers how the Act defines hospital managers, the functions of hospital managers, how hospital managers' functions may be delegated and the scrutiny of documents and the rectification of errors.

Under the Domestic Violence, Crime and Victims Act 2004[1] (DVCVA), victims of serious violent and sexual offences have the right to receive certain information about key stages in a part 3 patient's progress and treatment.

---

[1] Domestic Violence, Crime and Victims Act 2004. http://www.legislation.gov.uk/ukpga/2004/28

The chapter on offences describes the specific offences created by the Act, and the provisions which protect people who undertake actions under, or purporting to be under, the Act.

Transfer of patients between jurisdictions: chapters 34-38
On occasions it is necessary to transfer patients to different parts of the United Kingdom, the Channel Islands or the Isle of Man or abroad. These chapters look at the provisions within the Act which govern whether, and if so how, this may be done. Transfers between England and Wales are included in chapter 10.

References to legislation

iv. When this Reference Guide refers to parts, sections or schedules, it means sections or schedules of the Act itself, unless otherwise specified. When it refers to secondary legislation under the Act it means the following:

The HGT Regulations (or HGT Regulation X or Y)	The Mental Health (Hospital, Guardianship and Treatment) (England) Regulations 2008 (No. 1184)[2]
The AMHP Regulations	The Mental Health (Approved Mental Health Professionals) (Approval) (England) Regulations 2008 (No. 1206)[3]
The Conflict of Interest Regulations	The Mental Health (Conflicts of Interest) (England) Regulations 2008 (No. 1205)[4]
The Mutual Recognition Regulations	The Mental Health (Mutual Recognition) Regulations 2008 (No. 1204)[5]
The Nurses Order	Mental Health (Nurses) (England) Order 2008 (No. 1207)[6]
The Standing Rules	The National Health Service Commissioning Board and Clinical Commissioning Groups (Responsibilities and Standing Rules) Regulations 2012 (No. 2996)[7]

Figure 1: Clarifications of the Mental Health Act 1983: Code of Practice 2015

[2] The Mental Health (Hospital, Guardianship and Treatment) (England) Regulations. 2008 SI 2008/1184. http://www.legislation.gov.uk/uksi/2008/1184/pdfs/uksi_20081184_en.pdf
[3] The Mental Health (Approved Mental Health Professionals) (Approval) (England) Regulations. SI 2008/1206. http://www.legislation.gov.uk/uksi/2008/1206/pdfs/uksi_20081206_en.pdf
[4] The Mental Health (Conflicts of Interest) (England) Regulations. SI 2008/1205. http://www.legislation.gov.uk/uksi/2008/1205/pdfs/uksi_20081205_en.pdf
[5] The Mental Health (Mutual Recognition) Regulations. SI 2008/1204. http://www.legislation.gov.uk/uksi/2008/1204
[6] Mental Health (Nurses) (England) Order. SI 2008/1207. http://www.legislation.gov.uk/uksi/2008/1207
[7] The National Health Service Commissioning Board and Clinical Commissioning Groups (Responsibilities and Standing Rules) Regulations. SI 2012/2996. http://www.legislation.gov.uk/uksi/2012/2996

Code of Practice paragraph	Clarification
12.30 It is important that the patient's responsible clinician/s attend the Tribunal, supported by other staff involved in the patient's care, where appropriate, as their evidence is crucial for making the case for a patient's continued detention or CTO under the Act. Wherever possible the responsible clinician, and other relevant staff, should attend for the full hearing so that they are aware of all the evidence made available to the Tribunal and the Tribunal's decision and reasons.	The 'where appropriate' in the first sentence refers to 'other staff' rather than the responsible clinician.
15.16 It should also be borne in mind that a person who is removed to a place of safety may already be on a community treatment order (CTO) (chapter 29), conditional discharge (chapter 22) or leave of absence (chapter 27), or might be absent without leave (chapter 28) and that they may need to be recalled or returned to hospital. If it becomes apparent that this is the case, the professionals assessing the patient should make an effort to contact the patient's responsible clinician as soon as possible. 15.17 Where the person is known to be on a CTO and compulsory admission is indicated, the recall power should be used (see chapter 29). An application for detention should not be made in respect of a person who is known to be on a CTO.	These two paragraphs should be read in conjunction with chapter 16. They update paragraphs 10.54 and 10.55 in the 2008 Code and could have been located in new chapter 16 'Police powers and places of safety'.

<table>
<tr>
<td>29.46 The responsible clinician may recall a patient on a CTO to hospital for treatment if:
• the patient needs to receive treatment for mental disorder in hospital (either as an in-patient or as an out-patient), or
• there would be a risk of harm to the health or safety of the patient or to other persons if the patient were not recalled.

29.64 The CTO may be revoked if:
• the responsible clinician considers that the patient again needs to be admitted to hospital for medical treatment under the Act, **or**
• an AMHP agrees with that assessment, and also believes that it is appropriate to revoke the CTO.</td>
<td>Text in Act is correct and overrides Code text. Should be read as ‘and’ not ‘or’ in both cases.</td>
</tr>
<tr>
<td>39.4 The current regulations require that where the patient is to be admitted to an independent hospital and the doctor providing one of the medical recommendations is on the staff of that independent hospital, the other medical recommendation must be given by a doctor who is not on the staff of that independent hospital. That is, there will be a potential conflict if both doctors giving recommendations are on the staff of the independent hospital. It is also good practice for doctors on the staff of an NHS trust or NHS foundation trust to ensure that one of the recommendations is given by a doctor not on the staff of that trust.</td>
<td>The final word ‘trust’ in the last sentence of the paragraph should be read as hospital ie a single site hospital, rather than a multi-site trust.

Code paragraph 39.6 makes clear that no financial interest applies where an ‘assessor is paid a fee for making an application or giving a medical recommendation if it is paid regardless of the outcome of the assessment’.

Code paragraph IX and figure iii make clear the status of the Code and when departure is permitted.</td>
</tr>
</table>

Using the Act

The chapter in this section describes the structure of the Act and provides basic definitions for the terms used in the Act.

1: The Mental Health Act 1983 – the structure of the Act and definitions

Introduction

1.1 This chapter explains the structure of the Act and some of the most important definitions used in the Act and in this Reference Guide.

Purpose of the Act [section 1(1)]

1.2 Section 1 states that the Act concerns 'the reception, care and treatment of mentally disordered patients, the management of their property and other related matters'. As part 7 has now been repealed, the Act no longer deals with the management of patients' property.

Structure of the Act

1.3 The Act is divided into 10 parts as set out in figure 2.

Figure 2: Structure of the Mental Health Act 1983

Part	Sections	Heading	Particularly deals with
1	1	Application of the Act	Definition of mental disorder
2	2 to 34	Compulsory admission to hospital and guardianship	Detention in hospital Community treatment orders (CTOs) Guardianship (including procedures for admission, renewal, transfer and discharge for each of the above) Nearest relatives – definition and displacement

Part	Sections	Heading	Particularly deals with
3	35 to 55 (and schedule 1)	Patients concerned in criminal proceedings or under sentence	Powers of the courts to remand defendants to hospital while awaiting trial or sentence Powers of the courts to detain convicted offenders in hospital or make them subject to guardianship Transfer of patients from prison to hospital (and their return) Special restrictions on certain patients ('restricted patients') Conditional discharge of restricted patients by the Secretary of State Removal to hospital of certain other persons, eg those detained in immigration removal centres
4	56 to 64	Consent to treatment	Treatment for mental disorder without consent of patients detained in (or recalled to) hospital Safeguards for detained (and other) patients in respect of particular forms of treatment (eg medication, electro-convulsive therapy (ECT))
4A	64A to 64K	Treatment of community patients not recalled to hospital	Safeguards for CTO patients in relation to treatment for mental disorder while not recalled to hospital
5	65 to 79 (and schedule 2)	Mental Health Review Tribunals	Rights for patients (and nearest relatives) to apply to the appropriate tribunal for discharge Powers and duties of other people to refer cases to Tribunals Powers of Tribunals

Part	Sections	Heading	Particularly deals with
6	80 to 92	Removal and return of patients within the United Kingdom etc	Transfer of patients between England and Wales and Scotland, Northern Ireland, the Isle of Man and the Channel Islands Removal of patients to places outside the UK, Isle of Man or Channel Islands Patients who go absent across borders
8	114 to 122	Miscellaneous functions of local authorities and the Secretary of State	Approval of approved mental health professionals (AMHPs) Duty to provide after-care services Code of Practice
9	126 to 130L	Offences	Specific offences under the Act, including ill-treatment or neglect of patients
10	130A to 149	Miscellaneous and supplementary	Independent mental health advocacy (IMHA) Informal admission of patients to hospital Children and young people admitted to hospital Duties of hospital managers to give information to patients and nearest relatives Patients' correspondence Warrants to enter premises Detention in places of safety by the police Legal custody, conveyance and absconding Interpretation (ie definitions)

Meaning of part 2 and part 3 patients

1.4 People sometimes refer to 'part 2' and 'part 3' patients – and this Reference Guide uses these short-hand terms.

1.5 Broadly, part 2 patients are people who have been made subject to some form of compulsory measure under the Act in their own interests or to protect other people, without the involvement of the criminal courts. They are also termed 'civil patients'.

1.6 Part 3 patients are those who have been made subject to a compulsory measure under the Act by the criminal courts, or who have been transferred to hospital from prison or another type of custody, eg an immigration removal centre. They are also termed 'forensic patients'.

Definition of mental disorder [section 1(2)]

1.7 Mental disorder is defined for the purposes of the Act as 'any disorder or disability of the mind'.

Exclusion from the definition of mental disorder: alcohol or drug dependence [section 1(3)]

1.8 Dependence on alcohol or drugs is not considered to be a mental disorder for the purposes of the Act. This means that it is never possible, for example, to detain a person in hospital simply because they are dependent on alcohol or drugs.

1.9 People who are dependent on alcohol or drugs are not completely outside the scope of the Act, as they may well also have a mental disorder which is within the definition in the Act. Alcohol or drug dependence is often accompanied by, or associated with, other kinds of mental disorder.

1.10 It is only dependence on alcohol or drugs which is excluded. Other disorders associated with the use (or stopping the use) of alcohol or drugs are not excluded, even if they arise from (or are suspected to arise from) alcohol or drug dependence.

1.11 'Drugs' is not defined in the Act but can be taken to include psychoactive substances like certain solvents as well as medicines and illicit drugs.

Learning disability qualification [sections 1(2A), (2B) and (4)]

1.12 The Act defines a learning disability as a 'state of arrested or incomplete development of mind which includes significant impairment of intelligence and social functioning'.

1.13 Under the Act, a learning disability is, in general, regarded as a mental disorder because it is a disability of the mind.

1.14 For the specific purposes of the provisions set out in figure 3, a learning disability can only be considered a mental disorder if it is associated with 'abnormally aggressive or seriously irresponsible conduct' on the part of the person concerned.

Figure 3: Provisions to which the learning disability qualification applies

Sections	Which deal with
3, 20	Criteria for detention in hospital for medical treatment on the basis of an application for admission to hospital
7, 37	Criteria for guardianship under the Act
17A, 17E, 20A, 72(1)(b)	Criteria for CTO
35, 36, 37, 38, 45A, 51	Detention in hospital by the courts
47, 48, 50, 51, 52, 53	Transfer from prison to detention in hospital (and vice versa)
72(1)(b), (1)(c) and (4)	Criteria for discharge by the Tribunal from detention in hospital for treatment, and from CTOs and guardianship

1.15 One effect of this learning disability qualification is that people cannot be detained for treatment (rather than assessment) solely on the basis of a learning disability if they do not show abnormally aggressive or seriously irresponsible behaviour. Nor can they become CTO patients or be made subject to guardianship in the absence of such behaviour.

Diplomatic status

1.16 The Act does not apply to anyone who enjoys diplomatic immunity in the UK by virtue of section 2 and schedule 1 of the Diplomatic Privileges Act 1964.[8] This exemption is not limited to accredited diplomats may also extend to their spouses and children. Any mental health professional encountering such a case should immediately contact the Foreign and Commonwealth Office – Diplomatic Missions and International Organisations Unit, Protocol Directorate who will be able to confirm the person's diplomatic status. At the time of publication the contact number is 020 7008 1012.

Definition of medical treatment and medical treatment for mental disorder [section 145(1) and (4)]

[8] Diplomatic Privileges Act 1964. http://www.legislation.gov.uk/ukpga/1964/81

1.17 Throughout the Act, 'medical treatment' includes nursing, psychological intervention and specialist mental health habilitation, rehabilitation and care, as well as medication and other forms of treatment which might more normally be regarded as being 'medical'.

1.18 The difference between habilitation and rehabilitation is that the habilitation means equipping someone with skills and abilities they have never had, whereas rehabilitation means helping them recover skills and abilities they have lost.

1.19 When the Act is talking about medical treatment for mental disorder, it means medical treatment for the purpose of alleviating, or preventing a worsening of, the disorder or one or more of its symptoms or manifestations.

1.20 For example, in the criteria that must be met for detention for treatment under section 3 (see paragraph 8.2), there is a requirement that appropriate medical treatment must be available for the patient. By definition, that means there must be appropriate treatment available which is for the purpose of alleviating, or preventing a worsening of, the patient's mental disorder or one or more of its symptoms or manifestations.

1.21 'Symptoms' and 'manifestations' include the way a disorder is experienced by the individual concerned and the way in which the disorder manifests itself in the person's thoughts, emotions, behaviour and actions.

Definition of patient [section 145]

1.22 The Act uses 'patient' to mean a person who is, or appears to be suffering from mental disorder. This sometimes means the Act uses 'patient' where another term (like 'service user' or 'client') would almost certainly be used in practice. For instance, 'patients' subject to guardianship may not, in fact, be receiving much, if any, healthcare at a given time. This Reference Guide uses patient in the same way as the Act.

Definition of nearest relative [section 26]

1.23 People described in the Act as 'nearest relatives' have various rights in relation to patients who are – or might be – subject to compulsory measures under the Act. The meaning of nearest relative in the Act is described in chapter 2 of this Reference Guide. For the purposes of the Act it may not be the same as the patient's closest relative, their next of kin or carer.[9]

1.24 Patients do not necessarily have a nearest relative. Even if they do, it may not always be easy to identify accurately who that person is. The legislation

[9] The Code of Practice seeks to promote the role of carers, as defined in the Care Act 2014 (http://www.legislation.gov.uk/ukpga/2014/23), especially when these are not the same as the nearest relative. Professionals should aim to identify carers as well as the nearest relative and, if agreed by the patient, involve them in discussions. However, as the Act does not include the term carer it is not referred to in this Reference Guide, unless specified under other pieces of legislation.

recognises these difficulties. When it requires people to consult, inform or notify nearest relatives, the Act and the regulations typically refer to 'the person (if any) who appears to [the person in question] to be the nearest relative'. This Reference Guide normally refers to this as 'the person the [decision-maker] thinks is the nearest relative'.

1.25 Restricted patients (see paragraph 1.39), patients remanded to hospital by the courts under sections 35 or 36, and patients subject to interim hospital orders under section 38, do not have a nearest relative for the purposes of the Act.

1.26 Nearest relatives may delegate most of their functions. If they do so, most references in the legislation, and this Reference Guide, to nearest relatives should be read as being references to the person who has been authorised by the nearest relative to act on their behalf.

1.27 In certain circumstances, an acting nearest relative can be appointed by the county court in the place of the person who would otherwise be the nearest relative. When the Act, and this Reference Guide, refers to the nearest relative, it includes an acting nearest relative, unless it says otherwise.

1.28 For further detail on these points and nearest relatives generally, see chapter 2.

Definition of NHS and independent hospitals [sections 34 and 145]

1.29 The Act sometimes distinguishes between NHS hospitals and independent hospitals by calling the former 'hospitals' and the latter either 'independent hospitals' or 'registered establishments'. Sometimes (especially in part 2) the Act uses hospital to mean both NHS and independent hospitals.

1.30 The Act calls independent hospitals 'registered establishments' when they are hospitals as defined by section 275 of the National Health Service Act 2006[10] used for the carrying on of a regulated activity within the meaning of part 1 of the Health and Social Care Act 2008[11] which relates to the assessment or medical treatment of mental disorder and in respect of which there is a person or persons registered as a service provider under chapter 2 of that part. When referring to other independent hospitals, or to independent hospitals generally, the Act uses 'independent hospital'. This Reference Guide uses the term 'independent hospital' throughout to cover both registered establishments and other independent hospitals.

1.31 When the Act uses 'hospital', it means a specific hospital, not, for example, an NHS trust (which may have several hospitals). What constitutes a distinct hospital is a matter of fact. But there is no reason in principle why one building, or set of buildings, cannot contain more than one hospital, especially if they are the responsibility of different managers.

---

[10] National Health Service Act 2006. http://www.legislation.gov.uk/ukpga/2006/41
[11] Health and Social Care Act 2008. http://www.legislation.gov.uk/ukpga/2008/14

Definition of high security psychiatric hospital

1.32 A few provisions in the Act only apply to 'high security psychiatric hospitals'. These are hospitals particularly for the treatment of patients who are detained under the Act and who require this treatment under special security because of their dangerous, violent or criminal propensities (see section 4 of the National Health Service Act 2006). At the time of publication, there are three such hospitals – Ashworth, Broadmoor and Rampton – all of which are constituent parts of NHS trusts.

Definition of hospital managers [section 145]

1.33 The managers of hospitals have various powers and duties under the Act. In this context, 'managers' does not mean the management team of the hospital, but the people or body whose hospital it is, as set out in figure 4.

Figure 4: Identification of hospital managers

For a hospital which is	The managers are
Vested in a NHS trust	The NHS trust as a body
Vested in an NHS foundation trust	The NHS foundation trust as a body
Vested in a local health board (LHB) in Wales	The LHB as a body
An independent hospital	The person or persons registered as a service provider under Chapter 2 of part 1 of the Health and Social Care Act 2008 in respect of the regulated activity (within the meaning of that part) relating to the assessment or medical treatment of mental disorder carried out by the hospital

1.34 For the most part, hospital managers do not have to perform their functions personally, eg by decision of the board of an NHS trust, but may delegate them to officers, ie members of their staff), and, in some cases, to other people.

1.35 Hospital managers' functions under parts 2, 3 and 6 of the Act can be delegated in accordance with the regulations, or, in the cases of discharge decisions under section 23, in accordance with section 23 itself (see paragraphs to 31.7 to 31.17 and 26.7 and 26.8 in particular). Hospital managers' functions in respect of patients' correspondence under section 134 of the Act may be delegated in accordance with regulation 29 of the Mental Health (Hospital, Guardianship and Treatment) (England) Regulations 2008 (see paragraph 5.9).[12]

[12] The Mental Health (Hospital, Guardianship and Treatment) (England) Regulations. SI 2008/1184 http://www.legislation.gov.uk/uksi/2008/1184/pdfs/uksi_20081184_en.pdf

1.36 Hospital managers may delegate their other functions under the Act in any way they can normally delegate their functions – which will depend on the constitution of the body concerned and (in the case of NHS trusts and NHS foundation trusts) the relevant NHS legislation.

Meaning of 'detained' and 'liable to be detained'

1.37 The Act sometimes, but not always, distinguishes between people who are detained and those who are 'liable to be detained'. This latter term includes people who are actually detained, eg people who are in hospital and would be stopped from leaving if they tried to, and people who could lawfully be detained but who, for some reason, are not, eg because they have been given leave of absence from hospital. 'Liable to be detained' includes certain part 3 patients who have been conditionally discharged from detention in hospital, but who may be recalled if necessary (see chapter 27). It does not include patients who are subject to CTOs, even though they too may be recalled.

1.38 Unless otherwise stated, this Reference Guide uses 'detained' and 'subject to detention' to include all people who are liable to be detained, not just those who actually are detained, except patients who have been conditionally discharged, who are referred to as 'conditionally discharged patients'.

Meaning of restricted patient

1.39 Restricted patients are mentally disordered offenders (or sometimes people awaiting trial) who have become detained patients under part 3 of the Act and who are subject to special restrictions on (amongst other things) their discharge from hospital. By definition, all conditionally discharged patients are restricted patients (see chapter 21).

Meaning of AMHP, approved clinician and responsible clinician

1.40 Two terms for professionals with particular responsibilities under the Act recur throughout the Act and this Reference Guide: 'approved mental health professional' (or AMHP) and 'approved clinician'. These are explained in chapter 30. Unless the context demands otherwise, references in the legislation to AMHPs are to AMHPs acting on behalf of a local authority.

1.41 'Responsible clinician' is used frequently, although its meaning varies. For detained patients, it generally means the approved clinician with overall responsibility for their case (see paragraph 9.27).

Meaning of registered medical practitioner

1.42 Where the Act refers to 'registered medical practitioner', this Reference Guide uses 'doctor'. Both mean a person who is fully registered as a medical practitioner under the Medical Act 1983.[13]

Meaning of doctor approved under section 12

1.43 A doctor approved under section 12 means a doctor who has been approved by the Secretary of State or a person with whom the Secretary of State has entered into agreements under section 12ZA or 12ZB ('approving bodies') (or the Welsh Ministers) as having special experience in the diagnosis or treatment of mental disorder – see chapter 32. Doctors who are approved clinicians are automatically treated as being approved under section 12.

1.44 Approval under section 12 is primarily of significance in the context of making recommendations in support of applications for detention or guardianship under part 2 of the Act (see chapters 8 and 28 respectively) and evidence about the suitability of defendants and offenders for detention or guardianship under part 3 (see chapters 14 to 20).

Meaning of community treatment orders and CTO patients

1.45 The Act refers to people being given 'community treatment orders' (CTOs) and therefore becoming 'community patients'.

1.46 This Reference Guide refers to 'CTO' and 'CTO patients', to avoid confusion with the large majority of patients receiving healthcare services in the community who are not subject to any special measures under the Act.

Meaning of Secretary of State

1.47 When the Act refers to the Secretary of State, it means any Secretary of State (broadly speaking, a Cabinet Minister). Where the function concerned is, exercised by a particular Secretary of State, this Reference Guide names that Secretary of State. Responsibilities can and do move between Secretaries of State from time to time, without requiring any change in the legislation.[14]

Meaning of 'in writing' and use of electronic communication

1.48 Where the Act itself requires information to be recorded or given in writing, the use of electronic means to record or communicate the information is not sufficient. The record must be made, or the information communicated, in hard copy.

1.49 The same applies to requirements in the regulations to record or give information in writing, unless the regulations specifically say otherwise.

---

[13] Medical Act 1983. http://www.legislation.gov.uk/ukpga/1983/54

[14] This is different to the Code of Practice, where Secretary of State refers to the Secretary of State for Health unless specified.

Meaning of 'sent', 'delivered', 'furnished' and similar terms (service of documents) [regulation 3]

1.50 In general, where documents – other than notices recalling CTO patients to hospital – are required to be 'sent', 'delivered', 'furnished' (or other similar terms) to people under part 2 or part 3 of the Act, or the regulations, they may be:

- delivered by hand to the intended recipient (whether that is an individual or an organisation)
- delivered by hand to any person authorised by the recipient
- sent by pre-paid post to an organisation at its registered or principal address
- sent by pre-paid post to the recipient's usual or last known address, or
- delivered using an internal mail system operated by the recipient (eg a hospital's internal mail system), provided the recipient agrees to the use of its system for that purpose.

1.51 There are some exceptions to this rule, which are set out in regulation 3. In particular:

- applications for detention in hospital must be delivered by hand to an officer of the hospital managers authorised to receive them – see paragraph 8.65
- reports by doctors and approved clinicians temporarily detaining patients under the 'holding powers' in section 5 of the Act may only be furnished by hand to an authorised officer or sent using the hospital managers' internal mail system (with their agreement) – see paragraph 8.74, and
- nearest relatives may only serve orders discharging patients from detention or CTOs (and notice of their intention to do so) in certain specific ways – see paragraphs 27.14 and 26.107.

1.52 There are some cases in which the regulations allow other methods to be used, eg some documents and written information can be provided by electronic means where the recipient agrees.

1.53 Where the regulations say that pre-paid post may be used, they also say when the documents concerned are to be deemed to have been served, should that be in dispute. Specifically, unless something different can be shown:

- documents sent by first class post, or its equivalent, are deemed to have been served on the recipients on the second business day following the day of posting (eg on Wednesday, if posted on Monday), and
- documents sent by second class post, or its equivalent, are deemed to have been served on the recipients on the fourth business day following the day of posting (eg on Friday, if posted on Monday).

1.54 For these purposes, 'business days' means Mondays to Fridays, excluding public holidays.

1.55 The rules for serving notices recalling CTO patients to hospital – and when they are deemed to have been served – are different and are set out separately in regulation 6. See paragraph 26.34.

1.56 There are no specific rules about how documents and written information under other parts of the Act (eg written information for patients under sections 132 and 132A about the Act and their rights) must be furnished, nor when they are considered to have been served.

Glossary of key terms

1.57 There is a glossary of key words and phrases used in this Reference Guide at Annex A. This should be used in conjunction with Annex A in the Code of Practice.[15]

Statutory forms

1.58 This Reference Guides refers in various places to numbered forms which must be used to make applications, medical recommendations and to record various other decisions and events. These forms are set out in schedule 1 to the Mental Health (Hospital, Guardianship and Treatment) (England) Regulations 2008 (No. 1184).[16] If the regulations say that a particular statutory form must be used, a form whose wording corresponds to the up-to-date version of that form in schedule 1 must be used.

1.59 A list of the statutory forms in the regulations is at Annex B.

[15] Mental Health Act 1983: Code of Practice. Department of Health. 2015. https://www.gov.uk/government/publications/code-of-practice-mental-health-act-1983
[16] Mental Health (Hospital, Guardianship and Treatment (England) Regulations SI 2008/1184.

Protecting patients' rights and autonomy

This group of chapters addresses the issues of particular importance for empowering patients, carers, nearest relatives and others with a legitimate interest in matters relating to care and treatment under the Act. It provides guidance on the nearest relatives including the identification and appointment of an acting nearest relative by the court. It also describes the role and activities of independent mental health advocates and the roles of the Care Quality Commission and the Tribunal. The limited circumstances in which correspondence to or from patients may be withheld is explained.

2: The nearest relative

Introduction

2.1 This chapter describes the provisions of the Act dealing with the identification and displacement of a patient's nearest relative. It also covers the powers of nearest relatives to delegate their functions to other people.

The significance of the nearest relative in the Act

2.2 The Act confers various rights on patients' nearest relatives in connection with detention, community treatment orders (CTO) and guardianship under the Act. In addition to any rights they may have if they are also a carer, a donee of a lasting power of attorney, court appointed deputy, private guardian etc,[17] the nearest relative has the following rights under the Act. These are summarised in figure 5.

Figure 5: The rights of the nearest relative

The nearest relative can require the local authority (verbally or in writing), in which the 'patient' is living, to arrange for an approved mental health professional (AMHP) to 'consider the patient's case' including whether there is a need for compulsory admission to hospital. The local authority must inform the nearest relative in writing, of the reasons if no application for admission is made (section 13(4), Code 14.36 and 14.102).
The nearest relative can make an application (section 11(1)), provided there are valid medical recommendation(s), for the person's compulsory admission to hospital either for assessment (section 2 – form A1) or for treatment (section 3 – form A5) or in an emergency (section 4 – form A9). The nearest relative, if the applicant, must have seen the 'patient' within 14 days (24 hours if section 4) before making an application (section 11(5)). The Code of Practice (paragraph 14.30) notes that AMHPs are 'usually a more appropriate applicant'. 'If the nearest relative is the applicant, any AMHP, and other professionals involved in the assessment of the patient, should give advice and assistance. They should not assist in a patient's detention unless they believe it is justified and lawful' (Code 17.11). If the nearest relative does make the application, eg where the AMHP disagrees with need or urgency for compulsory admission and the person is detained in hospital under section 2 or section 3, the hospital managers must request the relevant local authority to provide them with a social circumstances report (section 14).

[17] For guidance on attorneys and deputies see chapter 7 the Code of Practice.

The nearest relative may make an application (section 11(1)), provided there are two valid medical recommendations, for the person to be received into guardianship (section 7). The nearest relative would complete form G1.

The nearest relative can be consulted, (section 11(4)(b)), whenever practicable, by an AMHP before a decision is made about a patient's possible compulsory admission to hospital for assessment (section 2) or for treatment (section 3).

While there is no requirement for the nearest relative to be informed and consulted when a CTO is being considered, the Code 29.10 notes that 'consultation at an early stage with the patient and those involved in the patient's care will be important, including family and carers'.

The nearest relative can formally object ((section 11(4), Code 14.65) to the making of an application by an AMHP for admission for treatment (section 3) or guardianship (section 7). If the nearest relative took this step, compulsory admission to hospital or reception into guardianship could not proceed at that time. The mental health professionals would in turn give urgent consideration to seeking the 'displacement' of the nearest relative in an application to the County Court (section 29(3)(c)).

The nearest relative can order a patient's discharge (section 23)

- from detention (section 2 or section 3)
- or from a community treatment order (CTO) (section 17A) but only where the CTO followed detention under section 3. This would also discharge the suspended section 3 underpinning the CTO.

The nearest relative must give 72 hours notice in writing to the hospital.[18] An illustrative standard letter for this purpose is given in the Code of Practice, paragraph 32.25. The nearest relative's order may be barred if within the 72 hours, the patient's responsible clinician provides a written report (M2) that they consider that the patient, if so discharged, 'would be likely to act in a manner dangerous to other persons or to himself' (section 25; regulation 25(1) (a) and (b), Mental Health Regulations 2008, and Code 32.20 – 32.25). The barring report prevents the nearest relative from ordering discharge at any time in the six months following the date of the report (section 25(1)(b), section 25(1A)). If the patient were detained under section 2 the nearest relative cannot take the matter further. If the patient is detained under section 3 or on a CTO following section 3, then the nearest relative may, within 28 days of the barring report being issued, apply to the Mental Health Tribunal for the patient's discharge instead (section 66(1)(g), section 66(2)(d)). For the situation when the matter is considered by the hospital managers panel, see Code 38.20.

The nearest relative can order a patient's discharge (section 23) from guardianship (section 7). There is no power for the responsible clinician to bar discharge.

[18] K (by his litigation friend, L) v Hospital Managers of the Kingswood Centre, Court of Appeal. Full reference and hyperlink.

Although they cannot order the discharge of a part 3 CTO patient, the nearest relative can apply to the Tribunal instead, in certain circumstances.
The nearest relative should be given 7 days notice, if practicable, by the hospital before a patient is discharged from detention under sections 2 or 3 or from a CTO (section 133). This duty does not apply if the patient or the nearest relative has requested that this information should not be given.
The functions of the nearest relative can be delegated to another person (Reg. 24, Mental Health Regulations, 2008, Code 5.5). There is no statutory form. Delegation must be in writing and could be an ordinary letter, eg 'I [insert name] of [insert address] being the nearest relative of [insert patient's name and address] for the purposes of the Mental Health Act 1983, hereby delegate my powers of nearest relative to [insert name] of [insert address]. I confirm that [insert name] has consented to act as the nearest relative of [insert patient's name].' As delegation could be time limited or until further notice, it is important that this issue is clearly addressed. It must also be signed and dated. Authorisation may be transmitted electronically (provided the new person is willing to receive it in that format). Delegation is not completed until received (and accepted), by the new person. The nearest relative must give notice of the delegation to the patient; the managers of the hospital if the person is detained and/or subject to a community treatment order; the local social services authority (and the private guardian, if any) if the person is subject to guardianship.
Nearest relatives can apply to the First-tier Tribunal if they have been displaced by the County Court on the grounds of either an unreasonable objection to detention or guardianship (section 29(3)(c)) or exercising their power of discharge (section 23) from detention or a CTO (including where it is considered the nearest relative is likely to do so) 'without due regard to the welfare of the patient or the interests of the public' (section 29(3)(d)). Application can be made once in the first year following displacement and once in each subsequent year (section 29(6), section 66(1)(h), section 66(2)(g)). The acting nearest relative has a separate power to make an application.
The patient or the nearest relative can apply to the Mental Health Tribunal for the patient's discharge when the patient is subject to an unrestricted hospital order (section 37) in the period between 6 and 12 months after the making of the hospital order and in any subsequent period of one year.
The nearest relative can, in addition to the patient's own right, apply to the Mental Health Tribunal for discharge when the patient is subject to a guardianship order (section 37) within the first 12 months of the order and in any subsequent 12 month period (section 69(1)(b)(ii)).

2.3 The rights and role of the nearest relative of detained patients were identified in R (on the application of M) v Secretary of State for Health.[19]

Patients who do not have a nearest relative for the purposes of the Act

2.4 Restricted patients, including conditionally discharged patients, do not have a nearest relative for the purposes of the Act. Nor do patients remanded to hospital under section 35 or 36, nor patients subject to interim hospital orders under section 38.

2.5 This is because there is nothing in the Act to say that the provisions in part 2 which deal with the identification of a nearest relative apply to these groups of patients. By contrast, part 1 of Schedule 1 specifically says that the provisions do apply to people subject to unrestricted hospital orders, hospital directions to which limitation directions no longer apply, or unrestricted transfer directions under part 3 ('unrestricted part 3 patients').

Meaning of relative in the Act [section 26(1), (6) and (7)]

2.6 'Relative' is defined for the purposes of part 2 the Act as anyone who is a patient's:

- husband, wife or civil partner
- son or daughter
- father or mother
- brother or sister
- grandparent
- grandchild
- uncle or aunt, or
- nephew or niece.

2.7 This includes relationships both of the 'whole blood' and the 'half-blood', ie with, or through, half-siblings.

2.8 It also includes relationships established through adoption, eg adoptive parent and child, adoptive aunt and nephew, but not step-relationship.

2.9 It includes the relationship of a father and a patient under 18 who is not born to parents who are married or in a civil partnership[20] (and any relationship established through such a relationship, eg between uncle and niece) only if the father has obtained 'parental responsibility' for the child within the meaning of section 3 of the Children Act 1989.

2.10 'Husband', 'wife' and 'civil partner' include people living with a patient as if they were husband, wife or civil partners, provided they have done so for at

---

[19] R (on the application of M) v Secretary of State for Health. 2003. EWHC 1094 (Admin). http://www.bailii.org/ew/cases/EWHC/Admin/2003/1094.html

[20] The section 26(2) requirement of parental responsibility only applies to patients under 18 who are not born to parents who are married or in a civil partnership.

least six months (or, when the patient is currently a hospital in-patient, they had lived together for at least six months before the patient's admission to hospital).

2.11 'Relative' also includes people who are not (in the usual sense) relatives but who are living ('ordinarily residing') with a patient and have done so for at least five years (or, when the patient is currently a hospital in-patient, had lived with the patient for at least five years before the patient's admission to hospital).

Identification of the nearest relative [section 26(3) – (5)]

2.12 The general rule is that the nearest relative is the person who comes first in the list of relatives described above (with people who are only relatives because they have lived with the patient for at least 5 years coming at the bottom of that list).

2.13 Men and women take equal priority – so sons and daughters come in the same place in the list. So do husbands, wives, civil partners and people who are treated as if they were husbands, wives and civil partners under the Act (see paragraph 2.10).

2.14 Where two or more people come in the same place in the list, the elder or eldest takes precedence (eg the elder parent, or eldest sibling).

2.15 There are several exceptions to the general rule, as follows:

- a relative who ordinarily lives with or cares for the patient takes precedence over other relatives
- a relative of the full-blood (eg a full brother or sister) takes precedence over one of the half-blood (eg a half-brother or half-sister) within any category of relatives, regardless of age
- a husband, wife or civil partner, or someone treated as such under the Act, who is permanently separated from the patient, whether by agreement or a court order, is not eligible to be the nearest relative
- a husband, wife or civil partner, or someone treated as such under the Act, who has deserted, or been deserted by, the patient is also not eligible to be the nearest relative. Desertion means that one party has left the marriage or partnership without the other's agreement, and
- otherwise, a legal husband, wife or civil partner takes precedence over anyone who is treated as such because they lived with the patient as if they were married or civil partners, and over anyone who is only treated as a relative because they have lived with the patient for at least 5 years.

2.16 In addition:

- no-one under 18 can be the nearest relative, unless they are the patient's mother, father, husband, wife or civil partner, or treated as such, and

- only patients who are not themselves ordinarily resident in the UK, the Channel Islands or the Isle of Man can have a nearest relative who also does not live in any of those places.

2.17 The box at the end of this chapter summarises how these rules are to be used to identify a patient's nearest relative.

Automatic change of nearest relative

2.18 The identity of the nearest relative will change if the current nearest relative dies, or if, for example, the nearest relative is a spouse or civil partner and the marriage or civil partnership ends.

2.19 It may also change for some other reason not directly involving the existing nearest relative, eg that the patient marries, or another relative reaches the age of 18, or comes to live in the UK, and therefore becomes eligible to be the nearest relative.

Exception from normal rules for children and young people in care [section 27]

2.20 The rules about the identity of nearest relatives do not apply to children or young people in the care of a local authority by virtue of a care order, or interim care order, under the Children Act 1989,[21] or where the rights and powers of their parent are vested in the local authority by virtue of section 16 of the Social Work (Scotland) Act 1968.[22]

2.21 In those cases, the local authority in question will be deemed to be the patient's nearest relative in preference to anyone except their husband, wife or civil partner, or someone who is treated as such under the Act.

Exception from normal rules for children and young people subject to guardianship under legislation for the protection of children [section 28]

2.22 If a guardian, or special guardian, has been appointed for a child or young person under 18 under sections 5 or 14A of the Children Act 1989,[23] that person, or all of them if there is more than one, will normally be deemed to be the nearest relative to the exclusion of anyone else, regardless of the normal rules. 'Guardian' here does not include a guardian appointed under the Act itself.

2.23 Similarly, if a residence order, as defined in section 8 of the Children Act 1989,[24] is in force in relation to a child or young person under 18, the person named in the order will be deemed to be the nearest relative to the exclusion of anyone else.

---

[21] Children Act 1989. http://www.legislation.gov.uk/ukpga/1989/41
[22] Social Work (Scotland) Act 1968. http://www.legislation.gov.uk/ukpga/1968/49
[23] Children Act 1989. http://www.legislation.gov.uk/ukpga/1989/41
[24] Children Act 1989. http://www.legislation.gov.uk/ukpga/1989/41

2.24 In both cases a person will not be deemed to be the nearest relative if they would automatically be ineligible under section 26(5) to be the patient's nearest relative. This means anyone who:

- is the patient's husband, wife or civil partner, or treated as such under the Act, but who is permanently separated from the patient by agreement or a court order, or who has either deserted, or been deserted by, the patient
- is under 18, and not the patient's mother, father, husband, wife or civil partner, or treated as such under the Act, or
- does not live in the UK, the Channel Islands or the Isle of Man, unless the patient is not also ordinarily resident in any of those places.

Delegation of rights of nearest relatives [section 32(2) and regulation 24]

2.25 It is open to nearest relatives of part 2 patients to delegate their functions by authorising someone else to exercise their rights on their behalf.

2.26 The same applies to nearest relatives of unrestricted part 3 patients, but with one exception. They may not delegate their right under section 69 to apply to the Tribunal on behalf of a restricted part 3 patient.

2.27 Nearest relatives may not delegate their functions to:

- the patient
- a person who, under section 26(5), is not eligible to be the patient's nearest relative – see paragraph 2.15, or
- a person who would currently be the nearest relative, were it not for an order of the court displacing them under section 29 (unless that order was given on the grounds that, at the time, no nearest relative could be identified) – see paragraph 2.37 onward.

2.28 Otherwise, nearest relatives may delegate their functions to anyone who is willing to undertake the role on their behalf. This includes people who were displaced only on the grounds that no nearest relative could, at the time, be identified.

2.29 Nearest relatives may delegate their functions at any time, whether or not a question of admission to hospital or guardianship has already arisen. Likewise, they may revoke the delegation at any time.

2.30 While the delegation is in force, only the person to whom the rights have been delegated may exercise them. The actual nearest relative may revoke the authorisation at any time.

2.31 Authorisations and revocations take effect when they are received by the person to whom the rights are delegated.

2.32 When making or revoking an authorisation delegating their rights, nearest relatives must immediately notify the patient.

2.33 If the person delegating the rights is the nearest relative of someone who is already subject to compulsory measures under the Act, they must also notify the relevant authority of the delegation or its revocation as set out in figure 6.

Figure 6: Authorities to be notified by nearest relatives when they delegate functions or revoke delegation

Patient who is	Authority to be informed of the delegation or its revocation
Detained in hospital (or liable to be detained, even if not actually detained)	The managers of the hospital in which the patient is liable to be detained
A CTO patient	The managers of the responsible hospital (see paragraph 26.6)
Subject to guardianship	The responsible local authority (see paragraph 28.18) and (if applicable) the private guardian

2.34 Authorisations and revocations (and notifications of either) must be in writing not only orally, but may be communicated electronically, eg as an email, if the recipient agrees.

2.35 Delegation lapses automatically on the death of the person who made it, or if that person ceases to be the nearest relative for any other reason. It also lapses on the death of the person to whom the functions have been delegated.

2.36 There are various duties in the Act and the regulations on hospital managers, local authorities, and other people to give information to nearest relatives, or to arrange for them to be given information. Where the nearest relative has delegated their functions to another person, the information should be given directly to that other person.

Appointment of acting nearest relatives where there is no nearest relative or where the nearest relative is to be displaced [section 29]

2.37 The rights of a nearest relative under the Act may only be removed and conferred on another person by the county court, or by another court on appeal. Likewise, only the county court, or another court on appeal, can appoint a nearest relative for someone who would otherwise not have one.

2.38 The county court may make an order directing that the functions of the nearest relative are to be exercised by another person, whether or not they are related to the patient and whether or not they would otherwise be eligible to be the patient's nearest relative. 'Person' in this context can include a local authority.

Applications to the county courts [section 29(1), (1A) and (2)]

2.39 An application for such an order may be made by:

- the patient
- any relative of the patient, as defined for the purposes of the Act (see paragraphs 2.6 to 2.11)
- any other person who lives with the patient or, if the patient is currently a hospital in-patient, was living with them before they were admitted, or
- an approved mental health practitioner (AMHP) acting on behalf of a local authority.

2.40 The application may, but does not have to, nominate someone whom the applicant would like to be appointed as the acting nearest relative. It may also contain more than one name from which the court will be invited to choose. The court can only appoint a person who is suitable and willing to act as nearest relative (see paragraph 2.49 below).

Grounds on which an application can be made [section 29(3)]

2.41 There are five grounds on which an application can be made, as set out in figure 7.

Figure 7: Grounds on which an application for an acting nearest relative may be made

Ground	Description	Section
1. No nearest relative	The patient has no nearest relative as defined in the Act, or it is not reasonably practicable to identify who the nearest relative is.	section 29(3)(a)
2. Incapacity of nearest relative	The nearest relative is incapable of acting as such by reason of mental disorder or some other health problem ('illness').	section 29(3)(b)
3. Unreasonable objection to application	The nearest relative has been acting unreasonably in objecting to an application for admission for treatment (under section 3) or for guardianship.	section 29(3)(c)
4. Use of power of discharge without due regard	The nearest relative has exercised the power to discharge the patient from detention, a CTO or guardianship, or is likely to do so, without due regard to the welfare of the patient or the interests of the public.	section 29(3)(d)
5. Unsuitability of nearest relative	The nearest relative is otherwise not a suitable person to act as nearest relative.	section 29(3)(e)

Effect of an application on a patient's detention for assessment under section 2 [sections 29(4) and 30(3)]

2.42 If an application is made on the third or fourth grounds above (unreasonable objection or use of power of discharge without due regard) while a patient is detained on the basis of an application for admission for assessment (section 2), the patient's maximum period of detention will be extended until at least the time at which the application to the court is finally disposed of. The application is only finally disposed of when it is withdrawn, when the time for appealing has passed, or – if there is an appeal – when that appeal is decided or withdrawn.

2.43 If the displacement order is ultimately made, and not reversed on appeal, the maximum period of detention will be extended for a further seven days starting with the day the application is disposed of. This allows time for an application for admission for treatment or for guardianship to be made, if appropriate.

2.44 Case law has established that there is a risk in these circumstances that patients' rights under article 5 of the European Convention on Human Rights[25] may be violated, because patients detained for assessment do not have the right to apply to the Tribunal after the first 14 days of their detention (see chapter 6).

2.45 Patients in this position may ask the Secretary of State for Health to refer their cases to the Tribunal under section 67 (see paragraph 6.56).

2.46 If patients lack capacity to make this request themselves, and no-one else is able to make it on their behalf, the House of Lords has ruled that managers of the hospital in which they are detained should consider asking the Secretary of State to make a reference if there is a risk that the patients' rights would otherwise be jeopardised. So should any local authority on whose behalf an AMHP was acting when making an application for the displacement of the nearest relative.[26]

2.47 This is particularly likely to be the case where the patient has not already had their case heard by the Tribunal, or where a significant period has passed since it was last heard. In any case, the managers will themselves normally have to refer a patient's case to the Tribunal if the patient has been detained in total for six months (see paragraph 6.42 onward).

An order appointing an acting nearest relative [section 29(1A)]

2.48 If the county court (or another court on appeal) decides to make an order, the order must specify who is to be the acting nearest relative. That must be:

---

[25] European Convention on Human Rights. http://www.echr.coe.int/Documents/Convention_ENG.pdf

[26] R (on the application of H) v Secretary of State for Health. 2005. UKHL 60; 4 All ER 1311.

- either the person, or one of the people, nominated in the application, if the court considers them to be a suitable (and willing) person to act as the patient's nearest relative, or
- if there is no such person, any other person whom the court considers is suitable, and willing, to do so.

2.49 If the application was made on the first, second or fifth grounds in figure 7 (no nearest relative, incapacity or unsuitability), the court may also specify the maximum period for which the order is to last.

2.50 One example of a way in which a court might use the power to time limit the order would be to specify that it should cease on the date when the eldest brother or sister of the patient reached 18 and would therefore normally become the nearest relative. The brother or sister could then take on the role of nearest relative without needing a further court order.

Interim orders

2.51 Case-law has established that the court may make an interim order appointing an acting nearest relative, pending its final decision.[27]

Duration of the order [sections 29(5) and 30(4) to (4B)]

2.52 Unless it is discharged by a court under section 30, a substantive order appointing an acting nearest relative order continues in effect as set out in figure 8.

2.53 In figure 8, a 'detained patient' means a patient detained in hospital on the basis of an application for admission under part 2, or a hospital order, hospital direction or transfer direction under part 3. It does not include people detained under the 'holding powers' in section 5, or those remanded to hospital under sections 35 or 36, or those subject to an interim hospital order under section 38.

Figure 8: Duration of orders appointing acting nearest relatives

Order made on the grounds of	Continues in force (unless discharged) until
Unreasonable objection to application (section 29(3)(c)) or **Use of power of discharge without due regard** (section 29(3)(d))	If the patient was not liable to be detained, a CTO patient or a guardianship patient on the date of the order, and has not since become one: • at the end of three months starting with the day of order Otherwise:

[27] R v Uxbridge County Court Ex p. Binns. 2000. MHLR 179.

Order made on the grounds of	Continues in force (unless discharged) until
	• when the relevant application for admission for treatment or application for guardianship under part 2, or order or direction under part 3 (other than under section 35, 36 or 38), ceases to have effect either because the patient is discharged, or for some other reason The order does not end as a result of the patient being discharged from detention onto a CTO, or being transferred to or from guardianship under section 19
No nearest relative (section 29(3)(a)) or **Incapacity of nearest relative** (section 29(3)(b)) or **Unsuitability of nearest relative** (section 29(3)(e))	The date (if any) specified in the order

Effect of an order appointing an acting nearest relative [section 29(6)]

2.54 While an order is in force, a patient's acting nearest relative is to be treated as if they were the patient's actual nearest relative.

2.55 Accordingly, they can exercise all of the rights of a nearest relative (including the power to delegate those rights to another person, as described at paragraph 2.25 onward). And where hospital managers and others are required to give information to nearest relatives, they must give that information to the acting nearest relative.

2.56 This applies even if the former nearest relative who was displaced would no longer be the nearest relative (eg because they have died, or because the patient has married or divorced, or entered or dissolved a civil partnership). The order has first to be discharged to allow the person who would otherwise now be the nearest relative to take over.

2.57 The same applies if the acting nearest relative dies. In that case no-one can exercise the rights of the nearest relative while the order remains in force, until the court discharges it, or varies it to appoint a new acting nearest relative.

Variation of an order appointing an acting nearest relative [section 30(2)]

2.58 The county court, or another court on appeal, may vary an order to appoint a different person as the acting nearest relative, if an application to that end is made by:

- the patient
- the current acting nearest relative, or
- an AMHP acting on behalf of a local authority.

2.59 As with the original application, if the court decides to vary the order, it must specify as the new acting nearest relative:

- either the person (or one of the people) nominated in the application, if the court considers them to be a suitable, and willing, person to act as the patient's nearest relative, or
- (if there is no such person) any other person whom the court considers is suitable, and willing.

Discharge of an order appointing an acting nearest relative [section 30(1) and (1A)]

2.60 The county court, or another court on appeal, may discharge an order appointing an acting nearest relative if an application to that end is made by someone is eligible to do so, as set out in figure 9.

Figure 9: People who may apply for the discharge of an order appointing an acting nearest relative

A person may apply for the discharge of the order if they are	In the following cases
The patient	All cases
The acting nearest relative	
The displaced nearest relative	If the original order was made on the first (no nearest relative) or second (incapacity) ground set out above, or (but only with the leave of the court) if the original order was made on the fifth ground (unsuitability)
Another person who would now be the nearest relative if the order had not been made (eg because the displaced nearest relative has died)	If the displaced nearest relative has died or would otherwise no longer be the nearest relative
Anyone who the Act treats as a relative of the patient (as described earlier in this chapter)	If the acting nearest relative dies

Procedure for applying to county court [section 31]

2.61 The Civil Procedure Rules, which are made by the Procedure Rules Committee, and the associated Practice Directions, govern the procedures which are to be followed in relation to applications to the court in respect of nearest relatives. See, in particular, part 8 of the Rules and the related Practice Directions.[28] The reference in the Act to the 'County Court Rules' is out of date and is now to be read as a reference to the Civil Procedure Rules.

Seven steps to identify the nearest relative

Determine whether there is a nearest relative

Step 1: Determine whether the patient has anyone who falls into one of the categories of the hierarchical list below. If there is no-one, the patient has no nearest relative.

Determine who the likely nearest relative is

Step 2: Identify whether there is anyone who falls into one of the categories in the hierarchical list with whom the patient ordinarily resides or by whom the patient is cared for (or, if the patient is currently a hospital in-patient, with whom the patient last ordinarily resided or by whom the patient was cared for before being admitted). If there is someone, skip to step 4.

Step 3: Identify all the people who meet the criterion in step 1 and then identify the one who comes highest in the hierarchical list as the likely nearest relative. If two or more people come equal first, identify the eldest as the likely nearest relative. Then skip to step 5.

Step 4: Identify all the people who meet the criterion in step 2 and then determine which one comes highest in the hierarchical list as the likely nearest relative. If two or more people come equal first, identify the eldest as the likely nearest relative.

Determine whether the likely nearest relative is actually the nearest relative

Step 5: Determine whether the patient is ordinarily resident in the UK, the Channel Islands or the Isle of Man. If not, skip to step 7.

Step 6: Is the likely nearest relative ordinarily resident in the UK, the Channel Islands or the Isle of Man? If not, return to step 2, but ignore the person who was previously the likely nearest relative. Repeat as necessary.

[28] Civil Procedure Rules – Rules & Practice Directions. http://www.justice.gov.uk/courts/procedure-rules/civil/rules

Determine the nearest relative.

Step 7: The likely nearest relative is indeed the nearest relative.

Note: Remember that there are special rules for certain children and young people. It is also good practice to involve carers, especially if the patient expresses a preference for their involvement, and they are different to the nearest relative as defined by section 26, see chapter 5 in the Code of Practice for further guidance.

Hierarchical list of potential nearest relatives
1st Husband or wife or civil partner (except one permanently separated from the patient by agreement or a court order, or who has deserted or been deserted by the patient)

2nd Person who qualifies as a relative by living with the patient as husband or wife or as if they were civil partners for at least six months (ie person treated as a husband, wife or civil partner under the Act)

3rd Son or daughter aged 18+

4th Father or mother

5th Brother or sister aged 18+

6th Half-brother or half-sister aged 18+

7th Grandparent

8th Grandchild aged 18+

9th Uncle or aunt aged 18+ of the whole blood

10th Uncle or aunt aged 18+ of the half-blood (eg half-sister of patient's mother)

11th Nephew or niece aged 18+ of the whole blood

12th Nephew or niece aged 18+ of the half-blood (ie child of a half-brother of the parent of the patient)

13th Other person aged 18+ who qualifies as a relative by having lived with the patient for at least five years

Note: Includes relationships made through adoption. Excludes step relationships.

Also excludes the relationship of a father and a child under 18 who is not born to parents who are married or in a civil partnership and any relationship established through such a relationship, eg between aunt and nephew, unless the father has parental responsibility for the child.

3: Code of Practice, Care Quality Commission and the general protection of patients

Introduction

3.1 This chapter describes the provisions of the Act in relation to the Code of Practice, general protection of patients and the role of the Care Quality Commission (CQC).

Code of Practice [section 118]

3.2 The Secretary of State must prepare, publish and from time to time revise, a Code of Practice. (Welsh Ministers must do the same for Wales.) This Reference Guide should be read in conjunction with the Code of Practice published in England in 2015.[29]

3.3 The Code must include guidance for doctors, approved clinicians, hospital and care home managers and staff, and approved mental health practitioners (AMHP) in relation to:

- the admission and detention of patients under the Act
- guardianship, and
- community patients.

3.4 The Code must include guidance for doctors and other professionals in relation to the medical treatment of patients suffering from mental disorder generally.

3.5 In particular, the Code must include a statement of the principles which the Secretary of State thinks should inform decisions made under the Act. The Act lists (in sections 118(2A) and (2B)) a number of matters which the statement of principles must address or to which the Secretary of State must have regard.

3.6 The Code must specify any particular medical treatments (apart from those already covered by section 57 – see chapter 23) which the Secretary of State thinks gives rise to special concerns and which should therefore not be given by doctors unless the patient in question has consented and a second opinion doctor (SOAD) has given a certificate approving it. At the time of

[29] Mental Health Act 1983: Code of Practice of Practice 2015. https://www.gov.uk/government/uploads/system/uploads/attachment_data/file/396918/Code_of_Practice.pdf

publication, no such treatments are specified in the Code (and none have ever been).

3.7 The people to whom the statutory guidance in the Code is addressed, as described above, are required to have regard to it when performing functions under the Act (see Code paragraphs II-V).

3.8 Before preparing the Code, or any revision to it, the Secretary of State must consult any organisations the Secretary of State thinks have an interest in it. CQC may at any time make proposals to the Secretary of State as to the content of the Code.

3.9 The Code, and any revision, must be laid before both Houses of Parliament. Within a specified period, either House can pass a resolution which would require the Secretary of State to withdraw the Code, or the revision, and bring forward a new one.

Care Quality Commission

3.10 CQC has the following functions conferred by the Health and Social Care Act 2008:

- registration functions
- review and investigation functions, and
- functions under the Mental Health Act 1983.

The main objective of CQC is to protect and promote the health, safety and welfare of people who use health and social care services. CQC's functions under the Mental Health Act 1983 are defined in chapter 4 of part 1 of, and Schedule 3 to, the Health and Social Care Act 2008.[30]

3.11 CQC registers all providers who carry on the regulated activity of assessment or medical treatment of people subject to the Act. A person may only be detained under the Act in an establishment which is registered with CQC to provide this regulated activity.

3.12 CQC will inspect registered providers against the relevant requirements of the Health and Social Care Act (Regulated Activities) Regulations 2014,[31] the Care Quality Commission (Registration) Regulations 2009[32] and, where appropriate, the Code of Practice.

3.13 CQC has integrated its monitoring functions under the Act with its registration function under the Health and Social Care Act 2008. The inspection of

---

[30] Health and Social Care Act 2008. http://www.legislation.gov.uk/ukpga/2008/14

[31] Health and Social Care Act (Regulated Activities) Regulations 2014. SI 2014/2936. http://www.legislation.gov.uk/uksi/2014/2936

[32] Care Quality Commission (Registration) Regulations. 2009. SI 2009/3112. http://www.legislation.gov.uk/uksi/2009/3112

providers registered with CQC to provide care and treatment to people subject to the Act will include review of how the Act is being applied.

General protection of patients [section 120]

3.14 Under the Act, the CQC is under a duty to keep under review and, where appropriate, investigate the exercise of the powers and discharge of the duties conferred by the Act in relation to the detention of patients, the reception of patients into guardianship, or to patients who are liable to be detained under the Act, community patients and patients subject to guardianship ('relevant patients').

3.15 The CQC must make arrangements for persons authorised by it to visit and interview in private patients who are detained in hospitals, and other 'relevant patients' in hospitals, other establishments registered under part 2 of the Care Standards Act 2000 (eg care homes and children's homes),[33] and, if access is granted, elsewhere.

3.16 CQC must make arrangements for such people to investigate any complaint:

> 'by anyone about the exercise of powers or the discharge of duties under the Act in respect of any patient who is, or has been, detained in a hospital, or any current or former 'relevant patient.'

3.17 The people carrying out an investigation on CQC's behalf can end the investigation if they consider it appropriate to do so, and the arrangements made by CQC may exclude matters from investigation in particular circumstances. Where complaints are made by Members of Parliament, they must be told the results of any investigation carried out.

3.18 For the purposes of the duty to keep the exercise of powers and discharge of duties under the Act under review and to investigate complaints, any person authorised by CQC has the right of access to patients in hospitals or other establishments at any reasonable time. They may visit, interview, and (if they are doctors or approved clinicians) examine, the patient in private. They may also require the production of and inspect any records relating to the detention or treatment of a person who is, or has been, detained under the Act or is or has been a community patient or a patient subject to guardianship. That might include admission documents, medical notes, records of seclusion, community treatment orders (CTO) and such like.

3.19 Hospital managers and local authorities must provide CQC with information (including documents and records) that it reasonably requests for or in connection with a review or investigation under the Act.

3.20 It is an offence under section 129 without reasonable cause to refuse authorised people access to a patient, records or premises, or in any way obstruct them in carrying out their functions.

---

[33] These are 'regulated establishments' in England, as defined by section 120(9) of the Act.

3.21 CQC may publish a report of a review or investigation it has carried out. It may direct a hospital manager or local authority to publish an action statement as to the action that is proposed to be taken as a result of a review or investigation.

Consent to treatment and second opinion doctors [section 119]

3.22 The CQC has the responsibility for appointing second opinion doctors (SOADs) and other people for the purposes of part 4 (and therefore, in practice, part 4A) of the Act. This includes the power to direct that a certificate issued by a SOAD is to cease to apply to any or all of the treatments it authorises from a specified date (see chapters 23 and 24).

3.23 If any treatments were ever to be specified in the Code of Practice as described in paragraph 3.6, CQC would also be responsible for appointing the necessary SOADs.

Reviewing decisions to withhold postal packets [section 134]

3.24 CQC is responsible, on request, for reviewing decisions by the managers of high security psychiatric hospitals to withhold patients' correspondence (see chapter 5).

Annual reports [section 120D]

3.25 CQC is required to publish an annual report on its activities in the exercise of its functions under the Act. CQC must send copies to the Secretary of State who must in turn lay a copy before each House of Parliament.

4: Independent mental health advocates

Introduction

4.1 This chapter describes the provisions in the Act relating to independent mental health advocate (IMHA) services.

Duty to arrange advocacy services [section 130A]

4.2 A local authority is required to make arrangements which it thinks reasonable for IMHAs to be available to help qualifying patients for whom the local authority is responsible.

Qualifying patients [section 130C]

4.3 Patients are eligible for advocacy services if they are:

- detained under the Act
- liable to be detained under the Act, even if not actually detained, including those who are currently on leave of absence from hospital or absent without leave, or those for whom an application or court order for admission has been completed
- conditionally discharged
- subject to guardianship, or
- community treatment order (CTO) patients

except:

- patients detained for assessment on the basis of an emergency application (section 4) until the second medical recommendation is received
- patients detained under the 'holding powers' in section 5, and
- patients detained in a place of safety under section 135 or 136.

4.4 Other patients ('informal patients') are eligible if they are:

- being considered for a treatment to which section 57 applies ('a section 57 treatment') – mainly neurosurgery for mental disorder (see paragraph 23.17), or
- under 18 and being considered for electro-convulsive therapy (ECT) or any other treatment to which section 58A applies ('a section 58A treatment') (see paragraph 23.42).

4.5 Informal patients who qualify because they are being considered for one of these treatments remain eligible until the treatment is finished, or stopped, or it is decided that they will not be given the treatment for the time being.

4.6 A local authority is responsible for a qualifying patient if:

- the patient is liable to be detained in the local authority's area
- the patient is subject to the guardianship of the local authority or a person who lives in the local authority's area
- the patient is on a CTO and the responsible hospital (the hospital whose managers have responsibilities in relation to the patient) is in the local authority's area, or
- in the case of a patient described in 4.4, the local authority is nominated as being responsible for arranging the patient's access to the services of an independent mental health advocate (IMHA) by:
    - the patient, if the patient has capacity or is competent to nominate the local authority
    - or if the patient lacks such capacity or competence, the patient's attorney or deputy, Court of Protection, or a person engaged in caring for the patient or interested in his welfare.

Principle of independence [section 130A(4)]

4.7 When making arrangements for advocacy, a local authority must have regard to the principle that advocates should, so far as is practicable, be independent of the professionals currently involved in the medical treatment of the patient they are helping. The Act describes this as being independent of 'any person who is professionally concerned with the patient's treatment'.

4.8 In this context, people are not to be considered to be professionally concerned with a patient's treatment if their only involvement with that treatment is acting as an advocate for the patient in connection with the treatment. Advocate here includes advocates under the Act, as well as independent mental capacity advocates (IMCAs) helping people under the Mental Capacity Act 2005,[34] and anyone else acting as a patient's representative.

4.9 The Secretary of State may make regulations about the criteria which people must meet to be eligible to be IMHAs.

The role of independent mental health advocates [section 130B]

4.10 The help which independent mental health advocacy services are to provide must include helping patients to obtain information about and understand the following:

- their rights under the Act

[34] Mental Capacity Act 2005. http://www.legislation.gov.uk/ukpga/2005/9/contents

- the rights which other people have in relation to them under the Act, eg any right their nearest relative has to discharge them
- the particular parts of the Act which apply to them, eg the basis on which they are detained, and which therefore make them eligible for advocacy
- any conditions or restrictions to which they are subject (eg as condition of leave of absence from hospital, as a condition of a CTO, or as a condition of conditional discharge)
- what, if any, medical treatment they are receiving, or which they might be given
- the reasons for that treatment, or proposed treatment, and
- the legal authority for providing that treatment, and the safeguards and other requirements of the Act which apply to that treatment.

4.11 The help which independent mental health advocacy services must provide also includes helping patients to exercise their rights, which can include representing them and speaking on their behalf. Independent mental health advocacy services are not designed to take the place of advice from, or representation by, qualified legal professionals.

Right of advocates to visit patients [section 130B(3)]

4.12 Advocates may visit and interview the patients they are helping in private. Anyone who prevents them doing so without reasonable cause would be guilty of the offence of obstruction under section 129 (see paragraph 38.13).

Duty of advocates to visit patients [section 130B(5) and (6)]

4.13 Advocates must comply with any reasonable request to visit and interview a patient, if the request is made by someone they think is the patient's nearest relative, or by an approved mental health professional (AMHP) or the patient's responsible clinician, if they have one.

4.14 Patients may refuse to be interviewed and do not have to accept help from an advocate if they do not want it.

Right of advocates to interview professionals and look at records [section 130B(3) and (4)]

4.15 Advocates have the right to visit and interview any person who is currently professionally concerned with a patient's medical treatment, provided it is for the purpose of supporting the patient.

4.16 They may require sight of records relating to a patient's detention or treatment in any hospital or after-care services provided under section 117 as well as any records made or held by a local authority which relate to the patient.

4.17 If the patient has capacity (or in the case of a child, is competent) to decide whether the advocate should see the records, advocates may only see them if the patient has consented.

4.18 Otherwise, where patients cannot consent (because they lack the capacity or, in the case of a child, the competence to do so), advocates may only access the records, if:

- it would not involve anyone going against a decision made on the patient's behalf in accordance with the Mental Capacity Act 2005 by a donee of a lasting power of attorney or a deputy, or a decision of the Court of Protection, and
- the person holding the records (the 'record-holder') thinks that:
  - the records may be relevant to the help which the advocate is providing to the patient, and
  - it is appropriate to let the advocate see them.

4.19 The Act allows the Secretary of State to make regulations setting out factors which record-holders should consider when deciding whether to allow access to records in these cases. At the time of publication, the Secretary of State has not made any such regulations.

Duty to inform patients about the availability of advocacy services [section 130D]

4.20 Certain people have a duty to take whatever steps are practicable to ensure patients understand that help is available to them from advocacy services and how they can obtain that help, as set out in figure 10. This must include giving the relevant information both orally and in writing.

Figure 10: Duty to provide patients with information about advocacy services

Type of patient	Steps to be taken by	As soon as practicable after
Detained patients	The managers of the hospital in which the patient is liable to be detained	The patient becomes liable to be detained
Patients liable to be detained, but not actually detained	The managers of the hospital in which the patient is liable to be detained	The patient becomes liable to be detained
Guardianship patients	The responsible local authority,[35] ie the local authority that is the patient's guardian or the local authority in which the person who is the patient's guardian lives	The patient becomes subject to guardianship

[35] Within the meaning of section 34(3) of the Act.

Type of patient	Steps to be taken by	As soon as practicable after
CTO patients	The managers of the responsible hospital	The patient becomes a CTO patient
Conditionally discharged patients	The patient's responsible clinician	The patient is conditionally discharged
Informal patients	The doctor or approved clinician who first discusses with the patient the possibility of them being given the section 57 treatment (or, for patients under 18, section 58A treatment) in question	That discussion (or during it)

Information for nearest relatives [section 130D(5) and (6)]

4.21 The person whose duty it is to inform the patient must also take whatever steps are practicable to give a copy of the written information to the person they think is the patient's nearest relative, unless the patient requests otherwise, or does not have a nearest relative. The information can be given to the nearest relative either when it is given to the patient or within a reasonable time afterwards.

4.22 The duty to give information to nearest relatives does not apply to informal patients or to patients, whether restricted or unrestricted, who are liable to be detained on the basis of an order or direction under part 3 of the Act , eg a hospital order or transfer direction, including those who have been conditionally discharged. It does apply to patients subject to guardianship orders under part 3 and to CTO patients who were formerly detained under part 3.

5: Patients' correspondence

Introduction

5.1 This chapter describes the provisions under which hospital managers may withhold post to and from detained patients and under which the Care Quality Commission (CQC) may review such decisions. The provisions for withholding post addressed to patients apply only to high security psychiatric hospitals.

Patients' correspondence [section 134]

5.2 Detained patients' post may be withheld from them or from the postal operator[36] (as the case may be) only in the circumstances described in figure 11, subject to the restrictions set out in paragraph 5.7 below. For these purposes, detained patients include patients detained under any provision of the Act, except patients on community treatment orders (CTOs) who have been recalled to hospital.

Figure 11: In which correspondence may be withheld

Patient detained in	**Outgoing post may be withheld if**	**Incoming post may be withheld if**
All hospitals	The addressee has requested that post from the patient should be withheld	May not be withheld
High security psychiatric hospitals only	It is likely to cause: • distress to the addressee or to any other person (not being on the staff of the hospital), or • danger to any person	It is necessary to withhold it: ▪ in the interests of the safety of the patient, or ▪ for the protection of other persons.

5.3 The Act refers to post as 'postal packets' which has the same meaning as in the Postal Services Act 2011, ie a letter, parcel, packet or other article transmissible by post. The power to withhold a postal packet also applies to anything contained in it.

5.4 A request from someone for post addressed to them to be withheld must be made in writing to:

---

[36] 'Postal operator' has the same meaning as in section 27 of the Postal Services Act 2011. http://www.legislation.gov.uk/ukpga/2011/5

- the hospital managers, or
- the approved clinician with overall responsibility for the patient's case.

5.5 The managers may open and inspect any letter or other postal packet in order to determine whether it is one which may, in principle, be withheld, and if so whether it, or anything contained in it, should in fact be withheld.

5.6 In hospitals other than high security psychiatric hospitals:

- it should never be necessary to open outgoing post for these purposes, but merely to check whether it is addressed to someone who has asked for it to be withheld, and
- incoming correspondence should not be opened or inspected at all for these purposes, as there is no power in the Act for the managers to withhold it from patients.

Correspondence not to be withheld [section 134(3) and (3A) and regulation 31]

5.7 Under no circumstances may the managers withhold post to or from:

- any Government Minister, any of the Welsh or Scottish Ministers, or the Counsel General to the Welsh Assembly Government
- a Member of either House of Parliament or a member of the National Assembly for Wales or the Scottish Parliament or the Northern Ireland Assembly
- any judge or officer of the Court of Protection, any Court of Protection Visitor, or any person asked by that Court for a report under section 49 of the Mental Capacity Act 2005 concerning the patient
- the Parliamentary Commissioner for Administration (the Parliamentary Ombudsman)
- the Scottish Public Services Ombudsman
- the Public Services Ombudsman for Wales
- the Health Service Commissioner for England (the Parliamentary and Health Service Ombudsman)
- a member (other than an advisory member) of the Commission for Local Administration in England (the Local Government Ombudsman)
- the Care Quality Commission (CQC)
- the First-tier Tribunal or the Mental Health Review Tribunal for Wales
- the NHS Commissioning Board, a clinical commissioning group (CCG), local health board, special health authority or local authority
- a Community Health Council (in Wales)
- a provider of probation services
- a provider of a patient advocacy and liaison service for the assistance of patients at the hospital in which the patient is detained and their families and carers, which is provided by an NHS trust, an NHS foundation trust, a CCG or the NHS Commissioning Board
- a provider of independent mental health advocacy services under the Act (see chapter 4), or independent complaints advocacy services under the

NHS Act 2006, the Local Government and Public Involvement in Health Act 2007[37] or the NHS (Wales) Act 2006, or independent mental capacity advocacy under the Mental Capacity Act 2005 for the patient
- the managers of the hospital in which the patient is detained
- the patient's legal adviser (if legally qualified and instructed by the patient to act on their behalf), or
- the European Commission of Human Rights or the European Court of Human Rights.

5.8 The Secretary of State for Health has the power to make regulations adding other independent advocacy services to the list above.

Procedure for inspecting correspondence [sections 134, 134A and regulation 29]

5.9 The functions of the managers in respect of correspondence must be discharged on their behalf by someone on the staff of the hospital appointed by them for that purpose ('an appointed person'). Different people may be appointed for different aspects of the managers' functions.

5.10 If a letter or other postal packet is opened but nothing is withheld, the appointed person who opened it must place a notice in it. That notice must state:

- that it has been opened and inspected
- that nothing has been withheld, and
- the name of the appointed person and the name of the hospital.

Inspection alone does not have to be recorded: this includes cases where the contents can be read without opening, eg in the case of a postcard.

5.11 Where a letter or other postal packet, or an item contained in it, is withheld, the appointed person who withheld it must make a record in a register kept for the purpose. The entry in the register must record:

- the fact that it or any item in it has been withheld
- the date and the grounds on which that was done
- a description of any item withheld, and
- the name of the appointed person.

5.12 If anything in a letter or other postal packet is withheld, but the rest of it is allowed to go on to the addressee, the appointed person must also place a notice in it before resealing it. That notice should state:

- that the letter or packet has been opened and inspected and an item or items withheld
- the grounds on which any item has been withheld, this is not required when it is withheld at the request of the addressee

[37] Section 223A of the Local Government and Public Involvement in Health Act 2007. http://www.legislation.gov.uk/ukpga/2007/28

- a description of any item withheld
- the name of the appointed person and the name of the hospital, and
- an explanation of the right to ask the CQC to review the decision and the steps the CQC may take as a result (see paragraphs 5.15 to 5.19).

The patient or, where applicable, the person who sent it, if known, must also be given the same information in writing within seven days.

5.13 Where a whole letter or packet is withheld, except at the request of the addressee, the patient and, where applicable, the person who sent it, if known, must be sent a written notice within seven days stating:

- that the letter or packet has been withheld
- the grounds on which it has been withheld
- a description of the contents of the letter or packet withheld
- the name of the appointed person who withheld it and the name of the hospital, and
- an explanation of the right to ask the CQC to review the decision and the steps CQC may take as a result.

5.14 In practice, because a patient can ask the CQC to review the decision within six months of receiving the notice, anything addressed to a patient which is withheld should be retained for at least six months, unless it is necessary to give it to the police or other similar body. After that – assuming the CQC is not in the process of reviewing the decision – it may be returned to the sender, if that can be done safely.

Care Quality Commission's power to review a decision to withhold post [section 134A and regulation 30]

5.15 The CQC must review any decision to withhold post, except when it is withheld at the request of the addressee, if the patient or the person by whom the post was sent applies to the CQC to review the decision within six months of when they receive written notice of the decision.

5.16 In the case of outgoing post, it is only the patient who may apply, but in the case of incoming mail, both the patient and the sender may apply.

5.17 The application need not be made in writing, but should be made in accordance with any guidance provided by the CQC. The applicant must provide the CQC with the written notice of the withholding, or a copy of it.

5.18 When reviewing a withholding decision, the CQC may require the relevant people to produce any documents, information and evidence, including what was withheld, which it reasonably requires.

5.19 The CQC can direct that what was withheld should no longer be withheld. The managers must comply with any such direction.

6: The Tribunal

Introduction

6.1 This chapter describes the two Tribunals which exercise functions under the provisions of the Act in England. Further information and guidance is published by the HM Courts and Tribunals Service, an executive agency of the Ministry of Justice. There is a description of the circumstances in which the First-tier Tribunal (and the Upper Tribunal on appeal) either may or must discharge patients. It describes the steps the Tribunal may take if it decides not to discharge certain patients. The chapter sets out the rights of patients and their nearest relatives to apply to the First-tier Tribunal under the Act. The chapter describes the duties of hospital managers to refer patients' cases to the First-tier Tribunal and the powers and duties of the Secretary of State to do so.

The First-tier Tribunal

6.2 The First-tier Tribunal is an independent judicial body established under the Tribunals, Courts and Enforcement Act 2007.[38] Among its many functions, the Health, Education and Social Care (HESC) Chamber of the First-tier Tribunal exercises powers under the Mental Health Act 1983 which, prior to 3 November 2008, belonged to the Mental Health Review Tribunal (MHRT)[39]. Specifically, it has the power to decide whether patients should continue to be detained (or be liable to be detained) under the Act, continue to be on a CTO, or remain subject to guardianship, as applicable.

6.3 The First-tier Tribunal's powers in these cases only apply to England. There is still an MHRT for Wales, established under section 65 of the Act.

6.4 The First-tier Tribunal does not review other people's decisions to detain patients or to make them subject to other forms of compulsory measures under the Act. It decides whether, at the time of the hearing, the patient concerned should remain subject to the relevant aspect of the Act.

6.5 In practice, cases under the Act typically involve making a balanced judgment on a number of serious issues such as the freedom of the individual, the protection of the public and the best interests of the patient. Tribunal hearings are normally in private and (for detained patients) usually take place in the hospital where the patient is detained.

6.6 In the case of detention and patients on a CTO, the burden of proof is on those who are detaining the patient, or keeping the patient liable to recall to

[38] Section 3 of the Tribunals, Courts and Enforcement Act 2007.
http://www.legislation.gov.uk/ukpga/2007/15

[39] See the Transfer of Tribunal Functions Order. 2008. SI 2008/2833 article 3 and Schedule 1.
http://www.legislation.gov.uk/uksi/2008/2833

hospital, to show that such steps are still justified. Patients are not required to prove that they should be discharged.

Upper Tribunal

6.7 The Upper Tribunal is also established under the Tribunals, Courts and Enforcement Act 2007. Its role in mental health cases is to determine appeals against decisions of the First-tier Tribunal. It also hears appeals against decisions of the MHRT for Wales.

Tribunal Rules and Practice Directions

6.8 The First-tier Tribunal and Upper Tribunal operate according to Rules made by the Lord Chancellor.[40]

6.9 Those Rules are supplemented by Practice Directions, which may be issued by the Senior President of Tribunals, by the President of the relevant chamber of the First-tier Tribunal or by the President of the Upper Tribunal.

6.10 The Rules and Practice Directions must be followed by people involved in Tribunal cases.

6.11 In most cases, there is a responsible authority which must provide the First-tier Tribunal with information and reports on the patient, in accordance with the Rules and Practice Directions.

6.12 The responsible authority is as set out in figure 12.

Figure 12: Authorities for the purposes of the Tribunal[41]

Patient	Responsible authority
Patients detained in hospital	The managers of the hospital.
CTO patients	The managers of the responsible hospital.
Guardianship patients	The responsible local authority.

6.13 For conditionally discharged patients, the Secretary of State for Justice is required to provide the names and addresses of the responsible clinician and any social supervisor in relation to the patient to the Tribunal, and upon being notified by the Tribunal, the responsible clinician and any social supervisor named are required to provide information and reports on the patient in

[40] The Rules are available at http://www.justice.gov.uk/tribunals/rules.

[41] The Tribunal Procedure (First-tier Tribunal)(Health, Education and Social Care Chamber) Rules 2008. SI 2008/2699. See rule 1(3).

accordance with the Rules and Practice Directions. The Secretary of State also provides the additional information specified in the Rules in respect of all restricted patients.

Reviews and appeals

6.14 Appeals to the Upper Tribunal may only be made on a point of law, and only with the permission of the First-tier Tribunal or the Upper Tribunal itself. Before deciding whether to grant permission to appeal, the First-tier Tribunal will first consider whether to review its own decision.

6.15 If it upholds an appeal, the Upper Tribunal may make a new decision itself, or it may remit the case back to the First-tier Tribunal to be heard again.

6.16 On appeal to the Upper Tribunal, the respondent is any person other than the appellant who was a party before the First-tier Tribunal or otherwise has a right of appeal against the decision of the First-tier Tribunal. In practice, this means that in unrestricted cases the responsible authority is the respondent in any case in which the patient (or, where relevant, the patient's nearest relative) seeks permission to appeal to the Upper Tribunal, and in cases involving restricted patients, the respondent is both the responsible authority and the Secretary of State for Justice.

6.17 This means that in practice, it is for the responsible authority and in restricted cases the Secretary of State to decide whether to oppose the request for review, the request for permission to appeal, or the appeal itself (as the case may be) and, if so, on what grounds.

6.18 Responsible authorities have the same right to appeal against decisions of the First-tier Tribunal as the patient and any other parties to the case.

Witness and information

6.19 A Tribunal has the power to obtain any information it thinks necessary, including the power to subpoena witnesses in accordance with the relevant Rules.

Representation

6.20 Patients are entitled to be represented at tribunal hearings. Patients are equally entitled not to have a legal representative, or to represent themselves. A legal representative can be very useful as they will explain the law to the patient and protect their best interests.

Legal aid

6.21 Legal Aid is available through the Legal Aid Agency to fund legal advice and representation for patients before the First-tier Tribunal, without requiring any assessment of the patients' means. Legal Aid for appeals to the Upper Tribunal is means-tested and subject to a merits test.

Administrative Justice Forum

6.22 The Administrative Justice Forum advises the Ministry of Justice on their oversight of the administrative justice and tribunals system. The forum provides a direct link between experts from across the administrative justice and tribunals system and the organisations that work with and represent its users. The forum brings an independent perspective to policy and practice in this important area of justice to inform the programme of work the Ministry of Justice will take forward to improve the system for users and taxpayers.

6.23 This forum provides a direct link between experts from across the administrative justice and tribunals system and the organisations that work with and represent its users, and advises the Ministry of Justice on their oversight of the administrative justice and tribunals system.

Patients' rights to make applications [section 66, 69 and 70]

6.24 Applications for discharge may be made to the Tribunal by patients as set out in the tables at the end of this chapter.

6.25 For applications by patients detained under part 2:

- patients detained for assessment (sections 2 or 4) – see figure 14
- patients detained for treatment (section 3) – see figure 15.

6.26 For applications by unrestricted patients detained under part 3:

- patients subject to unrestricted hospital orders (section 37 etc) – see figure 16
- patients subject to unrestricted transfer directions (sections 47 or 48) or hospital directions (section 45A) to which limitation directions no longer apply – see figure 17.

6.27 For applications by restricted patients detained under part 3:

- patients subject to restricted hospital orders (section 37 and 41 etc) – see figure 18
- patients subject to hospital and limitation directions (section 45A) – see figure 19
- patients subject to restricted transfer directions (sections 47, 48 and 49 etc) – see figure 20.

6.28 For applications by patients on a CTO:

- part 2 CTO patients – see figure 21
- part 3 CTO patients – see figure 22.

6.29 For applications by conditionally discharged restricted patients, see figure 23.

6.30 For applications by guardianship patients (both part 2 and part 3), see figure 24.

Nearest relatives' rights to make applications [section 66 and 69]

6.31 Applications for discharge may be made to the Tribunal by nearest relatives of patients as set out in the following figures:

- patients detained under part 2 – figure 25
- patients detained under part 3 (unrestricted patients only) – figure 26
- part 2 CTO patients – figure 27
- part 3 CTO patients – figure 22
- guardianship patients (part 3 only) – figure 28.

6.32 Nearest relatives may not make applications in respect of restricted patients.

Displaced nearest relatives' rights to make applications [section 66(1)(h)]

6.33 Figure 16 at the end of this chapter describes when former nearest relatives who have been displaced by the county court under section 29 may make applications to the Tribunal. This only applies to former nearest relatives who are displaced on the grounds that they have unreasonably objected to an application or have used (or were likely to use) their powers of discharge without due regard to the welfare of the patient or the interests of the public (see chapter 2).

Only one application per period [section 77]

6.34 Only one application may be made in any given period – but an application which is withdrawn in accordance with the Tribunal's Rules does not count.

6.35 For these purposes, where patients transfer from England to Wales a previous application to the Tribunal in one country counts as an application to the Tribunal in the other.

Applications to the Tribunal in Wales in respect of patients in England (and vice versa) [section 77(3) and (4)]

6.36 It may sometimes be necessary for applications to be made to the Tribunal in Wales even though the patient in question is in, or being cared for, in England (or vice versa). Applications are to be made as shown in figure 13 below.

Figure 13: Applications to the Tribunal

Patient is	Application to be made to Tribunal for the country in which
Liable to be detained in a hospital	The hospital is located
a CTO patient	the patient's responsible hospital is located
Conditionally discharged and not recalled to hospital	The patient is residing
Subject to guardianship	The patient is residing

6.37 The powers and duties of the MHRT for Wales to discharge patients are the same as those of the First-tier Tribunal in England.

Visiting and examination of patients in respect of applications [section 76]

6.38 Any doctor or approved clinician may be authorised by or on behalf of the patient, or anyone else entitled to make an application to the Tribunal, to advise on whether an application should be made, or to provide information on the patient's condition for the purposes of an application (or a reference made by the Secretary of State under section 67).

6.39 These authorised doctors or approved clinicians may visit and examine the patient in private at any time, and require any records relating to the patient's detention or treatment in any hospital, or relating to after-care services provided for the patient under section 117, to be produced for their inspection.

6.40 A person who refused, without reasonable cause, to let an authorised doctor or approved clinician see a patient in private, or inspect any records which they were entitled to see, would be guilty of the offence of obstruction under section 129 (see chapter 33).

Figure 14: By patients detained for assessment [section 66]

Applies to patients:

- detained for assessment on the basis of an application for admission for assessment under section 2
- detained for assessment on the basis of an emergency application under section 4, and
- treated as one of the above on transfer from outside England or Wales.

The patient may apply once during	Notes
The 14 days starting with the day on which the patient is admitted	In the case of a patient who is already in hospital, the day the patient is admitted means the day on which the application is received by the hospital managers. For patients transferred from outside England or Wales, it means the day on which they are treated as having been admitted to the hospital in England or Wales. The patient may not apply in the second 14 days of detention under section 2. So, for example, a patient admitted on 1 January must apply by the end of 14 January.

Note: If a patient's detention for assessment is extended under section 29 pending resolution of an application to the county court for the appointment of an acting nearest relative, the Secretary of State may – and in some circumstances should – be asked to refer the patient to the Tribunal under section 67 – see paragraph 6.40.

Figure 15: By patients detained for treatment under section 3 [section 66]

Applies to:

- patients detained on the basis of an application for admission for treatment under section 3
- patients treated as if they were detained on the basis of such an application following their transfer from guardianship, or from outside England or Wales, and
- former part 2 CTO patients detained again under section 3 following the revocation of their CTO.

If	The patient may apply once during	Notes
A patient is detained on the basis of an application for treatment (section 3)	The six months starting with the day on which the patient is admitted	For patients already in hospital, this means the day on which the section 3 application is received by the hospital managers. For patients transferred from outside England or Wales, it means the day they are admitted to hospital in England or Wales.
The patient's detention is renewed under section 20 or 21B	The period for which the detention is renewed	The first renewal period is six months. Subsequent periods are 12 months. The right to apply begins when the new detention period begins, not when the renewal report is made. A section 21B report only triggers a right to apply if it also serves as a section 20 renewal report.
The patient's community treatment order is revoked	The six months starting with the day the CTO was revoked	The hospital managers must also refer the case to the Tribunal as soon as the CTO is revoked.

Figure 16: By patients detained under unrestricted hospital orders [section 66 as applied by part 1 of Schedule 1, and section 69(2) to (5)]

Applies to patients:

- given an unrestricted hospital order by a court under section 37 or 51, including unrestricted hospital orders given to patients as a result of the Criminal Procedure (Insanity) Act 1964 or other legislation
- treated as if subject to an unrestricted hospital order following their transfer from a guardianship order or from detention outside England or Wales
- treated as if subject to an unrestricted hospital order because their restriction order has lapsed or been lifted, ie unrestricted patients who were previously restricted hospital order patients or were treated as such for any reason
- treated as if subject to an unrestricted hospital order as a result of a direction under the Repatriation of Prisoners Act 1984, or as result of any other legislation, or
- who are former part 3 CTO patients detained again on the basis of an unrestricted hospital order following the revocation of their CTO, ie those who were detained on the basis of a hospital order before being discharged onto a CTO, or who were treated as such for any reason.

If	**The patient may apply once during**	**Notes**
The patient's detention is renewed (section 20 or 21B)	The period for which the detention is renewed	The first renewal period is six months. Subsequent periods are 12 months. The right to apply begins when the new detention period begins, not when the renewal report is made. A section 21B report only triggers a right to apply if it also serves as a section 20 renewal report.
The patient's community treatment order is revoked	The six months starting with the day the CTO was revoked excluding any period during which less than six months has passed since the hospital order was first made (unless the patient would have been able to apply to the Tribunal during that period had they not become a CTO patient in the interim – see below)	The hospital managers must also refer the case to the Tribunal as soon as the CTO is revoked.

In addition, certain patients who are treated as having become subject to an unrestricted hospital direction may also apply to the Tribunal during the first six months before that order is renewed, as follows:

<table>
<tr><th>If</th><th>The patient may apply once during</th><th>Notes</th></tr>
<tr><td>A restricted patient's restriction order lapses or is lifted</td><td>Six months starting with the day on which the restriction order ceases to have effect</td><td>This includes the lifting of orders or directions under other legislation which are treated as if they were restriction orders.</td></tr>
<tr><td>A patient is transferred from guardianship order</td><td>Six months starting with the day of the transfer</td><td rowspan="3">This does not apply to people actually given unrestricted hospital orders by a court.</td></tr>
<tr><td>A patient is transferred from outside England or Wales</td><td>Six months starting with the day of admission to hospital in England as a result of the transfer</td></tr>
<tr><td>A patient is given a direction under Repatriation of Prisoners Act 1984</td><td>Six months starting with the day of the direction</td></tr>
</table>

Figure 17: Applications by patients detained under unrestricted transfer directions or hospital directions to which limitation directions no longer apply [section 66 as applied by part 1 of Schedule 1, and section 69(2)]

Applies to patients:

- given an unrestricted transfer direction under section 47 or 48 by the Secretary of State
- treated as if subject to an unrestricted transfer direction or hospital direction following their transfer from detention outside England or Wales
- treated as if subject to an unrestricted transfer direction because their restriction direction under section 49 has lapsed or been lifted, ie former restricted transfer direction patients including people treated as such for any reason
- treated as if subject to an unrestricted hospital direction because their limitation direction under section 45A has lapsed or been lifted, ie former hospital and limitation direction order patients including people treated as such for any reason
- treated as if subject to an unrestricted transfer direction as a result of a direction under the Repatriation of Prisoners Act 1984, or as a result of any other legislation, or
- who are former part 3 CTO patients detained again on the basis of an unrestricted transfer direction or hospital direction following revocation of their CTO, ie those who were detained on the basis of a hospital direction or transfer direction before being discharged onto a CTO, or who were treated as such for any reason.

If	The patient may apply once during	Notes
A patient becomes subject to an unrestricted transfer direction	The six months starting with the day on which the direction is given	In the case of a patient who is treated as if subject to a direction following transfer from detention outside England or Wales, this means the day on which the patient is admitted to hospital in England or Wales as a result of the transfer.
A restricted patient's restrictions lapse or are lifted	The six months starting on the day the restriction direction or limitation direction ceased to have effect	This includes the lifting of orders or directions under other legislation which are treated as if they were restriction directions or limitation directions.
The patient's detention is renewed (section 20 or 21B)	The period for which the detention is renewed	The first renewal period is six months. Subsequent periods are 12 months. The right to apply begins when the new

If	The patient may apply once during	Notes
		detention period begins, not when the renewal report is made. A section 21B report only triggers a right to apply if it also serves as a section 20 renewal report.
The patient's community treatment order is revoked	The six months starting with the day the CTO was revoked	The hospital managers must also refer the case to the Tribunal as soon as the CTO is revoked.

Figure 18: Applications by detained patients subject to restricted hospital orders [sections 69(2) and 70]

Applies to patients:

- given a hospital order by a court under section 37 or 51 together with a restriction order under section 41, including such orders given to patients as a result of the Criminal Procedure (Insanity) Act 1964 or under other legislation, or
- treated as if subject to restricted hospital orders following their transfer from detention outside England or Wales or as a result of a direction under the Repatriation of Prisoners Act 1984 or other legislation.

If	The patient may apply once during	Notes
The patient is detained in hospital under a restricted hospital order and has never been conditionally discharged	The period between the end of the six months starting with the day the order was made and the end of 12 months from that day, and each subsequent 12 month period	Example: patient given a restricted hospital order on 1 January 20154 can apply once between 1 July and 31 December 2015 and once between 1 January and 31 December each following year. For patients transferred from outside England or Wales, the day of the order means the day they were admitted to hospital in England or Wales as result of the transfer. For patients given a direction under the 1984 Act it means the date of that direction.
The patient has been conditionally discharged but then recalled called to hospital	The period between the end of the six months starting with the day of the patient's arrival at the hospital or unit to which they were recalled and the end of 12 months from that day, and each subsequent 12 month period	Example: patient recalled on 1 January 2009 arrives at relevant hospital on 2 January 2009. Can apply once between 2 July 2009 and 1 January 2010 and then once between 2 January 2010 and 1 January 2011 and so on each year. The Secretary of State must also refer the case to the tribunal when the patient is recalled.

In addition, certain patients who are treated as having become subject to a restricted hospital order may also apply during the first six months of that order, as follows:

If	The patient may apply once during	Notes
The patient was transferred from outside England or Wales under section 80B, 82 or 85	The period of six months starting with the day of admission to hospital in England as a result of the transfer	This does not apply to offenders transferred from the Isle of Man or any of the Channel Islands under section 84 having been found insane.
The patient was given direction under Repatriation of Prisoners Act 1984	The period of six months starting with the day of the direction	

Figure 19: Applications by detained patients subject to hospital and limitation directions [sections 69(2) and 70]

Applies to patients:

- given hospital and limitation directions by a court under section 45A, or
- treated as if subject to hospital and limitation directions following their transfer from detention outside England or Wales, as a result of a direction under the Repatriation of Prisoners Act 1984, or as a result of any other legislation.

If	The patient may apply once during	Notes
The patient is detained in hospital under hospital and limitation directions and has never been conditionally discharged	The period between the end of the six months starting with the day the directions were made and the end of 12 months from that day; and each subsequent 12 month period	Example: A patient given hospital and limitation directions on 1 January 2015 can apply once between 1 July and 31 December 2015 and once between 1 January and 31 December each following year. For patients transferred from outside England or Wales, the day the directions were made means the day they are admitted to hospital in England or Wales as result of the transfer.
The patient has been conditionally discharged but then recalled called to hospital	The period between the end of the six months starting with the day of their arrival at the hospital or unit to which they were recalled and the end of 12 months from that date, and each subsequent 12 month period	Example: A patient recalled on 1 January 2015 arrives at relevant hospital on 2 January 2015. Can apply once between 2 July 2015 and 1 January 2016 and then once between 2 January 2016 and 1 January 2017 and so on each year. The Secretary of State must also refer the case to the tribunal when the patient is recalled.

In addition, certain patients who are treated as having become subject to hospital and limitation directions may also apply during the first six months of those directions, as follows:

If	The patient may apply once during	Notes
The patient was transferred from outside England or Wales under section 80B, 82 or 85	The period of six months starting with the day of admission to hospital in England as a result of the transfer	

Figure 20: Applications by detained patients subject to restricted transfer directions [sections 69(2) and 70]

Applies to patients:

- given a transfer direction under section 47 or 48 together with a restriction direction under section 49, or
- treated as if subject to such a restricted transfer direction following their transfer from detention outside England or Wales, as a result of a direction under the Repatriation of Prisoners Act 1984, or as a result of any other legislation.

If	The patient may apply once during	Notes
The patient is detained under a restricted transfer direction and has never been conditionally discharged	The period of six months starting with the day the directions were made, the subsequent 6 months, and each subsequent 12 month period	Example: A patient given a restricted transfer direction on 1 January 2015 can apply once between then and 30 June 2015, once between 1 July and 31 December 2015 and once between 1 January and 31 December each following year. For patients transferred from outside England or Wales, the day the directions were made means the day they are admitted to hospital in England or Wales as result of the transfer.
The patient has been conditionally discharged but then recalled called to hospital	The period between the end of the six months starting with the day of their arrival at the hospital or unit to which they were recalled and the end of 12 months from that date, and each subsequent 12 month period	Example: A patient recalled on 1 January 2015 who arrives at the relevant hospital on 2 January 2015. Can apply once between 2 July 2015 and 1 January 2016 and then once between 2 January 2016 and 1 January 2017, and so on each year. The Secretary of State must also refer the case to the Tribunal when the patient is recalled.

Figure 21: Applications by part 2 CTO patients [section 66]

Applies to patients on a CTO who, immediately before becoming CTO patients, were:

- detained on the basis of an application for admission for treatment under section 3, or
- treated as if detained on the basis of such an application, following transfer from guardianship or from outside England or Wales.

If	The patient may apply once during	Notes
The patient becomes a patient on a CTO (or is treated as such on transfer from outside England or Wales)	The period of six months starting with the day the CTO is made (or treated as made)	In the case of patients transferred from outside England or Wales, they are treated as if their CTO was made on the day of their arrival at the place they are to reside in England or Wales.
The patient's CTO revoked	The period of six months starting with the day the CTO is revoked	The hospital managers must also refer the patient's case to the Tribunal as soon as possible after CTO is revoked.
The patient's CTO is extended (section 20A or 21B)	The period for which the CTO is extended	The first extension period is six months. Subsequent periods are 12 months. The right to apply begins when the new period begins, not when the extension report is made. A section 21B report only triggers a right to apply if it also serves as a section 20A extension report.

Figure 22: Applications by part 3 CTO patients and their nearest relatives [section 66 as applied by part 1 of Schedule 1 and modified by section 69(3) – (5)]

Applies to patients on a CTO who, immediately before being on a CTO, were:

- detained on the basis of a hospital order, unrestricted hospital direction, or transfer under part 3, or
- treated as if detained on the basis of such an order or direction, following transfer from outside England or Wales, or for any other reason, and
- the nearest relatives of such patients.

If	The patient and the nearest relative may each apply once during	Notes
A patient is discharged onto a CTO from an unrestricted hospital order which was given by a court within the previous six months	The period between the end of the six months starting with the day the hospital order was made and the six months starting with the day the CTO was made	Example: A patient given unrestricted hospital order on 1 January, and a CTO on 1 March can apply between 1 July and 31 August only. (But will be able to apply again if the CTO extended from 1 September). This only applies to patients who are actually given an unrestricted hospital order by a court. It does not apply to patients who are treated as having been given such an unrestricted hospital order and who therefore have the right to apply to the Tribunal before that order is first renewed (see Figure 20)
A patient becomes detained again under a unrestricted hospital order which was given by a court within the previous six months because the patient's CTO is revoked	The period between the end of the six months starting with the day the hospital order was given and the six months starting with the day the CTO was revoked	
Any other part 3 patient becomes an CTO patient	The period of six months starting with the day the CTO is made	This applies to patients who, before becoming patients on a CTO, were detained under unrestricted transfer directions or hospital directions, as well as unrestricted hospital order patients not covered by the rules above.
Any other part 3 patient's CTO is revoked	The period of six months starting with the day the CTO is revoked	
The patient's CTO is extended (section 20A or 21B)	The period for which the CTO is extended	The first extension period is six months. Subsequent periods are 12 months. The right to apply begins when the new period begins, not when the

If	The patient and the nearest relative may each apply once during	Notes
		extension report is made. A section 21B report only triggers a right to apply if it also serves as a section 20A extension report.

Figure 23: Applications by conditionally discharged restricted patients [section 75]

Applies to patients who have been:

- conditionally discharged from restricted hospital orders, hospital and limitation directions, or restricted transfer directions, or who are treated as such following their transfer from outside England and Wales, or
- conditionally discharged whilst treated as subject to such an order or direction, following their transfer from outside England or Wales, as a result of a direction under the Repatriation of Prisoners Act 1984, or as a result of other legislation.

If	The patient may apply once during	Notes
The patient is conditionally discharged and has not been recalled to hospital	The period between the end of the 12 months starting with the day of the conditional discharge and the end of two years from that date, and each subsequent two year period	Example: A patient conditionally discharged on 1 January 2015 can apply once between 1 January 2016 and 31 December 2016, and then once between 1 January 2017 and 31 December 2017 and so on. Where responsibility for a patient is transferred from outside England or Wales, the patient is treated as if conditionally discharged on the day of the transfer of responsibility.

For rights to apply if recalled to hospital, see figures 17 (restricted hospital orders), 18 (hospital and limitation directions) or 19 (restricted transfer direction) as appropriate.

Figure 24: Applications by guardianship patients [section 66 and 69(1)]

Applies to all patients subject to guardianship under the Act – both guardianship applications under part 2 and guardianship orders under part 3

If	The patient may apply once during	Notes
A patient is received into guardianship on the basis of an application for guardianship under part 2 (or treated as such on transfer from outside England or Wales)	The period of six months starting with the day on which the application is accepted (or deemed to have been accepted)	Where patients are transferred to guardianship from outside England or Wales, the application is deemed to have been accepted, or the order made (as the case may be) on the day of their arrival at the place they are to reside in England or Wales. Transfer from hospital to guardianship creates no new right to apply.
A guardianship order is made by a court under part 3 (or the patient is treated as if such an order had been made on transfer from outside England or Wales)	The period of six months starting with the day on which the order was made (or deemed to have been made)	
A patient's guardianship or guardianship order is renewed (section 20 or 21B)	The period for which guardianship is renewed	The first renewal period is six months. Subsequent periods are 12 months. The right to apply begins when the new period begins, not when the renewal report is made. A report under section 21B only triggers a right to apply if it also serves as a section 20A extension report.

Figure 25: Applications by nearest relatives of patients detained for treatment under section 3 [section 66]

Applies to nearest relatives of patients who are:

- detained on the basis of an application for admission for treatment under section 3, or
- who are treated as such following their transfer from guardianship or from outside England and Wales.

If	The nearest relative may apply once during
The responsible clinician bars a nearest relative's order for the discharge of a patient detained on the basis of an application for admission for treatment under section 3	The period of 28 days starting with the day on which they are informed of the report made by the responsible clinician which bars discharge.

This is the only case in which the nearest relative of a part 2 detained patient who has not been displaced (see Figure 16) may apply to the Tribunal.

The nearest relative has no right to apply if the responsible clinician bars the discharge of patient detained on the basis of an application for admission for assessment under section 2 or 4.

Figure 26: Applications by nearest relatives of unrestricted part 3 detained patients [section 69(1) and (3) to (5)]

Applies to nearest relatives of:

- patients detained under unrestricted hospital orders, unrestricted hospital directions or unrestricted transfer directions,
- patients treated as subject to such an order or direction for any reason; and
- former part 3 CTO patients detained again following revocation of their CTO.

If	The nearest relative may apply once during	Notes
The patient's detention is renewed (section 20 or 21B)	The period for which the detention is renewed	The first renewal period is six months. Subsequent periods are 12 months. The right to apply begins when the new detention period begins, not when the renewal report is made. A section 21B report only triggers a right to apply if it also serves as a section 20A extension report. Even where patients are permitted to apply during the first six months of their detention prior to its first renewal or their discharge onto a CTO, nearest relatives may not do so.
The patient's CTO is revoked	The six months starting with the day the CTO is revoked, excluding any period in which the patient could not apply – see Figure 6.3	The hospital managers must also refer the case to the Tribunal as soon as the CTO is revoked.

Figure 27: Applications by nearest relatives of part 2 CTO patients [section 66(1)(g)]

Applies to CTO patients who, immediately before becoming CTO patients, were:

- detained on the basis of an application for admission for treatment under section 3, or
- treated as if they were detained on the basis of such an application for any reason.

If	The nearest relative may apply once during
A responsible clinician bars a nearest relative's order for the discharge of a patient from CTO	The period of 28 days starting with the day on which they are informed of the report by the responsible clinician which bars discharge

This is the only case in which a nearest relative may apply for the discharge of a part 2 CTO patient.

For applications by nearest relatives of part 3 CTO patients, see Figure 22.

Figure 28: Applications by nearest relatives of guardianship patients [section 69(1)]

Applies only to patients subject to a guardianship order under part 3, and those who are treated as if they were following transfer from hospital or from outside England and Wales.

If	Nearest relatives may apply once during	Notes
A guardianship order is made by the court (or the patient is treated as if such an order had been made on transfer from outside England or Wales)	The period of 12 months starting with the day on which the order was made (or deemed to have been made) and in any subsequent period of 12 months	Where patients are transferred to a guardianship order from outside England or Wales, the order is deemed to be given on the day of their arrival at the place they are to reside in England or Wales.

Note: because nearest relatives of patients subject to guardianship under part 2 can discharge patients themselves, they do not have the right to apply to the Tribunal (unless displaced – see Figure 16).

Figure 29: Applications by displaced nearest relatives of part 2 detained patients, part 2 CTO patients and guardianship patients [section 66(1)(h)]

Applies to applications by nearest relatives who have been displaced by the appointment of an acting nearest relative by the county court on the grounds that:

- they have unreasonably objected to an application for admission for treatment or a guardianship application, or
- they have exercised, or are likely to exercise, their power of discharge without due regard to the welfare of the patient or the interests of the public.

In other words, nearest relatives displaced on the grounds in paragraphs (c) or (d) or section 29(3) – see chapter 2.

If they would otherwise have been the nearest relative of a patient who is	Nearest relatives may apply once during the	Notes
Detained on the basis of an application for admission for assessment or treatment under section 3, or	The period of 12 months starting with the day of the county court's order, and subsequently once in each 12 month period for which order is in force	Nearest relatives displaced on other grounds do not have a right to apply to the Tribunal. Displaced nearest relatives cannot make applications in respect of part 3 patients (whether detained, on CTO or subject to guardianship orders).
A part 2 CTO patient, or		
Subject to guardianship on the basis of an application under part 2		

Definitions

6.41 'Detained patients' means patients liable to be detained on the basis of an application for admission under part 2, or subject to a hospital order, hospital direction or transfer direction under part 3.

Hospital managers' duty to refer certain patients to the Tribunal after six months of first being detained [section 68]

6.42 Hospital managers must refer certain patients to the Tribunal if six months have passed since they were first detained (or transferred to detention from outside England and Wales) as set out in figure 17.

6.43 In that figure:

- ‘section 2 patient’ means a patient detained on the basis of an application for admission for assessment
- ‘section 3 patient’ means a patient detained on the basis of an application for admission for treatment
- ‘part 2 CTO patient’ means a section 3 patient who was then discharged onto a CTO
- ‘hospital order patient’ means a patient subject to an unrestricted hospital order
- ‘part 3 CTO patient’ means a hospital order patient who was then discharged onto a CTO
- ‘admission to hospital’ means the day the patient is treated as having been admitted to hospital on the basis of the relevant application or order (eg for patients who were already in hospital when an application under was made, it means the day the application was received by the hospital managers)
- a ‘relevant application or reference’ means an application or reference made by, or in respect of, the patient to the Tribunal (or the Mental Health Review Tribunal for Wales) – except one made by the patient, the patient’s nearest relative or the Secretary of State while the patient was detained under section 2 or section 4
- applications or references which are made, but then withdrawn, do not count as relevant applications.

Figure 30: Patients to whom the managers’ duty to refer at six months applies

Patient	Unless a relevant application or reference has already been made, a reference must be made after
Section 2 patient (whose detention is extended under section 29 because of an application to displace their nearest relative)	Six months from the date of admission to hospital for assessment under section 2 or 4
Section 3 patient	If originally admitted to hospital under section 2 or 4 – six months from the date of that admission Otherwise, six months from the date of admission to hospital under section 3
Part 2 CTO patient	
Hospital order patient or part 3 CTO patient, but only if transferred to the hospital order from a guardianship order	Six months from the date of the transfer from the guardianship order

6.44 If the patient is, at the time, a CTO patient, the duty to make a reference to the Tribunal falls on the managers of the responsible hospital. Otherwise, it falls on the managers of the hospital in which the patient is liable to be detained.

6.45 The effect of the duty described in figure 27 is that no patient originally detained under part 2 (and no part 3 patient who was originally given a guardianship order but then transferred to hospital) should wait more than six months from first being detained before their case is put to the Tribunal while they remain a detained or a CTO patient.

6.46 In addition, the managers' duty to refer applies even if patients have already had a Tribunal hearing as a result of an application or reference they, or someone else made while they were detained under section 2 or 4. Those applications and references are to be ignored by the managers when deciding whether the patient's case needs to be referred to the Tribunal after six months. In other words, it is only applications and references made while a patient is detained under section 3, or is a CTO patient, which are relevant.

6.47 There is one exception to this rule – an application made by a displaced nearest relative under section 66(1)(h) would be a relevant application even if it were made while the patient were still detained under section 2.

6.48 In all cases, applications or references which are made, but then withdrawn, do not affect the managers' duty to refer after six months.

Hospital managers' duty to refer certain patients to the Tribunal after three years (or one year) since their last Tribunal hearing [section 68(6)]

6.49 Hospital managers must refer the cases of detained patients (unless they are restricted patients) and CTO patients in the circumstances set out in figure 31.

Figure 31: Circumstances in which hospital managers must refer patients to the Tribunal after the first six months

Hospital managers must refer patients' cases to the Tribunal if:	
Patients aged 18 or over	A period of more than 3 years has passed without the patient's case being considered by the Tribunal (or the MHRT in Wales)
Patients under 18	A period of more than 1 year has passed without the patient's case being considered by the Tribunal (or the MHRT in Wales)

6.50 The three year period is three calendar years from the date of the last hearing, ie if the last hearing was on 1 June 2014, the three years will end on 31 May 2017. Similarly, the one year period is one year from the date of the last hearing.

6.51 In the case of unrestricted part 3 patients whose cases have never been heard by the Tribunal, the three year (or one year) period begins as set out in figure 32.

Figure 32: Unrestricted part 3 patients: start of the three year (or one year) period after which a referral may have to be made

If the patient	the 3 year (or 1 year) period runs from
Was previously a restricted patient	The date on which the patient's restrictions ended or were lifted
Was transferred from outside England or Wales	The date of the patient's admission to hospital in England or Wales, or the date on which they were treated as becoming a CTO patient in England or Wales (as the case may be)
Is neither of the above	The date of the hospital order or transfer direction

6.52 Again, if the patient is a CTO patient, the duty falls on the managers of the responsible hospital. Otherwise, it falls on the managers of the hospital in which the patient is liable to be detained.

Hospital managers' duty to refer patients on a CTO to the Tribunal if their CTO is revoked [section 68(7)]

6.53 Hospital managers must also refer the cases of patients whose CTOs are revoked, as soon as possible after the CTO is revoked.

6.54 The duty to refer falls on the managers of the hospital in which the patient is now detained, even if it was not previously the patient's responsible hospital.

Secretary of State's power to refer patients (except restricted patients) [section 67(1)]

6.55 The Secretary of State may at any time refer the case of a patient to the Tribunal. This includes patients who are detained in hospital, who are CTO patients or who are subject to guardianship under part 2. It also includes part 3 patients detained under unrestricted hospital orders, transfer directions or under hospital directions where the associated limitation direction is no longer in force, and patients who have been discharged from such an order or direction onto a CTO. It also includes patients subject to guardianship orders under part 3. It does not include restricted patients, who can be referred under section 71 instead – see below.

6.56 Anyone, including hospital managers, local authorities, nearest relatives and patients themselves, may request the Secretary of State for Health to consider making a reference to the Tribunal, by contacting the Department of Health.

6.57 Case law suggests that hospital managers and local authorities should consider doing so where a patient's rights under the European Convention on Human Rights might otherwise be jeopardised.[42]

6.58 A request for a reference should, in particular, be considered in any case where a patient's detention on the basis of an application for admission for assessment under section 2 is extended by virtue of section 29 pending the outcome of an application to displace the patient's nearest relative – especially if the patient has not yet had a Tribunal hearing, or a significant period has passed since the patient's last hearing.[43] Patients themselves have no right to apply to the Tribunal in such situations.

References by the Secretary of State in respect of restricted patients [section 71]

6.59 The Secretary of State for Justice may at any time refer the case of a restricted patient to the Tribunal. This includes patients who have been conditionally discharged.

6.60 The Secretary of State must refer a restricted patient's case to the Tribunal if the patient is detained in hospital and three years have passed without the patient's case having been considered by the Tribunal, or by the MHRT in Wales.

6.61 The Secretary of State must also refer to the Tribunal the case of every conditionally discharged patient recalled to hospital. The Secretary of State must make the reference to the Tribunal immediately, and in any case within one month of the patient arriving at, or being brought to, the hospital to which they are recalled.

References to the Tribunal in for Wales in respect of patients in England (and vice versa) [section 77(3)]

6.62 It may sometimes be necessary for references to be made to the Tribunal in Wales even though the patient in question is in, or being cared for, in England (or vice versa). References are to be made to the same Tribunal as an application by the patient would be made – see paragraph 6.36

Secretary of State's power to vary periods after which patients must be referred to the Tribunal [sections 68A and 71(3)]

6.63 The Secretary of State can reduce the six month, 3 year and 1 year periods described earlier in this chapter by making an order under section 68A or

[42] R (Modaresi) v Secretary of State for Health. 2013. UKSC 53. 2013. MHLO 63. http://www.bailii.org/uk/cases/UKSC/2013/53.html
[43] R (on the application of H) v Secretary of State for Health. 2005. UKHL 60; 4 All ER 131. http://www.bailii.org/uk/cases/UKHL/2005/60.html

71(3) (as applicable). At the time of publication, no such order has been made.

Visiting and examination of patients in respect of references [section 67(2) and 68(8)]

6.64 Any doctor or approved clinician may be authorised by or behalf of the patient in order to provide information for the purposes of a reference by the Secretary of State for Health under section 67 or by the hospital managers under section 68.

6.65 Authorised doctors or approved clinicians may visit and examine the patient in private at any time, and require any records relating to the patient's detention or treatment in any hospital, or relating to after-care services provided for the patient under section 117, to be produced for their inspection.

6.66 A person who refused, without reasonable cause, to let an authorised doctor or approved clinician see a patient in private, or inspect any records which they are entitled to see, would be guilty of the offence of obstruction under section 129 (see chapter 33).

Patients who are outside the remit of the Tribunal

6.67 The Tribunal does not deal with the discharge of the patients who are:

- detained under the 'holding powers' in section 5 (see paragraphs 8.71 to 8.85)
- remanded to hospital under sections 35 or 36 (see chapter 14)
- subject to an interim hospital order under section 38 (see chapter 18), or
- detained in a place of safety sections 135 or 136 (see chapter 7).

6.68 References in this chapter to 'any' or 'all' patients do not therefore include the patients listed above.

Powers in respect of detained patients except restricted patients [section 72]

6.69 The Tribunal may discharge any patient (other than a restricted patient) from liability to detention at any time as it sees fit.

6.70 As well as having this general discretion, the Tribunal must always discharge detained patients if the criteria in figure 33 are met.

Figure 33: Circumstances in which the Tribunal must discharge detained patients

<table>
<tr><th>Patient</th><th>The Tribunal must discharge if</th></tr>
<tr><td>Detained on the basis of an application for admission for assessment (section 2 or 4)</td><td>The Tribunal is not satisfied that:
• the patient is then suffering from mental disorder of a nature or degree which warrants detention in hospital for assessment (or assessment followed by medical treatment) for at least a limited period; and
• the patient's detention is justified in the interests of the patient's own health or safety or with a view to the protection of others</td></tr>
<tr><td>Detained on the basis of an application for admission for treatment (section 3)</td><td rowspan="2">The Tribunal is not satisfied that:
• the patient is then suffering from mental disorder of a nature or degree which makes it appropriate for the patient to be liable to be detained in hospital for medical treatment
• it is necessary for the health or safety of the patient or for the protection of other persons that the patient should receive such treatment
• appropriate medical treatment is available for the patient; and
• (if the nearest relative has applied to the Tribunal because the responsible clinician has barred discharge under section 25) the patient, if released, would be likely to act in a manner dangerous to other persons or themselves</td></tr>
<tr><td>Patients subject to a hospital order, hospital direction or transfer direction</td></tr>
</table>

6.71 When discharging patients from detention or a CTO, but not from guardianship, the Tribunal may direct that the discharge will take effect at a specified future date. This is commonly known as 'discharge on a future date' and is not to be confused with a deferred (provisional) conditional discharge which only applies to restricted patients. Otherwise, discharges by the Tribunal take effect immediately.

6.72 If the Tribunal decides not to discharge a patient from detention, it may recommend that the patient be granted leave of absence or be transferred to another hospital or into guardianship, with a view to facilitating the patient's discharge on a future occasion.

6.73 The Tribunal cannot discharge patients onto a CTO, and is not required to discharge patients from detention just because it thinks that a CTO might be appropriate for them. The Tribunal may recommend that the responsible clinician considers whether to discharge a patient onto a CTO.

6.74 The Tribunal's recommendations are not binding on hospital managers or responsible clinicians, although they must be considered. If its recommendations are not put into practice, the Tribunal may, if it wishes, further consider a patient's case, without the patient or anyone else having to make a new application. If the hospital manager or the responsible clinician do not put the recommendations in place, it is good practice that they put their reasons in writing and explain these to the patient, nearest relative and, if different, carer, (see paragraph 12.41 of the Code of Practice.)

Powers in respect of patients on a CTO [section 72]

6.75 The Tribunal may discharge any patient from a CTO at any time as it sees fit, even if the patient is recalled to hospital at the time.

6.76 The Tribunal must always discharge CTO patients if the criteria in the figure 34 are met.

Figure 34: Circumstances in which the Tribunal must discharge patients from a CTO

The Tribunal must discharge patients on a CTO if
The Tribunal is not satisfied that: • the patient is then suffering from mental disorder of a nature or degree which makes it appropriate for the patient to receive medical treatment • it is necessary that the patient should receive such treatment for the patient's health or safety or for the protection of other people • it is necessary that the responsible clinician should be able to exercise the power to recall the patient to hospital • appropriate medical treatment is available for the patient, and • (if the nearest relative has applied to the Tribunal because the responsible clinician has barred discharge under section 25) the patient, if discharged from a CTO, would be likely to act in a manner dangerous to other persons or themselves. In determining whether the responsible clinician needs to have the power of recall, the factors the Tribunal must consider include the same factors which the responsible clinicians must always consider when deciding if a CTO should be made in the first place (see paragraph 26.13).

6.77 The Tribunal cannot discharge patients from detention onto a CTO. Nor can it order the release of a CTO patients who is detained temporarily as a result of being recalled to hospital (without at the same time discharging then from the CTO itself).

Powers in respect of guardianship patients [section 72]

6.78 The Tribunal has discretion to discharge a patient from guardianship in any case.

6.79 The Tribunal must discharge guardianship patients if the criteria in figure 35 are met.

Figure 35: Circumstances in which the Tribunal must discharge patients from guardianship

The Tribunal must discharge guardianship patients if
The Tribunal is satisfied that: • the patient is not then suffering from mental disorder, or • it is not necessary that the patient should remain subject to guardianship in the interests of the welfare of the patient or for the protection of other people.

Powers in respect of patients subject to restriction orders [section 73]

6.80 The Tribunal has no general discretion to discharge restricted patients. It may only discharge them where it is required by the Act to do so.

6.81 The Tribunal must discharge patients who are subject to a restriction order (other than patients who have been conditionally discharged and not recalled to hospital) if it is not satisfied that the criteria for continued detention for treatment under a hospital order are met (see figure 34).

6.82 The discharge must be conditional, unless the Tribunal is satisfied that it is not appropriate for the patient to remain liable to be recalled to hospital for further treatment, ie to be made subject to conditional discharge.

6.83 If the patient is to be discharged absolutely, the discharge takes effect immediately. The Tribunal cannot defer an absolute discharge.

6.84 Where the Tribunal is required to discharge a restricted patient conditionally it may, but does not have to, impose conditions with which the patient is to comply. The Secretary of State for Justice may impose conditions and vary those imposed by the Tribunal.

6.85 Where the Tribunal makes a preliminary decision to order conditional discharge it may defer its final direction until arrangements have been made to its satisfaction for the discharge to take effect. This is commonly known as 'deferred conditional discharge'. But case law has established that the Tribunal may not defer a discharge in this way to enable the patient's progress to be tested in the interim.[44]

6.86 Where the Tribunal does defer conditional discharge, the primary care trust (or local health board in Wales) and local authority which are responsible for providing after-care under section 117 must use their best endeavours to put in place after-care which will allow the patient to be discharged subject to the conditions specified by the Tribunal *(Various cases).* See chapter 29 for more on after-care under section 117.

6.87 If such arrangements cannot be put in place, the Tribunal may reconvene and reconsider its decision. If it reconvenes, it may decide to vary the conditions it had in mind to impose, make an absolute discharge if it believes the criteria for that are now met, or decide that the conditions for neither absolute nor conditional discharge are met and that the patient should accordingly remain detained. It is unlawful for the Tribunal to defer conditional discharge if the purpose of the deferment is actually to secure the patient's admission to another hospital.[45]

6.88 See chapter 27 for a description of the effect of conditional discharge.

Powers in respect of patients subject to limitation directions or restriction directions [section 74]

6.89 As with other restricted patients, the Tribunal has no general discretion to discharge patients subject to hospital and limitation directions or restricted transfer directions.

6.90 In addition, because these patients are liable to resume serving their sentence of imprisonment, or its equivalent, if they no longer require treatment in hospital, special arrangements apply where the Tribunal believes that the criteria for discharge from detention are met.

6.91 The criteria for the discharge of patients subject to these directions are the same as those for patients subject to restricted hospital orders – see paragraphs 6.81 and 6.82.

6.92 Where the Tribunal decides that such a patient would be entitled to be discharged absolutely or conditionally if the patient were subject to a restriction order, as described above, it must inform the Secretary of State for Justice.

6.93 If the patient would be entitled to conditional discharge, the Tribunal may recommend that the patient continue to be detained in hospital, rather than

[44] R (on the application of the Secretary of State for the Home Office) v Mental Health Review Tribunal; PG as an Interested Party. 2002. EWHC Admin 2043. http://www.bailii.org/ew/cases/EWHC/Admin/2002/2043.html

[45] Secretary of State for the Home Office v Mental Health Review Tribunal for the Mersey Regional Health Authority. 1986. 3 All ER 233.

going to prison or other custodial institution, if the patient is not, in fact, discharged.

6.94 In the case of patients who are remand prisoners or other unsentenced prisoners subject to restricted transfer directions under section 48, the Secretary of State has no discretion. If the Tribunal has decided that such a patient would be entitled to be conditionally discharged and has made a recommendation for the patient's continued detention in hospital, the patient remains detained and subject to the restriction direction or limitation direction. Otherwise, the Secretary of State must issue a warrant directing the person's return to prison, or any other place of detention in which the patient could have been detained but for being in hospital.

6.95 In the case of a sentenced prisoner subject to hospital and limitation directions or a restricted transfer direction under section 47, the Secretary of State has the discretion to agree to the patient's discharge.

6.96 In these cases, the Secretary of State has 90 days from being informed of the Tribunal's findings in which to give notice that the patient may be discharged. If the Secretary of State does not do so, the patient must be returned to prison, or its equivalent, unless the Tribunal has recommended that the patient remain in hospital if not conditionally discharged.

6.97 Where sentenced prisoners subject to hospital and limitation directions or transfer directions remain in hospital only as a result of a recommendation by the Tribunal, they have the right to apply to the Parole Board for release once they have served the minimum period set by the court (the 'tariff' period) in the same way as other prisoners. If that point has already been reached when the Tribunal recommendation is first acted on, the Secretary of State will refer their case automatically to the Parole Board.

Powers in respect of conditionally discharged patients [section 75]

6.98 When considering applications by conditionally discharged patients, or references in respect of them from the Secretary of State for Justice, the Tribunal may discharge the restriction order, limitation direction or restriction direction to which they are subject. If it does so, patients are automatically discharged from the underlying hospital order, hospital direction or transfer direction as well.

6.99 If the Tribunal decides not to discharge a conditionally discharged patient, it may vary the conditions to which the patient is subject, or impose new conditions.

Assessment, transport and admission to hospital

This group of chapters is concerned with the ways in which civil (part 2) patients may be admitted to hospital, the circumstances in which patients may be transferred between hospitals if that becomes necessary as part of their care and treatment and how patients who are absent without leave may be returned.

7: Police powers and places of safety

Introduction

7.1 This chapter describes the provisions in the Act concerned with powers of entry to premises and with the powers of the police to take people who appear to have a mental disorder to a place of safety.

Approved mental health professionals' power of entry and inspection [section 115]

7.2 Approved mental health professionals (AMHPs), when acting as such on behalf of a local authority, may at all reasonable times enter and inspect any premises, including care homes and private dwellings, in which a mentally disordered patient is living, if the AMHP has reasonable cause to believe that the patient is not 'under proper care'.

7.3 If asked to do so, AMHPs must produce an authenticated document confirming that they are AMHPs. The relevant document is issued by local authorities for this purpose.

7.4 If AMHPs are refused entry to premises or required to leave without reasonable cause, the person who does so might be committing an offence of obstruction under section 129. AMHPs do not have any power to force entry to premises or to remain on them if the occupier insists they leave. If necessary, they may be able to obtain a warrant under section 135 (see below).

Warrants to search for and remove patients not receiving proper care [section 135(1)]

7.5 An AMHP acting on behalf of a local authority may apply to a magistrate for a warrant authorising a police officer to enter specific premises, by force if necessary. The application should be made to a magistrate for the area where the premises are located.

7.6 Magistrates can issue warrants if satisfied, on the basis of information provided (on oath) by an AMHP, that there is reasonable cause to suspect that someone believed to be suffering from mental disorder:

- has been or is being ill-treated, neglected, or 'kept otherwise than under proper control', or
- is living alone and unable to care for themselves.

7.7 A warrant can be issued even if the person's name is not known.

7.8 The warrant gives a police officer the right to enter any premises specified in the warrant, by force if necessary, to search for the person, and (if it is thought fit) to remove the person concerned to a place of safety with a view to an application for detention or guardianship being made under part 2 of the Act, or other arrangements being made for the person's treatment or care.

7.9 The police officer must be accompanied by an AMHP and a doctor.

7.10 A place of safety for these purposes means:

- residential accommodation provided by an local authority (under part 1 of the Care Act 2014)[46]
- a hospital, including an independent hospital
- a police station
- a care home, or
- any other suitable place where the occupier is willing temporarily to receive the patient.

7.11 A person who is removed to a place of safety on the basis of a warrant may be detained there for a maximum of 72 hours. Within that period they may be transferred to one or more other places of safety by a police officer, an AMHP acting on behalf of a local authority or by anyone authorised by a police officer or AMHP.

7.12 The maximum 72 hour period begins at the time of arrival at the first place of safety. Transfers between places of safety must happen within this timeframe.

Warrant to search for and remove patients who are liable to be taken or returned under the Act [section 135(2)]

7.13 Magistrates can issue a warrant to allow the police to enter premises and remove people who are liable to be taken or returned to hospital or any other place, or to be taken into custody, under the Act because, for example, they have gone absent without leave. This also applies to people who may be taken into custody under equivalent legislation having gone absent without leave from Scotland.

7.14 A warrant may be applied for by a police officer or any other person who is authorised to take or return the patient to any place or take them into custody. A magistrate may issue a warrant, if satisfied on the basis of the information provided by that person, on oath, that:

- there is reasonable cause to believe that the patient in question is to be found on premises within the magistrate's area, and
- admission to the premises has been refused or is expected to be refused.

[46] The Care Act 2014. http:// http://www.legislation.gov.uk/ukpga/2014/23/contents/enacted

7.15 The warrant gives a police officer the right to enter any premises specified in the warrant, by force if necessary, and remove the patient. The purpose of this is to return the patient to where they ought to be. The police officer may (but does not have to) be accompanied by a doctor or any person authorised to take or retake the patient, or both.

Power of police to remove mentally disordered persons from public places to places of safety [section 136]

7.16 The police also have an emergency power under the Act in relation to people whom they find in a place to which the public have access who appear to be suffering from mental disorder and to be in immediate need of care or control. Any police officer can remove such a person to a place of safety, as described in paragraph 7.10. Removal may take place if the police officer believes it is necessary in the interests of that person, or for the protection of others.

7.17 For these purposes, 'a place to which the public have access' includes places to which members of the public have open access, access if a payment is made or access at certain times of the day. It does not include private premises, such as the person's own place of residence or private homes belonging to others in which case a section 135 warrant is needed. It is not appropriate to encourage a person outside in order to use section 136 powers. Section 135 should be used if the person is in private premises.

7.18 People removed to a place of safety can be detained there for a maximum of 72 hours so that they can be examined by a doctor and interviewed by an AMHP, in order that any necessary arrangements can be made for their treatment or care.

Related material

Standards on the use of section 136 of the Mental Health Act 1983 (England and Wales). Royal College of Psychiatrists CR159. 2011. http://www.rcpsych.ac.uk/usefulresources/publications/collegereports/cr/cr159.aspx

8: Applications for detention in hospital

Introduction

8.1 This chapter describes the procedures for detaining patients in hospital under part 2 of the Act.

Criteria for admission for assessment [section 2]

8.2 Patients may be detained in hospital for assessment on the grounds that they:

- are suffering from mental disorder of a nature or degree which warrants their detention in hospital for assessment, or for assessment followed by medical treatment, for at least a limited period, and
- ought to be so detained in the interests of their health or safety, or with a view to the protection of others.

8.3 Case law has established that here (and in section 3) 'nature' refers to the particular mental disorder from which the patient is suffering, its chronicity, its prognosis, and the patient's previous response to receiving treatment for the disorder. 'Degree' refers to the current manifestation of the patient's disorder.[47]

8.4 Detention for assessment under section 2 is for up to 28 days. It cannot be renewed, although in certain cases it may be extended while an application is made to the county court to replace the patient's nearest relative (see paragraph 2.42 onward).

8.5 Although there must be an intention to assess the patient's needs if the criteria above are to be met, a patient detained for assessment may also be treated. Indeed, treatment may form part of the assessment.

Criteria for admission for treatment [section 3]

8.6 Patients may be detained in hospital for medical treatment on the grounds that:

- they are suffering from mental disorder of a nature or degree which makes it appropriate for them to receive medical treatment in hospital
- it is necessary for their health or safety, or for the protection of others, that they should receive that treatment
- that treatment cannot be provided unless they are detained under section 3, and

[47] R v Mental Health Review Tribunal for the South Thames Region Ex p. Smith. 1999. C.O.D. 148

- appropriate medical treatment is available for the patient.

8.7 For these purposes, mental disorder does not include learning disability, unless that learning disability is associated with abnormally aggressive or seriously irresponsible conduct on the part of the patient concerned (see paragraph 1.11 onward and Code paragraphs 20.4-20.17).

8.8 Appropriate medical treatment means medical treatment which is appropriate in the patient's case, taking into account the nature and degree of the patient's mental disorder and all other circumstances of the case. Available means that appropriate treatment is actually available for the patient. It is not enough that appropriate treatment exists in theory for the patient's condition. See paragraph 1.17 onward for the definition of medical treatment in the Act and the meaning of medical treatment for mental disorder.

8.9 Detention for treatment under section 3 is for up to six months initially and may be renewed (see paragraphs 25.29-25.35).

8.10 These criteria require that it is appropriate and necessary for the patient to receive medical treatment in hospital, section 3 cannot be used if the intention is to admit and detain the patient for a purely nominal period during which no necessary and appropriate treatment will be given.[48]

8.11 The Code of Practice gives guidance on when it is appropriate to use section 2 rather than section 3 (or vice versa). The conditions for section 2 admissions are not quite so stringent as those for section 3 admissions because assessment may well be used for the purpose of determining whether the more stringent conditions apply. The powers under section 2 can only be used for the limited purpose for which they were intended. They cannot be used to further detain patients for the purposes of assessment beyond the 28 days period. Nor can they be used as a temporary alternative to detention under section 3 merely to allow an application to be made to the county court under section 29 for an order to appoint an acting nearest relative in place of a nearest relative who objects to the use of section 3[49] – see paragraphs 8.23 to 8.30.

Applications for admission to hospital [sections 2, 3 and 11]

8.12 In order for a patient to be detained in hospital for assessment or treatment under part 2 of the Act, an application for admission to hospital must be made to the managers of the hospital in question.

8.13 An application may be made by the patient's nearest relative, or by an approved mental health professional (AMHP) acting on behalf of a local authority.

---

[48] R v Hallstrom ex p. W; R v Gardner, ex p. L 1986. 2 All ER 306.

[49] R v Wilson, ex p. Williamson. 1996. C.O.D. 42

8.14 An application under section 2 is known as an 'application for admission for assessment'. An application under section 3 is known as an 'application for admission for treatment'.

Applications in respect of wards of court [section 33]

8.15 An application in respect of a ward of court cannot be made without leave of the High Court (section 33(1)).

Duty on local authority to arrange for AMHP to consider making application for admission to hospital [section 13]

8.16 Local authorities must arrange for an AMHP to consider a patient's case on their behalf, if they have reason to believe that an application for admission to hospital may need to be made in respect of a patient who happens, at the time, to be within their area. It does not matter whether the patient lives in the area.

8.17 In addition, local authorities must arrange for an AMHP to consider the case of a patient who lives in their area if required to do so by the patient's nearest relative. If AMHPs decide not to make an application in these cases, they must give the nearest relative their reasons in writing.

8.18 In certain cases, local authorities must also arrange for an AMHP to consider the case of a patient who is in a hospital outside their area. This applies where the patient concerned is already detained for assessment on the basis of an application made by an AMHP acting on behalf of the local authority in question. If that local authority has reason to think that an application for admission for treatment may now be needed for the patient, it is that local authority, rather than the one for the area in which the hospital is, or where the patient lives, which is under a duty to arrange for an AMHP to consider making the further application.

8.19 The fact that an AMHP is acting on behalf of a local authority does not make it unlawful for them to make an application outside the area of that local authority. And the fact that one local authority has a duty to arrange for an AMHP to consider a patient's case on its behalf, does not prevent another local authority from doing so instead, if it wishes.

Duty on clinical commissioning groups to give local authorities notice of hospitals having arrangements for special cases [section 140]

8.20 Clinical commissioning groups (CCGs) must keep local authorities whose areas overlap (wholly or partly) with their own informed of the hospital or hospitals where arrangements are in force for the reception of patients in case of special urgency or the provision of accommodation and facilities designed to be specially suitable for patients under the age of 18 (see also Code paragraphs 14.77-14.86).

Duty on AMHPs to inform nearest relatives of applications for admission for assessment [section 11(3)]

8.21 Where the application is one for admission for assessment, AMHPs must take whatever steps are practicable to inform the person, if any, whom they think is the patient's nearest relative:

- that the application is about to be, or has been, made, and
- of the nearest relative's power to discharge the patient under section 23 (see paragraphs 27.10 to 27.16).

8.22 This must be done either before, or within a reasonable time after the application is made. Although the duty falls on the AMHP making the application, the actual giving of the information need not necessarily be undertaken by the AMHP personally.[50]

Nearest relative's power to object to an application for admission for treatment and AMHP's duty to consult [section 11(4)]

8.23 An AMHP may make an application for admission for assessment even though the nearest relative objects.

8.24 An AMHP may not make an application for admission for treatment under section 3 if the patient's nearest relatives may lodge their objection either with the AMHP directly, or with the local authority on whose behalf the AMHP is acting. The objection does not have to be made in any particular form,provided it is clearly an objection to the proposed application being made.

8.25 AMHPs must therefore consult the person, if any, whom they think is the nearest relative before making the application.

8.26 AMHPs do not have to consult the nearest relative if, in the circumstances, they think it is not reasonably practicable or that it would involve unreasonable delay.

8.27 For practical reasons, it may not always be possible to identify, locate and contact the nearest relative within a reasonable time. It will also not be reasonably practicable to consult with the nearest relative where – in all the circumstances – the detrimental impact of that consultation on the patient's rights under article 8 of the European Convention on Human Rights to privacy and family life means it would not be justified and proportionate. Consultation with the nearest relative that interferes with the patient's article 8 rights may be justified to protect the patient's article 5 rights.[51]

---

[50] R v South Western Hospital Managers, ex p. M. 1994 1 ALL E.R. 161.

[51] TW v Enfield Borough Council. 2014. EWCA Civ 362. http://www.bailii.org/ew/cases/EWCA/Civ/2014/362.html

8.28 Consultation with the nearest relative can precede the obtaining of the two medical recommendations which are needed to support the application (as described below)[52] and in suitable circumstances, AMHPs can carry out their duty to consult through the medium of another person.[53]

8.29 Case law also requires that nearest relatives should be given sufficient information about the proposed application and the reasons for it to enable them to form an opinion about whether to object to the application being made.

8.30 If the nearest relative objects, the AMHP cannot make the application. An unreasonable objection by a nearest relative is one of the grounds in section 29(3) for the county court, on application, to transfer the powers of the nearest relative to another person (see chapter 2).

Duty of the AMHP to be satisfied that detention in hospital is the most appropriate course of action [section 13(2)]

8.31 Before making an application (whether for admission for assessment or treatment), AMHPs must interview the patient 'in a suitable manner', eg taking account of the patient's age and understanding, and any learning disability, autism spectrum disorder or hearing or linguistic difficulties the patient may have.

8.32 AMHPs must also be satisfied that detention in a hospital is the most appropriate way of providing the care and medical treatment the patient needs. In making that decision, AMHPs are required to consider 'all the circumstances of the case'. In practice, that might include the past history of the patient's mental disorder, the patient's present condition and the social, familial, and personal factors bearing on it, the other options available for supporting the patient, the wishes of the patient and the patient's relatives and carers, and the opinion of other professionals involved in caring for the patient.

8.33 In principle, an application can be made even if the patient has only recently been discharged from detention under the Act.

8.34 In general, an AMHP cannot lawfully apply for the admission of a patient who has recently been discharged by the Tribunal if the AMHP is aware of that fact.

8.35 In such cases, AMHPs can only properly make applications if they have formed a reasonable and bona fide opinion that there was information not known to the Tribunal which puts a significantly different complexion on the case compared with that which was before the Tribunal.[54] See chapter 6 for more about the Tribunal.

---

[52] Re Whitbread (Times Law Report) 14 July 1997

[53] R v South Western Hospital Managers, ex p. M. 1994. 1 All ER 161

[54] R v East London and City Mental Health NHS Trust Ex. p Brandenburg 2003. UKHL 58. http://www.publications.parliament.uk/pa/ld200203/ldjudgmt/jd031113/east-1.htm

Duty on AMHPs to make applications in certain circumstances [section 13(1A)]

8.36 AMHPs must make an application if they think that an application ought to be made and, taking into account the views of the relatives and any other relevant circumstances, they think that it is 'necessary or proper' for them to make the application, rather than the nearest relative.

8.37 This does not affect the rules about consultation with nearest relatives described above, or nearest relatives' right to object to an application for admission for treatment.

Medical recommendations [section 12]

8.38 An application must be supported by written recommendations from two doctors who have personally examined the patient, as shown in figure 36.

Figure 36: Medical recommendations

One doctor	Other doctor
Approved under section 12	*If the doctor approved under section 12 does not have previous acquaintance with the patient:* If practicable, a doctor who has previous acquaintance with the patient
	Otherwise: Any doctor

8.39 Doctors are approved under section 12 if they have been approved by the Secretary of State or approving bodies listed on the gov.uk website (or the Welsh Ministers) as having special experience in the diagnosis or treatment of mental disorder. Doctors who are approved clinicians are automatically treated as being approved under section 12. See chapter 30 for more information on approvals.

8.40 At least one of the doctors should, if practicable, have had previous acquaintance with the patient. Preferably, this doctor should have treated the patient personally, but case law has established that previous acquaintance need not involve personal acquaintance, provided the doctor in question has some knowledge of the patient and is not 'coming to them cold'.[55]

[55] Mental Capacity Act 2005. http://www.legislation.gov.uk/ukpga/2005/9/contents

8.41 The two doctors may examine the patient jointly or separately. No more than five clear days must elapse between the days of the two examinations. For example, if the first doctor examines the patient on 1 January, the second doctor must examine the patient no later than 7 January – see paragraph 8.60.

8.42 Medical recommendations in support of an application for admission for assessment must state that, in the doctor's opinion, the criteria described at paragraph 8.2 are met.

8.43 Recommendations for applications for admission for treatment must state that, in the doctor's opinion, the criteria described in paragraph 8.6 are met, and must in particular explain why the patient cannot be treated without being detained in this way, eg as an outpatient, or as a voluntary in-patient, or in accordance with the Mental Capacity Act 2005.

8.44 Recommendations may be made separately by each doctor, or as a joint recommendation signed by both.

8.45 The recommendations must be signed on or before the day the application is signed. In principle, this means a recommendation could be signed after the application itself is signed. In practice, an application could not be acted on until the necessary recommendations are signed, because it would not be founded on the required recommendations.

Emergency applications for admission for assessment [section 4]

8.46 In exceptional cases, it may be necessary to admit patients for assessment as an emergency before obtaining a second medical recommendation.

8.47 An emergency application ('section 4 application') must state that it is of urgent necessity that the patient should be admitted and detained for assessment, and that compliance with the normal procedures would involve undesirable delay. This must be confirmed by the doctor making the medical recommendation.

8.48 The doctor giving the recommendation does not have to be approved under section 12. If practicable, the doctor should be one who has had previous acquaintance with the patient (see paragraph 8.40).

8.49 An emergency application can be used to detain patients in hospital for no more than 72 hours, unless during that period a valid second medical recommendation is received by the hospital managers.

8.50 The second medical recommendation will only be valid if the two recommendations together would be sufficient to support an ordinary application for admission for assessment (except for the fact that the second recommendation may well, by necessity, have been signed after the date on which the application was signed).

8.51 The 72 hour period runs from the time the patient is admitted to hospital. If the patient is already in hospital, it runs from when the application is received by, or on behalf of, the hospital managers.

8.52 If a second medical recommendation is received within the 72 hour period, patients are treated as if they had been admitted originally on the basis of an ordinary application for admission for assessment. In other words, they may be detained for up to 28 days from the day they were admitted, not the end of the 72 hour period. This is often referred to as 'converting' the application from section 4 to section 2, but the Act does not use that term.

8.53 If a second medical recommendation is not received within the 72 hour period, the authority to detain the patient expires and the patient must be allowed to leave the hospital if that is what the patient wants to do.

8.54 If the relevant criteria are met, there is nothing to prevent an application for admission for treatment being made under section 3 while a patient is detained under section 4, but two new medical recommendations would be required.

Conflicts of interest [section 11(1) and 12A and Conflicts of Interest regulations]

8.55 AMHPs may not make an application if they have a potential conflict of interest as defined in the Mental Health (Conflicts of Interest) (England) Regulations 2008[56] and described in figure 37. An application made by an AMHP who had a potential conflict of interest would be invalid and would not provide any authority for the patient's detention. See also Code of Practice chapter 39.

[56] Mental Health (Conflicts of Interest) (England) Regulations. 2008. SI 2008/1205. http://webarchive.nationalarchives.gov.uk/+/www.dh.gov.uk/en/Healthcare/Mentalhealth/InformationontheMentalHealthAct/DH_106630

Figure 37: Potential conflicts of interest for AMHPs

<table>
<tr><th colspan="2">AMHPs have a potential conflict if any of the following apply:</th></tr>
<tr><td colspan="2">The AMHP has a financial interest in the outcome of the decision whether or not to make the application</td></tr>
<tr><td>The AMHP employs</td><td rowspan="3">The patient, or

either of the doctors making the recommendations on which the application is based</td></tr>
<tr><td>The AMHP directs the work of</td></tr>
<tr><td>The AMHP is closely involved in the same business venture (which includes being a partner, director, other office-holder or major shareholder) as</td></tr>
<tr><td>The AMHP is the wife, ex-wife, husband, ex-husband, civil partner, ex-civil partner, mother, father, sister, brother, half-sister, half-brother, daughter, son, aunt, uncle, grandmother, grandfather, grandson, granddaughter, first cousin, nephew, niece, mother-in-law, father-in-law, daughter-in-law, son-in-law, sister-in-law, brother-in-law, grandmother-in-law, grandfather-in-law, granddaughter-in-law, grandson-in-law, (including adoptive and step-relationships) of</td><td rowspan="2">The patient, or

Either of the doctors making the recommendations on which the application is based</td></tr>
<tr><td>The AMHP is living as if wife, husband or civil partner with</td></tr>
<tr><td colspan="2">The AMHP and both the doctors making the recommendations on which the application is based are members of the same team organised to work together for clinical purposes on a routine basis (but see paragraph 8.58 for urgent cases)</td></tr>
<tr><td colspan="2">The AMHP and the patient are members of the same team organised to work together for clinical purposes on a routine basis (but see paragraph 8.58 for urgent cases)</td></tr>
</table>

8.56 Similarly, doctors may not give a medical recommendation if they have a potential conflict of interest, as described in figure 38. An application which relied on a recommendation made by a doctor who had a potential conflict of interest would be invalid.

Figure 38: Potential conflicts of interest for doctors

<table>
<tr><th colspan="2">Doctors have a potential conflict if any of the following apply.</th></tr>
<tr><td colspan="2">The doctor has a financial interest in the outcome of the decision whether or not to give a recommendation</td></tr>
<tr><td>The doctor employs</td><td rowspan="3">The patient, or

The other doctor making a recommendation on which the application is based, or

The applicant (whether an AMHP or the nearest relative)</td></tr>
<tr><td>The doctor directs the work of</td></tr>
<tr><td>The doctor is closely involved in the same business venture (which includes being a partner, director, other office-holder or major shareholder) as</td></tr>
<tr><td>The doctor is employed by</td><td rowspan="2">The nearest relative (if the nearest relative is the applicant)</td></tr>
<tr><td>The doctor works under the direction of</td></tr>
<tr><td>The doctor is the wife, ex-wife, husband, ex-husband, civil partner, ex-civil partner, mother, father, sister, brother, half-sister, half-brother, daughter, son, aunt, uncle, grandmother, grandfather, grandson, granddaughter, first cousin, nephew, niece, mother-in-law, father-in-law, daughter-in-law, son-in-law, sister-in-law, brother-in-law, grandmother-in-law, grandfather-in-law, granddaughter-in-law, grandson-in-law (including adoptive and step-relationships) of</td><td rowspan="2">The patient, or

The other doctor making a recommendation on which the application is based, or

The applicant (whether an AMHP or the nearest relative)</td></tr>
<tr><td>The doctor is living as if wife, husband or civil partner with</td></tr>
<tr><td colspan="2">Both doctors and the AMHP making the application are members of the same team organised to work together for clinical purposes on a routine basis (but see paragraph 8.58 for urgent cases)</td></tr>
<tr><td colspan="2">The doctor and the patient are members of the same team organised to work together for clinical purposes on a routine basis (but see paragraph 8.58 for urgent cases)</td></tr>
<tr><td colspan="2">The doctor is on the staff of an independent hospital to which the patient's admission is being considered and so is the other doctor making a recommendation</td></tr>
</table>

8.57 Among the effects of this are that:

- only one of the recommendations in support of an application for admission to an independent hospital may be made by a doctor on the staff of that hospital, and
- three professionals involved in an application may not all be in the same clinical team, as described above, nor may any of the professionals involved be in the same clinical team as the patient.

8.58 The latter rule about membership of the same clinical team does not apply if the AMHP or doctor concerned thinks that it is of urgent necessity that an application be made and a delay would involve serious risk to the health or safety of the patient or others. In other words, in urgent cases it is possible for all three professionals to be from the same clinical team, and for any or all of them to be from the same clinical team as the patient.

8.59 Note that 'in-law' relationships include relationships based on civil partnerships as well as marriage. They do not include relationships based on people living together as if they were married or in a civil partnership.

Time limits in respect of making applications [sections 6, 11 and 12]

8.60 Certain time limits apply in respect of applications under sections 2 and 3, as set out in figure 39.

Figure 39: Time limits for applications under sections 2 and 3

Action	Time limit	Example
Application	The applicant must personally have seen the patient within the period of 14 days ending on the date of the application	If the applicant last saw the patient on 1 January, the application must be signed on or before 14 January
Examination for purposes of medical recommendation for application	No more than 5 clear days must have elapsed between the days on which the separate examinations took place (where relevant)	If the first doctor examined the patient on 1 January, the second doctor's examination must take place on or before 7 January

Medical recommendations in support of applications	Must be signed on or before the date of application	If the application is signed by the nearest relative or AMHP at noon on 1 January, the medical recommendation must be signed by the doctor(s) concerned before midnight on that day
Conveyance and admission of patient to hospital in pursuance of application	Patients can only be conveyed and admitted to hospital within the period of 14 days starting with the day on which the patient was last examined by a doctor for the purposes of the application	If the patient was last examined on 1 January, the patient can only be taken to or admitted to hospital if that happens on or before 14 January. The application must also have been signed before they can be taken to hospital

Time limits for emergency applications [section 4]

8.61 Some of the time limits for emergency applications are shorter. The time limits for emergency applications are described in figure 40.

Figure 40: Time limits for emergency applications under section 4

Action	Time limit	Example
Application	The applicant must personally have seen the patient within the 24 hours prior to making of the application (ie signing the properly completed form)	If the applicant last saw the patient at noon on 1 January, the application must be signed before noon on 2 January
Medical recommendation in support of application	Must be signed on or before the date of application	If the application is signed by the nearest relative or AMHP at noon on 1 January, the medical recommendation must be signed by the doctor concerned before midnight on that day

Conveyance and admission of patient to hospital in pursuance of the application	The patient can be conveyed and admitted to hospital only within the period of 24 hours starting at the time when the patient was last examined by the doctor for the purposes of the application, or the making of the application (whichever is earlier)	If the patient was last examined at noon on 1 January, and the application is signed in the interim, the patient can only be taken to or admitted to hospital if that happens before noon on 2 January If the application was signed at 9am on 1 January, before the patient was examined at noon, the patient can only be taken to or admitted to hospital if that happens before 9am on 2 January
Second medical recommendation (to 'convert' the emergency application into a section 2 application).	Must be signed by the doctor and received by (or on behalf of) the hospital managers within 72 hours of the patient being admitted in pursuance of the application	If the patient was admitted to hospital at noon on 1 January, the second recommendation must be signed and received before noon on 4 January

Forms to be used for making the application [regulation 4]

8.62 The forms are to be used for applications and medical recommendations are set out in figure 41.

Figure 41: Forms to be used for applications and medical recommendations

	Application for admission for assessment (section 2)	**Application for admission for treatment (section 3)**	**Emergency application for assessment (section 4)**
Application by nearest relative	Form A1	Form A5	Form A9
Application by AMHP	Form A2	Form A6	Form A10
Single medical recommendation	Form A4	Form A8	Form A11
Joint medical recommendation	Form A3	Form A7	

8.63 If doctors making recommendations have examined the patient in Wales they must use the equivalent Welsh form on which to make their recommendations. If doctors are making a joint recommendation, and one of them examined the patient in England and one in Wales, then they may use either the English or Welsh form.

8.64 Applications to hospitals in Wales must be made in accordance with the Welsh regulations (which will always involve using a Welsh application form).

Procedure to be used for making the application [regulations 3 and 4]

8.65 An application must be addressed to the managers of the hospital to which the applicant wants the patient admitted. Applications must be served by delivering them to an officer of the managers of the hospital to which admission is sought who is authorised to receive them. This means that the application should be delivered to the hospital in which the patient is to be detained.

Transport ('conveyance') of patients to hospital [sections 6, 137 and 138]

8.66 A duly completed application for admission provides the authority for the applicant, or anyone authorised by the applicant, to take and convey the patient to the hospital named in the application in order for the patient to be admitted and detained there within the time periods described in figures 39 and 40.

8.67 An application cannot be considered duly completed without the necessary medical recommendations. It is essential that the application and recommendations are signed and dated, and where relevant indicating the time, by people qualified to do so before any action is taken on the basis of them.

8.68 Patients being taken and conveyed to hospital on the basis of an application for admission are considered to be in legal custody and the applicant, or the person authorised by the applicant, as the case may be, may take steps accordingly to prevent the patient absconding. If patients abscond while being taken to hospital they may be retaken within the 14 days or 24 hour period during which they could be conveyed to hospital originally (as described earlier in this chapter).

8.69 For further information on legal custody and absconding, see chapter 11.

Applications in respect of patients already in hospital [section 5(1)]

8.70 Applications for admission for assessment or treatment may be made in respect of patients who are already in hospital. This includes applications for admission for treatment in respect of patients who are already detained on the basis of an application for admission for assessment. It is not possible to make further applications for assessment in respect of patients who are already detained on the basis of such an application.

Holding powers pending applications in respect of patients already in hospital [sections 5(2) and 5(4)]

8.71 In certain circumstances, hospital in-patients may be detained temporarily in the hospital pending the making of an application, as described below.

8.72 This does not apply to patients who are already detained on the basis of an application under the Act, nor to patients in respect of whom a community treatment order (CTO) under the Act is in force – see chapter 26.

Holding power of doctor or approved clinician in charge of patient's treatment [section 5 and regulations 3 and 4]

8.73 In-patients, whether or not they are already being treated for mental disorder, may be detained in a hospital for up to 72 hours if the doctor or approved clinician in charge of their treatment reports that an application for admission under section 2 or 3 ought to be made.

8.74 This report must be made on form H1 and must then be furnished to the hospital managers. That can be done in one of two ways. The report may either be:

- delivered personally to an officer of the hospital managers authorised to receive such reports on behalf of those managers, or
- sent to the hospital managers using their internal mail system (provided that the managers have agreed to the use of the internal mail system for this purpose).

8.75 The managers may authorise any officer to agree on their behalf to the use of their internal mail system. The 72 hour period during which the patient may be detained begins at the time the report is delivered in person to an authorised officer of the managers or when it is put into the managers' internal mail system.

8.76 The doctor or approved clinician in charge of a patient's treatment may nominate one, but only one, other doctor or approved clinician on the staff of the same hospital to exercise the holding power on their behalf in their absence. They may nominate different deputies for different patients.

8.77 The identity of the doctor or approved clinician in charge of a patient's medical treatment will depend on the particular circumstances. There may be more than one person who could reasonably be said to be in charge of a patient's treatment, for example where a patient is already receiving treatment both for physical and mental disorder. A professional who is treating the patient under the direction of another professional should not be considered to be in charge.

8.78 Doctors and approved clinicians who make reports under section 5(2) do not have to detain patients personally. Patients may only be detained in the hospital in which they were in-patients when the report was made.

Nurses' six hour holding power [section 5(4) and (5), regulations 3 and 4, and nurses order]

8.79 Nurses 'of the prescribed class' may authorise the detention for up to six hours of an patient who is already being treated for mental disorder in the hospital as an in-patient if they think that:

- the patient is suffering from mental disorder to such a degree that it is necessary for the patient's health or safety, or for the protection of others, for the patient to be immediately restrained from leaving the hospital, and
- it is not practicable to secure the immediate attendance of a doctor or an approved clinician for the purpose of furnishing a report under section 5(2) (as described above).

Nurses may not authorise the detention of patients who are not already receiving in-patient treatment for mental disorder in the hospital.

8.80 A nurse of the prescribed class means a nurse registered in the register of qualified nurses and midwives maintained by the Nursing and Midwifery Council as follows:

- registered in sub-part 1 of the register, whose entry includes an entry to indicate the nurse's field of practice is mental health nursing (Registered Nurse Mental Health Level 1)
- registered in sub-part 1 of the register, whose entry includes an entry to indicate the nurse's field of practice is learning disabilities nursing (Registered Nurse Learning Disabilities Level 1)
- registered in sub-part 2 of the register, whose entry includes an entry to indicate the nurse's field of practice is mental health nursing (Registered Nurse Mental Health Level 2), or
- registered in sub-part 2 of the register, whose entry includes an entry to indicate the nurse's field of practice is learning disabilities nursing (Registered Nurse Learning Disabilities Level 2).

8.81 The authority to detain the patient begins when the nurse records the necessary opinion that the criteria above are met, using form H2. It ends either six hours later, or on the arrival at the place the person is being detained of a doctor or approved clinician entitled to make a report on the patient under section 5(2), if that is earlier.

8.82 The record made by the nurse must be delivered to the hospital managers, or someone authorised to act on their behalf, as soon as possible, either by the nurse or by someone authorised by the nurse.

8.83 The period for which a patient has already been detained as a result of a nurse's decision under section 5(4) counts as part of the maximum 72 hours for which they may be detained in total if the doctor or approved clinician concerned then decides to make a report under section 5(2).

8.84 Nurses who make reports under section 5(4) do not have to detain patients personally. Patients may only be detained in the hospital in which they were inpatients when the report was made.

Example

A patient starts preparing to leave a psychiatric ward at noon on 1 May against the advice of the ward staff. The psychiatrist in charge of the patient's treatment is not immediately available. A level 1 nurse decides that the patient needs to be detained until the psychiatrist, or nominated deputy, can attend and makes a record under section 5(4) to that effect at five past noon. The patient may now be detained in the hospital until five past six o'clock that evening at the latest.

The psychiatrist arrives at five o'clock and, after talking to the nurse and the patient, thinks that an application for admission for treatment should be made because the patient needs further treatment which could not otherwise be given. Before contacting an AMHP to come and interview the patient, the psychiatrist makes a report to the hospital managers under section 5(2).

Even though the report is given to the person authorised by the managers to receive it at half past five on 1 May, the patient can be detained, pending a decision on an application, only until 72 hours after the nurse made the original record under 5(4), ie until five past noon on 4 May.

Admission to hospital on the basis of an application [section 6 and regulation 4]

8.85 An application for admission, properly completed and delivered, provides the authority for hospital managers to detain patients, provided the patient is admitted within the relevant time limit described earlier in this chapter.

8.86 The Act places no obligation on a hospital to admit a patient merely because an application has been made.

8.87 The managers must record the time and date of admission using form H3, which must then be attached to the application. The managers may authorise officers to make the necessary records on their behalf.

8.88 Where patients are already in hospital, they are treated as having been 'admitted' when the application is received by or on behalf of the managers.

Circumstances in which an application may not be acted on [section 6(3)]

8.89 The managers may detain a patient on the basis of an application which appears to them, or in practice a person authorised on their behalf to receive it, to be duly made and founded on the necessary medical recommendations.

8.90 A document cannot be regarded as a proper application or medical recommendation if, for example:

- an application is not accompanied by the correct number of medical recommendations
- the application and the recommendations do not all relate to the same patient
- an application or recommendation is not signed at all, or is signed by someone not qualified to do so, or
- an application does not specify the correct hospital.

8.91 The managers do not have to seek further proof that the signatories are who they say they are or that they have the qualification to make the application which they have signed to say they have. Nor do they need to seek further proof for any factual statement or opinion contained in the document.

8.92 For example, the managers do not need to check that signatories who state they are registered medical practitioners are in fact, registered, or seek independent verification of the time when the patient was last examined or that there was sufficient urgency to justify the making of an emergency application.

8.93 If an application is discovered to be fundamentally flawed because of the sorts of error set out above (or for any other reason), there is no authority for the patient's detention because fundamentally defective applications cannot be retrospectively validated.[57]

8.94 In these circumstances, authority for the patient's detention can only be obtained if the patient is already in hospital). Any new application must, of course, be accompanied by medical recommendations which comply with the Act. But this does not exclude the possibility of one of the two existing medical recommendations being used, if the time limits and other requirements of the Act can still be complied with.

[57] Re S-C (Mental Patient: Habeas Corpus). 1996. 1 All ER 532, CA.

Effect of admission on previous applications [section 6(4)]

8.95 The admission of patients on the basis of an application for treatment, but not assessment, automatically causes any previous application for admission, or for guardianship, to cease to have effect.

Effect of admission for treatment on patients on community treatment orders or subject to guardianship [section 6(4)]

8.96 Because patients on CTOs can be recalled to hospital for treatment if required, it should not be necessary to make applications for their detention. In practice, this may happen if the people making the application do not know that the patient is on a CTO.

8.97 An application for admission for assessment under section 2 or 4 does not affect the patient's CTO. Nor does an application for admission for treatment under section 3 if, before going onto a community treatment order (CTO), the patient had been detained on the basis of a hospital order, hospital direction or transfer direction under part 3 of the Act.

8.98 Because an application for admission for treatment automatically ends any previous application for admission, it would also bring to an end a patient's CTO, if before going onto the CTO, the patient had been detained under section 3. In that case, a new CTO would have to be made for the patient when they no longer needed to be detained in hospital. For more on CTOs, see chapter 26.

8.99 Once a patient subject to guardianship is admitted for treatment, the guardianship ceases. For more on guardianship, see chapter 28.

9: Detention in hospital

Introduction

9.1 This chapter describes the main provisions of the Act which apply to patients while detained in hospital. Patients' correspondence, transfer between hospitals, and medical treatment, are covered separately in chapters 5, 10 and 23 respectively.

Patients to whom this chapter applies

9.2 Figure 42 sets out the groups of detained patients to whom this chapter primarily applies, together with the terms used in the chapter to describe them.

Figure 42: Patients to whom this chapter primarily applies

Patients	Terms used in this chapter
Patients detained on the basis of an application for admission for assessment or treatment and those who are treated as such, eg having been transferred from guardianship or from outside England or Wales	'Patients admitted on the basis of an application' or 'part 2 patients'
Which includes: Part 2 patients detained on the basis of an application for admission for treatment under section 3 (and those who are treated as such, eg having been transferred from guardianship or from outside England or Wales)	'Patients detained for treatment under part 2'
Patients detained in hospital on the basis of a hospital order, a hospital direction or a transfer direction (and those who are treated as such, eg having been transferred from a guardianship order or from outside England or Wales)	'Part 3 patients'

Patients	Terms used in this chapter
Which includes: Part 3 patients who are subject to a restriction order, limitation direction or a restriction direction and patients treated as if they are, eg when committed to hospital under section 44, and	'Restricted patients'
Part 3 patients who are not restricted patients. This includes patients who were originally restricted patients but whose restrictions have since ended or been lifted	'Unrestricted part 3 patients'

9.3 Unless stated otherwise, this chapter does not apply to patients:

- detained under the 'holding powers' in section 5 – see chapter 8
- remanded to hospital under section 35 or 36 – see chapter 14
- subject to interim hospital orders under section 38 – see chapter 18
- detained in a hospital as a place of safety pending formal admission under a hospital order (section 37) or hospital and limitation directions (section 45A) – see chapters 15 and 16, or
- detained in a hospital as a place of safety pending assessment under section 135 or 136 – see chapter 7.

Paragraphs which do apply to some or all of the patients above include: the rules on when time limits for detention start (9.5); duties on hospital managers to give patients information (9.10 to 9.20); accommodation for children and young people (9.21 to 9.24); responsible clinicians (9.27 to 9.29).

9.4 This chapter does not apply to patients on community treatment orders (CTOs), even when recalled to hospital. It does apply to patients who have had their CTOs revoked, and so have ceased to be CTO patients and become part 2 or part 3 detained patients again (see chapter 26).

Start of period of detention [sections 2, 5 and 20]

9.5 The maximum periods for which patients may be detained are described in the earlier chapters. Those periods begin as set out in figure 43.

Figure 43: Time at which detention periods start

Authority to detain	Time runs from
Section 5(4)	The time at which the relevant nurse makes a record of the need for the patient to be prevented from leaving (see paragraph 9.5)
Section 5(2)	The time at which the doctor or approved clinician in charge of the person's treatment furnishes the necessary report to the hospital managers (see paragraph 8.74) – unless section 5(4) was used first, in which case the period runs from the time the nurse make the record under that section
Part 2 patients	The day on which the patient is admitted to hospital Where patients are already in hospital, they are treated as having been 'admitted' when the relevant application was received by or on behalf of the managers For patients admitted on the basis of an emergency application (section 4), the 72 hour initial period runs from the time of admission
Part 3 patients	The date of the relevant hospital order, hospital direction or transfer direction (even if the patient is not admitted until sometime later)
Remands and interim hospital orders under part 3	The date of the relevant remand or interim hospital order (even if the patient is not admitted until sometime later)
Detention in a place of safety under section 135 or 136.	The time at which the patient is first detained at a place of safety. If the place of safety is a hospital, the patient may not necessarily have been formally 'admitted' in the normal way

Record of admission or detention [regulation 4]

9.6 The managers are required to record the time and date of the admission of part 2 patients using form H3. If the patient is already in hospital, that means the time and date that the managers receive the application.

9.7 If a patient is admitted on the basis of an emergency application under section 4, the managers must also use the same form H3 to record when they receive the second medical recommendation (see paragraph 8.49 onward).

9.8 Form H3 must be attached to the application.

9.9 There is no requirement to use form H3 to record the admission of other patients (eg Part 3 patients).

The duty of hospital managers to provide information [section 132]

9.10 Section 132 places a duty on hospital managers to provide certain information to patients who are detained in their hospitals and to their nearest relatives.

9.11 With one exception, this applies to all patients detained in hospital under the Act, regardless of the provision under which they are detained. The exception is that the duty does not apply to CTO patients recalled to hospital in respect of whom a more limited duty applies instead – see paragraphs 26.44 and 26.45. The duty in section 132 does apply to such patients if their CTOs are subsequently revoked and they become detained patients again as a result.

9.12 Section 132 requires the hospital managers to take whatever steps are practicable to ensure that patients understand:

- which section of the Act for the time being authorises their detention and the effects of that section, and
- their right to apply to the Tribunal, if applicable.

9.13 This action must be taken as soon as practicable after the patient's detention begins and again as soon as practicable if the patient becomes detained under a different provision of the Act.

9.14 Hospital managers must also to take whatever steps are practicable to ensure that patients who have been detained understand the relevant effects, if any, of the following sections of the Act:

- sections 23, 25 and 66(1)(g), which deal with the power of responsible clinicians, hospital managers and nearest relatives to discharge patients (see chapter 27)
- part 4 of the Act, which deals with consent to treatment (see chapter 23)
- section 118, which deals with the Code of Practice (see chapter 3)
- section 120, which deals with the general protection of patients (see chapter 3), and
- section 134, which deals with patients' correspondence (see chapter 5).

9.15 In particular, the intention is that patients should understand the means by which their detention can be ended and the various safeguards in place to protect their interests, including those concerning consent to treatment.

9.16 The steps taken must include providing the necessary information both orally and in writing.

9.17 The managers must take whatever steps are practicable to give or send a copy of the written information to the person they think is the patient's nearest relative, unless the patient requests otherwise, or does not have a nearest relative. This must be done either at the same time, or within a reasonable time afterwards.

9.18 Steps to inform or involve nearest relatives may not be practicable, even if physically possible, if the detrimental impact of this on the patient would breach the patient's rights under article 8 of the European Convention of Human Rights (ECHR) to privacy and family life. Consultation with the nearest relative that interferes with the patient's article 8 rights may be justified to protect the patient's article 5 ECHR right to liberty[58] – see guidance in chapter 2 of the Code of Practice.

9.19 For more information on the identification of a patient's nearest relative, see chapter 2. By definition, restricted patients do not have a nearest relative for the purposes of the Act. Nor do patients remanded to hospital under section 35 or 36, or subject to an interim hospital order under section 38.

Information about independent mental health advocates (IMHAs) for detained patients [section 130D]

9.20 Hospital managers must also take steps to provide information about IMHAs, where relevant (see chapter 4).

Children and young people [section 131A]

9.21 Hospital managers are required to ensure that where a child or young person aged under 18 is admitted to, or remains in, hospital for mental health treatment, that child or young person's environment in the hospital is suitable, having regard to their age, subject to their needs). This applies to all in-patient mental health services, including highly specialised services. Clinical commissioning groups (CCGs) are required to notify local authorities in their area of the hospital that are designed to be specifically suitable for patients under 18.

9.22 In other words, hospital managers must ensure that the child or young person's environment is suitable for a person of their age. Accommodation in an environment which would not normally be suitable for a person of that age is permissible if the patient's individual needs make such alternative accommodation necessary, or more appropriate.

---

[58] TW v Enfield Borough Council. 2014. EWCA Civ 362. http://www.bailii.org/ew/cases/EWCA/Civ/2014/362.html

9.23 This duty applies to all children and young people admitted to hospital for treatment for mental health treatment, whether or not they are detained under the Act. It does not form part of the criteria for detention under the Act, but, in practice, a hospital should not agree to accept a detained patient for whom it cannot provide appropriate accommodation.

9.24 In deciding how to fulfil their duty, the managers must consult a person who appears to them to have knowledge or experience of cases involving patients under 18 which makes them suitable to be consulted. Typically, this will mean that a child or adolescent mental health services (CAMHS) professional will assess the suitability of the environment and be involved in decisions about the patient's accommodation, care and facilities for education in the hospital.

Social report [section 14]

9.25 When patients are admitted to hospital on the basis of an application for admission made by their nearest relative, rather than an approved mental health professional (AMHP), the managers of the hospital must inform the local authority for the area where the patient lived immediately before admission as soon as practicable.

9.26 As soon as practicable, that local authority must then arrange for an AMHP to interview the patient on its behalf and provide a report on the patient's social circumstances, which must be sent to the hospital managers.

Responsible clinicians [section 34]

9.27 All part 2 and part 3 patients (as defined for this chapter in figure 42) must have a responsible clinician to perform various functions under the Act. The same applies to patients remanded under section 36, or subject to an interim hospital order under section 38 (see chapters 14 and 18 respectively).

9.28 The responsible clinician is the approved clinician who has overall responsibility for the patient's case. Having overall responsibility for the patient's case does not mean that the responsible clinician must personally supervise all the medical treatment provided to the patient under the Act. Responsible clinicians come from a number of different professions and may not be professionally qualified to take personal responsibility for each particular type of treatment their patient is receiving.

9.29 The functions of the responsible clinician may not be delegated, but the patient's responsible clinician may change from time to time and the role may be occupied on a temporary basis in the absence of the usual responsible clinician.

10: Transfer of patients

Introduction

10.1 This chapter describes the provisions of the Act which allow patients to be transferred between hospitals, or between detention in hospital and guardianship, within England and Wales. Transfers to or from places outside England and Wales are dealt with in chapters 34 to 38.

Patients to whom this chapter applies

10.2 As in chapter 9:

- 'part 2 patients' means patients detained on the basis of an application for admission for assessment or treatment including those who are treated as such, eg having been transferred from guardianship or from outside England or Wales
- 'part 3 patients' means patients detained in hospital on the basis of a hospital order, a hospital direction or a transfer direction including those who are treated as such, eg having been transferred from a guardianship order or from outside England or Wales), and
- 'restricted patients' means part 3 patients who are subject to a restriction order, limitation direction or restriction direction including patients treated as if they are, eg when committed to hospital under section 44, and 'unrestricted part 3 patients' means those who are not.

10.3 Patients remanded to hospitals by the courts under section 35 or 36, or subject to interim hospital orders under section 38, may not be transferred under the provisions described in this chapter. Nor, with the exception of patients transferred from or between high security psychiatric hospitals by the Secretary of State, may patients detained under the 'holding powers' in section 5 or detained in hospitals as places of safety pending admission to hospital under part 3 be transferred under the arrangements described in this chapter.

10.4 For the transfer of patients detained under sections 135 or 136 between places of safety, see chapter 7.

Transfers from England to Wales and vice versa – applicable regulations [section 19 and regulation 10]

10.5 The references to regulations in this chapter are to the regulations in force in relation to England. Those regulations apply to transfers between hospitals within England and to transfers from England to Wales.[59]

---

[59] Mental Health (Hospital, Guardianship and Treatment) (England) Regulations. SI 2008/118

10.6 Transfers from Wales to England are governed by the equivalent Welsh regulations instead. Refer to guidance issued by the Welsh Government for details of what is required by those regulations.

Transfer of patients detained in hospital [section 19 and regulation 7]

10.7 Hospital managers may arrange for part 2 and unrestricted part 3 patients to be transferred between different hospitals at any time.

10.8 Managers may only transfer restricted patients with the consent of the Secretary of State for Justice. That includes transferring restricted patients to a different unit within the same hospital, if the patient's hospital order, hospital direction or transfer direction specifies a particular unit.

10.9 Subject to getting the consent of the Secretary of State for Justice in the case of restricted patients, the legislation does not require hospital managers to follow any particular process when transferring patients between different hospitals, or units, under their own management.

10.10 To transfer a patient to any other hospital, the managers must give an authority for the transfer using form H4. They must also be satisfied that arrangements have been made for the admission of the patient to the new hospital within a period of 28 days starting with the day on which the authority for transfer is signed, ie before the end of 28 January if the authority were to be signed on 1 January.

10.11 There is no minimum period which must pass before patients may be transferred from one hospital to another under the Act. Patients may not be transferred from a hospital until they have been admitted to and detained in that hospital.

10.12 Hospital managers may authorise any officer to authorise transfers on their behalf. 'Officer' can include clinical as well as administrative staff, including a patient's responsible clinician.

Transfers of NHS patients detained in independent hospitals [regulation 7]

10.13 If an NHS patient is detained in an independent hospital, an authorisation to transfer the patient to a hospital under different managers, but not the same managers, may also be given by an officer of the relevant NHS body[60] who has been authorised by that body to do so.

10.14 In other words, the relevant NHS body can authorise the patient's transfer without the agreement of the managers of the independent hospital. For

[60] For these purposes, the NHS body could be a clinical commissioning group, NHS trust, NHS foundation trust, NHS Commissioning Board (known as NHS England), special health authority, local health board or the Welsh Ministers.

restricted patients, the agreement of the Secretary of State for Justice is still required.

10.15 As with the power to discharge such patients, the relevant NHS body is the one which has contracted for the patient's care in that hospital.

Transport of patients who are being transferred [regulation 11 and section 137(1) and 138]

10.16 When hospital managers give an authority for transfer using form H4, it also provides the authority for the patient to be conveyed to the new hospital by an officer of the managers of either hospital, or by any person authorised by the managers of the new hospital.

10.17 In both cases, the authority is valid for 28 days starting with the day on which it was given.

10.18 Patients being transferred between hospitals under the same managers, when no form H4 is required, may be conveyed by an officer of those managers or by any other person authorised by them.

10.19 In all cases, patients are deemed to be in legal custody while being conveyed, which means that the person conveying them can take steps to stop them absconding, and retake them if they do (see chapter 11). If they abscond while being transferred, they are also treated as if they were absent without leave (AWOL) from both hospitals – which affects who may take them into custody and allows them to be returned to either hospital (see chapter 11).

Effect of transfer between hospitals [section 19]

10.20 When patients are transferred to another hospital, they are treated as if they had been detained in that hospital all along, and the application, order or direction on which their detention is based is to be read accordingly.

10.21 This means that the various powers and duties of the hospital managers transfer along with the patient to the managers of the new hospital (if the managers are different).

10.22 The transfer takes effect when the patient is admitted to the new hospital. If the patient has already been admitted to that new hospital, eg by being there on leave of absence from the first hospital, it takes effect when the new managers receive the authority for the transfer.

10.23 A transfer between hospitals does not affect patients', or their nearest relatives', rights to apply to the Tribunal, nor give them any new right to do so.

Records of admission [regulation 7]

10.24 Where hospital managers authorise the transfer of a patient to a hospital under different managers, the managers of the new hospital must record the time and date of the patient's admission to that hospital using form H4. If the patient is already in the hospital, that will be the time at which the managers receive the authority. The record may be made by an officer authorised by the managers to do so.

10.25 No particular form is required to be used in other cases, eg transfers between hospitals under the same managers or transfers from hospital to guardianship.

Information for patients transferred between hospitals and their nearest relatives [section 132 and regulation 26(1)(a)]

10.26 The managers of the hospital to which a patient is to be, or has been transferred, must take whatever steps are reasonably practicable to arrange for the person they think is the patient's nearest relative to be informed of the transfer, unless the patient has requested otherwise, or does not have a nearest relative. If the patient does not wish their nearest relative to be informed, managers will need to consider whether doing so would interfere with the patient's right to respect for their privacy and family life under article 8 of the European Convention on Human Rights (ECHR) to an extent that would not be justified and proportionate in the particular circumstances of the case. It may be justifiable to inform the nearest relative to continue to enable their involvement to benefit the patient and protect the patient's article 5 ECHR right to liberty.[61]

10.27 This should be done, if practicable, before the transfer, or as soon as possible afterward. Information given to nearest relatives must be in writing, but may be communicated by electronic means, (eg email, if the nearest relative agrees.

10.28 Hospital managers' duty under section 132 to give detained patients (and, where relevant, their nearest relatives) information about the Act and their rights under it applies when patients are admitted to a new hospital in the same way as it does when they are first detained (see paragraph 9.10 onwards.)

Transfer from guardianship to hospital [sections 19, 66 and 68 and regulations 8 and 11]

10.29 Patients may also be transferred to detention in hospital from guardianship. This must be authorised by the responsible local authority using form G8. The authorisation can only be given if an approved mental health professional (AMHP) acting on behalf of a local authority has, in effect,

[61] TW v Enfield Borough Council. 2014. EWCA Civ 362. http://www.bailii.org/ew/cases/EWCA/Civ/2014/362.html

made an application for admission for treatment under section 3 (see chapter 28).

10.30 The patient must be admitted to hospital no later than the end of the 14 days starting with the day that the patient was last examined by a doctor for the purposes of giving a medical recommendation in support of the AMHP's application. They may be conveyed to hospital by an officer of the local authority, or anyone else authorised by the local authority, and are deemed to be in legal custody while being conveyed (see paragraph 10.19).

10.31 Part 2 patients transferred under these procedures are treated as if they had been admitted to the hospital in question under an application for admission for treatment at the time when they were first received into guardianship (not the date of their actual admission as a result of the transfer). Patients who were subject to guardianship orders under part 3 are treated on their admission as if they are now subject to an unrestricted hospital order made on the same date as the guardianship order.

10.32 When the patient is admitted to hospital on transfer from guardianship, the hospital managers, or an officer authorised by them, must record the patient's admission in part 2 of the form G8 which authorised the transfer and attach it to the application for admission. If the patient happens already to be in the hospital, the patient is treated as having been admitted on receipt of the authority for the transfer.

10.33 Admission on transfer from guardianship gives a patient a right to apply to the Tribunal (see chapter 6). It also places a duty on the hospital managers to refer the patient's case to the Tribunal if they do not apply to the Tribunal themselves, and no-one else applies or makes a reference on their behalf, during the six months starting with the day of their admission as a result of the transfer (see chapter 6).

Transfer from hospital to guardianship [section 19 and regulation 7]

10.34 Hospital managers, or an officer authorised by them, may authorise the transfer of part 2 and unrestricted part 3 patients to guardianship using form G6. They must first consult the local authority which would become responsible for the patient, which must agree to the transfer and specify the date on which it is to take place. The hospital managers must record the local authority agreement and the date the local authority has specified for the transfer on the form G6. If the proposed guardian is not the local authority, that person must record their agreement on the same form before the transfer can take effect.

10.35 If the managers give the authorisation, the transfer takes effect on the date specified by the local authority. On that date, the patient ceases to be liable to be detained. Part 2 patients are then treated as if their application for admission were in fact an application for guardianship which had been accepted by the local authority on the date they were admitted to hospital on the basis of the original application for admission. Unrestricted part 3 patients are treated as if their hospital order, hospital direction or transfer direction were in fact a guardianship order made on the same day as the original order or direction.

10.36 Authorisation for an NHS patient to be transferred to guardianship from an independent hospital may also be given by, or on behalf of, the relevant NHS body,[62] instead of the managers of the independent hospital. As with other transfers from independent hospitals, the relevant NHS body is the one which has contracted with the independent hospital for the patient's care in that hospital.

10.37 An authorisation for transfer to guardianship does not give anyone any authority to convey the patient in question anywhere. If the patient did not go to the place, if any, the new guardian requires them to live, they would be considered AWOL and so could be taken to that place in accordance with section 18. For further information on that, and on guardianship generally, see chapter 28).

10.38 Restricted patients may not be transferred to guardianship.

[62] For these purposes, the NHS body could be a clinical commissioning group, NHS trust, NHS foundation trust, NHS Commissioning Board (NHS England), special health authority, local health board or the Welsh Ministers

11: Legal custody, absconding and returning

Introduction

11.1 This chapter describes the provisions in the Act which relate to keeping patients in legal custody and returning them if they abscond.

Custody under the Act [section 137(2)]

11.2 A police officer, or other constable, or any other person required or authorised under the Act to convey or detain any person, or take them into custody, has for those purposes, all the 'powers, authorities, protection and privileges' of a constable acting within the constable's own area. This means, for example, that they may use reasonable force to stop the person escaping, to secure the conveyance or arrest the person.

11.3 The police should only be asked to assist in returning a patient to hospital if necessary. If the patient's location is known, the role of the police should, wherever possible, only be to assist a suitably qualified and experienced mental health professional in returning the patient to hospital.

People deemed to be in legal custody [section 137(1)]

11.4 Section 137 says that wherever people are required or authorised by or under the Act to be taken, removed or returned to a particular place, or to be detained temporarily in a place of safety, they are deemed to be in legal custody. This includes, for example:

- patients being conveyed to hospital to be admitted on the basis of an application for admission under part 2 (see paragraphs 8.66 to 8.69)
- patients on escorted leave from hospital (see paragraph 9.34)
- patients being taken under section 18 to the place they are required to reside as a condition of leave of absence from hospital, because they have not gone there themselves (see paragraphs 9.51 to 9.58)
- guardianship patients being taken under section 18 to the place they are required to reside, because they have not gone there themselves (see paragraph 9.56)
- people being conveyed between hospitals when being transferred under section 19 or 123 (see chapter 10)
- patients detained under part 3 of the Act being taken to or from court
- people being detained in a hospital (or elsewhere) as a place of safety after being taken from a public place by the police under section 136 (see chapter 7), and

- patients who are being taken back to hospital (or any other place) having gone absent without leave.

Patients who abscond from legal custody [section 138]

11.5 The Act distinguishes between people who are absent without leave (AWOL) and those who have absconded in other circumstances.

11.6 Rules on returning patients who are AWOL from:

- hospital while detained in or recalled to hospital
- the place they are required to live as a condition of leave of absence from hospital, and
- where they are required to live by their guardian

are described in chapters 9, 26, and 28 and are largely to be found in section 18 of the Act. See in particular paragraphs 25.21 to 25.28 (detained patients), paragraphs 26.67 to 26.70 (patients on a community treatment order (CTO) recalled to hospital) and paragraphs 28.90 to 28.95 (guardianship patients).

11.7 The rules for returning patients who have absconded in other circumstances are largely dealt with in section 138, and are described below.

11.8 When someone who is deemed to be in legal custody as a result of section 137 absconds, they can be returned by:

- any police officer, or other constable
- any approved mental health professional (AMHP) acting on behalf of an local authority, or
- by the person in whose custody they were when they absconded.

11.9 If, at the time they absconded, they were liable to be detained in hospital, were a patient on a CTO who had been recalled to hospital, or a guardianship patient, they may also be returned by anyone who could do so if they had gone AWOL. For example, a patient who was liable to be detained in hospital could also be returned by anyone with written authorisation to do so given by the managers of the hospital in question.

11.10 For these purposes, patients being transferred between hospitals are treated as if they were detained in (and therefore AWOL from) both hospitals, so that people with written authorisation from either set of managers may retake them.

11.11 Similarly, patients:

- being transferred to detention in hospital in England or Wales from Scotland, Northern Ireland, the Isle of Man or any of the Channel Islands, or

• subject to hospital orders or hospital directions who are being detained in a place of safety pending admission to the hospital specified in the order or direction, or while being taken from court to that place of safety or from it to the relevant hospital are treated as if they had already been admitted to the hospital in question. That means they can be retaken by anyone authorised by the managers of the hospital in question. It also means that they are treated as if they were AWOL from the hospital for the purposes of calculating the period during which they may be taken into custody and taken to the hospital.

Time limits for returning patients who are AWOL or who have absconded from legal custody under the Act [sections 18 and 138]

11.12 The time limits for returning patients who go AWOL or otherwise abscond in England or Wales are summarised in figure 44.

11.13 Where the police are asked for help in returning a patient, they must be informed of the time limit for taking them into custody. They should also be told immediately if a patient is found or returned.

Figure 44: Summary of time limits for returning patients who are absent without leave or otherwise liable to be retaken

A patient who, at the time of absconding, was (or is treated as):	May not be returned after:
Liable to be detained on the basis of a nurse's record under section 5(4)	6 hours starting at the time the nurse made the record
Liable to be detained on the basis of the report of a doctor or an approved clinician under 5(2)	72 hours starting at the time the doctor or approved clinician furnished the report, or If the patient was first held under section 5(4) following a record made by a nurse, 72 hours starting at the time the record was made
Being conveyed to hospital on the basis of an application for admission for assessment or treatment under section 2 or 3	14 days starting with the day the patient was last examined by a doctor for the purposes of a medical recommendation in support of the application

<table>
<tr><th>A patient who, at the time of absconding, was (or is treated as):</th><th>May not be returned after:</th></tr>
<tr><td>Being conveyed to hospital on the basis of an emergency application under section 4</td><td>24 hours starting at the time the patient was last examined by a doctor for the purposes of the medical recommendation in support of the application</td></tr>
<tr><td>Detained on the basis of an emergency application under section 4, where the second medical recommendation has not yet been received</td><td>72 hours starting at the time the patient was admitted (or treated as admitted) to the hospital on the basis of the emergency application</td></tr>
<tr><td>Detained on the basis of an application for admission for assessment under section 2 (or under section 4, where the second medical recommendation has since been received)</td><td>28 days starting with the day the patient was admitted (or treated as admitted) on the basis of the application</td></tr>
<tr><td>Detained on the basis of an application for admission for treatment under section 3</td><td rowspan="2">The later of:

six months starting with the day the patient went absent, or

the date on which the authority under which they were detained at the time they went absent is due to expire (ignoring any possibility of it being renewed or replaced by a different authority and any extension allowed because of the patient's absence)</td></tr>
<tr><td>Liable to be detained on the basis of an unrestricted hospital order, hospital direction or transfer direction under part 3</td></tr>
<tr><td>A patient on a community treatment order who had been recalled to hospital</td><td>The later of:

six months starting with the day the patient went absent, or

the date on which the community treatment order is due to expire (ignoring any possibility of it being extended or revoked and any extension allowed because of the patient's absence)</td></tr>
</table>

<table>
<tr><th>A patient who, at the time of absconding, was (or is treated as):</th><th>May not be returned after:</th></tr>
<tr><td>Subject to a restriction order, limitation direction or restriction direction (whether or not conditionally discharged)</td><td>The restriction order, limitation direction or restriction order ceases to have effect (which may not be until the patient dies)</td></tr>
<tr><td>Subject to guardianship on the basis of an application for guardianship under part 2</td><td rowspan="2">The later of:

six months starting with the day the patient went absent, or

the date on which the authority under which the patient was subject to guardianship at the time the patient went absent is due to expire (ignoring any possibility of it being renewed and any extension allowed because of the patient's absence)</td></tr>
<tr><td>Subject to a guardianship order under part 3</td></tr>
<tr><td>Detained in a place of safety under section 135 or 136</td><td>The earlier of:

72 hours from the time the patient absconded, or

the period for which the patient may be detained, ie 72 hours' from the start of the patient's detention in the place of safety</td></tr>
<tr><td>Subject to a remand under section 35 or 36 or an interim hospital order under section 38</td><td>No time limit is specified. The patient may be arrested by any police officer (or other constable), and when arrested must be brought before the court that made the remand or interim hospital order as soon as practicable</td></tr>
<tr><td>Being conveyed in England or Wales en route to Scotland, Northern Ireland, the Isle of Man or any of the Channel Islands, in accordance with a transfer warrant</td><td>The period during which the patient could be retaken if no transfer was being attempted. This is because, until the transfer is complete, they remain subject to detention or guardianship in England</td></tr>
</table>

A patient who, at the time of absconding, was (or is treated as):	May not be returned after:
Being conveyed in England or Wales en route from detention in Scotland, Northern Ireland, in accordance with a transfer warrant (or its equivalent) or from the Isle of Man under section 84, but yet to arrive at the hospital to which they are to be admitted	The end of the period during which the patient could be retaken if they had already been admitted to hospital in England or Wales and had then gone AWOL. This will vary depending on the type of application, order(s) or direction(s) to which they would be treated as subject on completion of the transfer
Being conveyed from the Isle of Man or any of the Channel Islands, in accordance with a transfer under section 85, but yet to arrive at the hospital to which they are to be admitted.	The end of the period during which they could be retaken had they absconded while still in the Isle of Man or the relevant Channel Island

Patients who go absent without leave or abscond from England or Wales to Scotland, Northern Ireland, the Isle of Man or the Channel Islands

11.14 Under the rules described in figure 45, patients who can be taken into custody and taken to any place in England or Wales can also be taken into custody and returned from outside England or Wales. The precise detail of the arrangements varies according to the jurisdiction and should be checked with the relevant authorities if necessary.

11.15 These arrangements do not apply to patients subject to guardianship (so a guardian's powers are effectively in abeyance while patients are outside England or Wales).

Figure 45: Retaking of patients who abscond to Scotland, Northern Ireland, the Isle of Man or the Channel Islands

A person (other than one subject to guardianship) who could be taken into custody in England and Wales may be taken into custody and returned by		**in accordance with**
Scotland	• a (Scottish) constable • a mental health officer as defined in the Mental Health (Care and Treatment) (Scotland) Act 2003 • a member of staff of any hospital in Scotland • anyone authorised by the patient's responsible clinician (or equivalent)	The Mental Health (Absconding patients from other jurisdictions) (Scotland) regulations 2008
Northern Ireland	• a constable or officer of the Police Service of Northern Ireland • an Northern Ireland approved social worker • anyone who could do so in England or Wales	Section 88
IoM / Channel Islands	• anyone authorised under local legislation	The applicable local legislation

Patients absent without leave while on escorted leave to Scotland

11.16 A detained patient who has been granted escorted leave of absence under section 17 to go to Scotland and who escapes from custody while in Scotland may be retaken in Scotland in accordance with the Mental Health (cross- border visits) (Scotland) Regulations 2008.[63]

11.17 A detained patient who has been granted escorted leave of absence under section 17 to go to Northern Ireland and who escapes from custody while in Northern Ireland may be retaken in Northern Ireland in accordance with sections 18, 88, 137 and 138 of the Act.

11.18 Escorted leave means that the patient has been given leave of absence from hospital on condition that the patient remains in someone's custody while away from the hospital (see paragraphs 25.4 to 25.8).

11.19 At the time of publication, it is not possible to grant escorted leave of absence to Northern Ireland, the Isle of Man or any of the Channel Islands.

[63] Mental Health (cross-border visits) (Scotland) Regulations. SI 2008/181 http://www.legislation.gov.uk/ssi/2008/181

Patients who go AWOL or abscond overseas [section 40(6)]

11.20 The Act does not permit patients to be retaken outside the UK, the Isle of Man or the Channel Islands. In certain cases, under the Extradition Act 2003,[64] patients who are convicted offenders or accused of a crime may be extradited back to England, if the necessary warrants have been issued. The effect of section 40(6) is that if a patient subject to a restricted hospital order is detained overseas under extradition arrangements, the patient is treated as having been taken into custody under section 18 when first held on the basis of the extradition warrant in the country in question, rather than when returned to the UK. If the patient's restriction order is for a fixed period (see paragraph 21.15), that may affect whether it is still in force when the patient returns to England or Wales.

Patients on escorted leave etc from Scotland, Northern Ireland, Isle of Man or Channel Islands [section 17(6) and (7), 137 and 138]

11.21 A patient can be kept in custody, conveyed to a particular place or detained in a place of safety in England or Wales, if that is a condition of leave of absence from hospital granted under equivalent legislation in Scotland, Northern Ireland, the Isle of Man or any of the Channel Islands.

11.22 In each case, section 137 means they are deemed to be in legal custody while being escorted, conveyed or detained in England and Wales. As a result, if they abscond while in England or Wales, they may be retaken, under section 138, by the person authorised to keep the patient in custody in England, by a police officer, or other constable, or by an AMHP, for as long as they could be retaken under the legislation in the jurisdiction from which they are on leave.

Patients absent without leave etc from Scotland, Northern Ireland, Isle of Man or Channel Islands [section 87 and 89]

11.23 In some circumstances, patients who have gone AWOL, or otherwise absconded, under the equivalent legislation in Scotland, Northern Ireland, the Isle of Man or any of the Channel Islands, may be taken into custody in England or Wales and then be taken or returned to where they ought to be, as described in figure 46.

11.24 This does not apply to patients subject to guardianship.

11.25 The periods during which patients who have gone AWOL or otherwise absconded in Scotland, Northern Ireland, the Isle of Man or any of the Channel Islands vary according to the period allowed for retaking them in the jurisdiction from which they have absconded. The period may well not be the same as it is for patients subject to similar forms of detention, or other

[64] Extradition Act 2003. http://www.legislation.gov.uk/ukpga/2003/41

compulsory measures, in England. Advice should be sought from the relevant authorities in the jurisdiction in question, if necessary.

Figure 46: Retaking of patients who have absconded to England and Wales (other than guardianship patients)

A person who could be taken into custody under		**May be taken into custody in England and Wales and returned by**
Scotland	Sections 301, 302 or 303, or regulations made under section 290 or 310 of the Mental Health (Care and Treatment) (Scotland) Act 2003	• a police officer (or other constable) • an AMHP • a mental health officer (as defined in the Scottish legislation) • a member of staff of any hospital in Scotland • a member of staff of an establishment in which the patient was required to live as a condition of a compulsory treatment order or compulsion order under Scottish legislation • anyone in whose charge the patient was to be kept as a condition of the equivalent of leave of absence under Scottish legislation • anyone else authorised by the patient's responsible medical officer • (where the patient was in the process of being removed from Scotland) anyone authorised under Scottish legislation to escort the patient See article 8 of the Mental Health (Care and Treatment) (Scotland) Act 2003 (Consequential Provisions) Order 2005[65]

[65] Mental Health (Care and Treatment) (Scotland) Act 2003 (Consequential Provisions) Order. 2003. SSI 2005/2078. http://www.legislation.gov.uk/uksi/2005/2078

A person who could be taken into custody under		May be taken into custody in England and Wales and returned by
Northern Ireland	Article 29 or 132, or article 29 as applied by article 31 of the Mental Health (Northern Ireland) Order 1986 ('the Order'[66])	• a police officer (or other constable) • an AMHP or a Northern Ireland approved social worker (ASW) • any officer on the staff of the relevant hospital in Northern Ireland • anyone else authorised by the authority responsible for that hospital • anyone in whose legal custody the patient was under article 31 of the Order when the patient absconded See section 87 of the Act
Isle of Man or Channel Islands	Provisions in the legislation of island in question which corresponds to sections 18 or 138	• a police officer (or other constable), or • an AMHP See section 89 of the Act

[66] Mental Health (Northern Ireland) Order 1986 NISI 1986/595. http://www.legislation.gov.uk/nisi/1986/595

Additional considerations for specific patients

These chapters set out how the Act regards three specific groups of patients – those under 18 years of age, informal patients (ie those who are not detained under the Act and are receiving treatment voluntarily),and patients who have been referred to hospital after coming into contact with the criminal justice system (part 3 patients). Part 3 patients may be sent to hospital by the courts or be transferred from prison or other forms of custody, eg immigration removal centres.

12: Children and young people under the age of 18

Introduction

12.1 This chapter summarises the provisions of the Act which relate specifically to children and young people, or which apply special rules to them. This includes rules which apply to wards of court.

12.2 The Code of Practice provides in chapter 19 that professionals, practitioners and others responsible for the care and treatment of children and young people should be familiar with other relevant legislation including the Children Acts 1989[67] and 2004,[68] the Mental Capacity Act 2005 and the Human Rights Act 1998[69] and should be aware of the United Nations Convention on the Rights of the Child.[70]

Consent to admission by patients aged 16 or 17 [section 131]

12.3 Young people aged 16 or 17 who have the capacity (as defined in the Mental Capacity Act 2005) to do so, may consent to their own admission to hospital for treatment for mental disorder (or to remaining in hospital for such treatment), even if a person with parental responsibility for them (under the Children Act 1989) does not agree, or wishes to discharge them.

12.4 Similarly, young people aged 16 or 17 who have the capacity to consent, but who do not do so, may not be admitted to, or kept in, hospital for treatment for mental disorder on the basis of consent provided by a person with parental responsibility for them.

Children and young people aged under 18 admitted to hospital for mental health treatment [sections 131A and 140]

12.5 Where a child or young person aged under 18 is admitted to, or remains in, hospital (whether compulsorily or not) for treatment for mental disorder, the managers of that hospital must ensure that the child or young person's environment in the hospital is suitable, having regard to their age, subject to their needs. The duty applies to persons who are detained in hospital, as a place of safety under sections 135 or 136 of the Act.

12.6 Hospital managers must ensure that the child or young person's environment is suitable for a person of their age. Accommodation in an environment which

---

[67] Children Act 1989. http://www.legislation.gov.uk/ukpga/1989/41
[68] Children Act 2004. http://www.legislation.gov.uk/ukpga/2004/31
[69] Human Rights Act 1998. http://www.legislation.gov.uk/ukpga/1998/42
[70] United Nations Convention on the Rights of the Child. http://www.unicef.org.uk/UNICEFs-Work/UN-Convention

would not normally be suitable for a person of that age is permissible if the patient's individual needs make such alternative accommodation necessary, or more appropriate, for the patient.

12.7 In deciding how to fulfil their duty, the managers must consult a person who appears to them to have knowledge or experience of cases involving patients under 18 which makes them suitable to be consulted. Typically, this will mean that a child or adolescent mental health professional will need be involved in decisions about matters such as the patient's accommodation, care and facilities for education in the hospital.

12.8 The Care Quality Commission (CQC) must be notified without delay if a person aged under 18 is placed on an adult psychiatric ward for longer than a continuous period of 48 hours (see chapter 3). See the CQC website for information on notification processes, including the appropriate form to be used http://www.cqc.org.uk/content/mental-health-notifications.

12.9 Section 140 of the Act places a duty on clinical commissioning groups to notify local authorities in their area of the arrangements that are in place for the provision of accommodation or facilities designed so as to be specifically suitable for persons aged under 18 (see para 8.20).

Electro-convulsive therapy (ECT) [section 58A]

12.10 Except in emergencies, no patient aged under 18 – whether or not they are subject to any kind of compulsory measure under the Act – may be given ECT or any other treatment to which section 58A applies unless it has been approved as being appropriate by a second opinion appointed doctor (SOAD).

12.11 Unless the treatment is authorised by the Act itself, it remains necessary for there to be legal authority to provide the treatment in addition to the SOAD's approval – see chapter 23.

Wards of court [section 33]

12.12 An application for admission to hospital may only be made in respect of a minor who is a ward of court ('a ward') with the leave of the court. Approved mental health professionals (AMHPs) are not required to consult the nearest relative under section 11 about an application to admit a ward to hospital for treatment (section 3), nor may the nearest relative block the application by objecting to it.

12.13 A ward may not be the subject of a guardianship application, nor may a ward be transferred from hospital to guardianship.

12.14 Where a ward is liable to be detained in hospital on the basis of an application for admission, or is a patient on a community treatment order (CTO), the powers of the nearest relative to discharge the patient, or to apply to the Tribunal (where applicable) may only be exercised with the leave of the court. They may also be exercised by the court itself.

12.15 Where a ward is a patient on a CTO, the provisions of part 2 of the Act apply subject to any order which the court makes in the exercise of its wardship jurisdiction (except during any period when the ward is recalled to hospital).

Children and young people in local authority care [section 27 and 116]

12.16 The Act contains two special provisions in relation to children or young people under the age of 18 in the care of a local authority by virtue of a care order, or where the rights and powers of their parent are vested in the local authority by virtue of section 16 of the Social Work (Scotland) Act 1968.[71]

12.17 The local authority in question will be deemed to be the patient's nearest relative in preference to anyone except their spouse or civil partner.

12.18 In addition, if any of these children or young people is suffering, or appears to be suffering, from mental disorder, ie is a 'patient' as defined in the Act, and is admitted to a hospital or a care home in England or Wales (for any reason), the local authority must arrange for visit to be made to them on its behalf.

12.19 The local authority must also 'take such other steps in relation to the patient while in the [hospital or care home] as would be expected to be taken by [the child or young person's] parent.' The same applies to people of any age who are subject to the guardianship of a local authority under the Act or where a local authority is temporarily exercising the function of being their nearest relative (see paragraph 2.24).

Children and young people under guardianship or special guardianship (otherwise than under the Act) [section 28]

12.20 If a guardian (or special guardian) has been appointed for a child or young person under 18, that person, or all them if there is more than one, will normally be deemed to be the nearest relative to the exclusion of anyone else. 'Guardian' here does not include a guardian appointed under the Act itself.

12.21 Similarly, if a child arrangement order (which replaces residence orders and contact orders section 12 of the Children and Families Act 2014 amends section 8 (1) of the Children Act 1989[72] is in force in relation to a child or young person under 18, the person named in the order will be normally be deemed to be the nearest relative to the exclusion of anyone else.

---

[71] Social Work (Scotland) Act 1968. http://www.legislation.gov.uk/ukpga/1968/49
[72] Children and Families Act 2014 amends section 8 (1) of the Children Act 1989 http://www.legislation.gov.uk/ukpga/2014/6/section/12/enacted

12.22 In both cases, a person will not be deemed to be the nearest relative if, by virtue of section 26(5), they are not eligible to be the patient's nearest relative (see paragraph 2.27).

Other provisions where particular rules apply to children or young people

12.23 Figure 47 summarises the other sections of the Act which make special provisions in respect of children or young people.

12.24 Local authorities should ensure that they arrange for visits to be made to:

a) children and young people looked after by them who are in hospital , whether or not they are under a care order, and
b) children and young people accommodated, or intended to be accommodated for 3 months or more by NHS-funded hospitals. Such visits must be undertaken in accordance with the Visits to Children in Long-Term Residential Care Regulations 2011.[73]

Figure 47: Other special rules affecting children or young people

Provision	Special rules affecting children or young people	See
Guardianship (sections 7 and 37)	No-one under the age of 16 may be made subject to guardianship under the Act	paragraph 28.17
Nearest relative (section 26)	A person under the age of 18 is to be disregarded when identifying a patient's nearest relative unless they are that patient's parent, spouse, civil partner (or they have been living as spouse or civil partner for at least six months)	Paragraph 2.15
Delegation of nearest relative's functions (regulation 24)	Nearest relatives cannot delegate their functions to anyone who is excluded by section 26(5) from being the patient's nearest relative. In practice, that means that (with very limited exceptions) nearest relatives cannot delegate to anyone under the age of 18	paragraph 2.27

[73] Visits to Children in Long-Term Residential Care Regulations. 2011. SI 2011/1010. http://www.legislation.gov.uk/uksi/2011/1010

Provision	Special rules affecting children or young people	See
Information for courts (section 39)	Clinical commissioning groups must respond to requests from courts for information about hospitals that could take people to whom they are considering giving hospital orders or interim hospital orders If the defendant is under the age of 18, the courts may also require information when considering remanding the defendant to hospital under sections 35 or 36 or (in the case of a magistrates' court) ordering a defendant's detention in hospital under section 44 when committing them to the Crown Court When requiring information about a person under the age of 18, the court may specifically ask about accommodation and facilities designed to be specially suitable for patients aged under 18	paragraph 141.14
Committal for restriction order (section 43)	A magistrates' court may not commit a person under 14 to the Crown Court with a view to a restriction order being imposed	paragraph 17.2
Treatment of community patients (not recalled to hospital) (section 64Aff)	The provisions for patients aged over and under 16 differ in some details	paragraphs 24.6 to 24.15
Managers' duty to refer cases to the Tribunal (section 68)	The duty of hospital managers to make a reference to the Tribunal if it has not heard the patient's case for three years applies after only one year if the patient is under 18	paragraph 6.49
Independent mental health advocates (section 130C)	Patients under 18 who are being considered for electro-convulsive therapy (or any other treatment to which section 58A applies) are eligible for help from an independent mental health act advocate, even though they are not detained or a patient on a CTO	paragraph 4.4

12.25 As explained in the figure above, a person's age sometimes makes a difference to the actions that a court can take under part 3 of the Act. A person's exact age may sometimes be in doubt. Section 55(7) says that section 99 of the Children and Young Persons Act 1933[74] – which deals with presumptions about, and determination of, people's ages in court proceedings – is also to apply to part 3 of the Act.

12.26 The flowcharts in chapter 19 of the Code of Practice set out the steps which need to be taken when making decisions about the medication of children and young people.

Figure 48: SOAD role in certification child and adolescent detained patients

The form to be used in certification is indicated in brackets.

Child or adolescent (patient under 18 years)		Consenting	Incapable	Refusing
Detained in hospital	ECT	SOAD certifies (T5)	SOAD certifies (T6)	Emergency treatment only (section. 62)
	Meds	Approved clinician in charge of the treatment in question usually certifies (T2) SOAD may also certify (T2)	SOAD certifies (T3)	SOAD certifies (T3)
CTO in community	ECT	SOAD certifies (CTO)	SOAD certifies (CTO 11)	Cannot be given
	Meds	SOAD certifies (T5)	SOAD certifies (CTO 11)	Emergency treatment only (section 64G)
Informal	ECT	SOAD certifies (T5)	SOAD certifies (T6)	Cannot be given

[74] Children and Young Persons Act 1933. http://www.legislation.gov.uk/ukpga/Geo5/23-24/12

Related material

- The Legal Aspects of the Care and Treatment of Children and Young People with Mental Disorders: a guide for professionals. National Institute for Mental Health in England. 2009. http://www.chimat.org.uk/resource/item.aspx?RID=94476
- Working Together to Safeguard Children: a guide to inter-agency working to safeguard and promote the welfare of children. Department for Children, Schools and Families. 2010. http://www.workingtogetheronline.co.uk/resources.html
- Procedure for the Transfer from Custody of Children and Young People to and from Hospital under the Mental Health Act 1983 in England. Department of Health and Youth Justice Board, 2011. https://www.gov.uk/government/uploads/system/uploads/attachment_data/file/215496/dh_128855.pdf

13: Informal patients

Introduction

13.1 This chapter summarises the provisions of the Act which apply to patients who are not subject to any form of compulsory measure under it ('informal patients').

Informal admission [section 131]

13.2 Nothing in the Act prevents people being admitted to hospital without being detained, and this is expressly stated in section 131. Compulsory admission under the Act has always been intended to be the exception, not the rule. Where it is possible to treat a patient safely and lawfully without detaining them under the Act, the patient should not be detained. Wherever possible a patient's independence should be encouraged and supported with a focus on promoting recovery wherever possible. (For further information see the least restrictive option and maximising independence guiding principle in the Code of Practice, especially Code of Practice paragraphs 1.2-1.6.)

13.3 The mental capacity of a person to consent to admission as an informal patient is likely to include consideration of (a) the relevance of the admission for the relevant purpose, (b) to stay in hospital whilst its purpose is carried out and (c) to the circumstances relating to a possible deprivation of liberty that might prevail during that admission.[75]

13.4 A patient who lacks capacity to consent to admission should not be admitted to hospital informally if the admission constitutes a deprivation of liberty.

Other provisions which apply to informal patients

13.5 The provisions set out in figure 49 also apply to informal patients.

Figure 49: Other provisions which apply to informal patients

Section	Provision	See
57 (and related aspects of 59 to 62)	Safeguards and restrictions in relation to the administration of neurosurgery for mental disorder ('psychosurgery') and certain other treatments	paragraphs 23.16 to 23.24

[75] AM v South London and Maudsley NHS Foundation Trust. 2013. UKUT 0365 (AAC). http://www.bailii.org/uk/cases/UKUT/AAC/2013/365.html

Section	Provision	See
58A (and related aspects of 59 to 62)	Safeguards in relation electro-convulsive therapy (ECT) etc for children and young people under 18	paragraph 23.41 onward
116	Local authorities' duty to arrange visits and take other steps in relation to guardianship patients who are admitted to a hospital or care home, also applies to any patient for whom the local authority is, for the time being, exercising the functions of nearest relative, and to certain children and young people in the local authority's care	paragraph 28.155 28.155
127	Offence of ill-treatment etc.	paragraph 38.7
130A to 130D	Independent mental health advocacy, in relation to sections 57 or 58A as above	paragraph 4.4

14: Remands to hospital

Introduction

14.1 This chapter describes the provisions in part 3 of the Act which enable the courts to remand defendants to detention in hospital. Chapters 14-22 concern patients concerned with criminal proceedings and relate particularly to Code of Practice chapter 22.

Remand to hospital for report [section 35]

14.2 The courts may remand defendants to hospital for the preparation of a report on their mental condition, as set out in figure 50.

Figure 50: Criteria for remand for report under section 35

Remand for report (section 35)		
May be exercised by	A magistrates' court or Crown Court	
in respect of a defendant who is	Where the power is being exercised by a magistrates' court:	Where the power is being exercised by the Crown Court:
	Convicted of an offence punishable on summary conviction with imprisonment, or Charged with (but not convicted of) such an offence, if the court is satisfied that the defendant did the act or made the omission charged *or* if the defendant has consented to the exercise of the power	Awaiting trial before that court for an offence punishable with imprisonment, or Who has been arraigned but has yet to be sentenced or otherwise dealt with for the offence (other than a person convicted – not merely accused – of murder)
If	The court is satisfied on the written or oral evidence of a doctor approved under section 12 that there is reason to suspect that the defendant is suffering from mental disorder, and The court is of the opinion that it would be impracticable for a report on the defendant's mental condition to be made if the defendant were remanded on bail	

and	The court is satisfied, on the written or oral evidence of the approved clinician who would be responsible for making the report, or some other person representing the managers of the relevant hospital, that arrangements have been made for the defendant to be admitted to that hospital within the 7 days starting with the day of the remand.

14.3 For these purposes, mental disorder does not include learning disability, unless that learning disability is associated with abnormally aggressive or seriously irresponsible conduct on the part of the patient concerned (section 1(2) and 2A).

14.4 The requirement that the doctor giving evidence about the defendant's mental disorder must be approved under section 12 is to be found in section 54(1), rather than section 35 itself.

14.5 Throughout the Act, the reference to an offence 'punishable on summary conviction by imprisonment' should not be read as excluding people under 18 who cannot be sentenced to imprisonment. Section 55(2) provides that such references should be construed without regard to any prohibition or restriction imposed by or under any enactment relating to the imprisonment of young offenders. Therefore where a magistrates' court has powers in relation to individuals charged or convicted with an offence punishable on summary conviction by imprisonment, the court's powers extend to those under 18.

14.6 Remand to hospital under section 35 provides an alternative to remanding defendants in custody for a medical report, in circumstances where it would not be practicable to obtain the report if they were remanded on bail, eg because they might decide to break a condition of bail that they should reside at a hospital, and the hospital would then be unable to prevent them from discharging themselves.

14.7 If a remand for report is made, the arrangements in figure 51 apply.

Figure 51: Duration, renewal and termination of remand for report under section 35

Initial duration	Remand is in the first instance for the period specified by the court, which may be up to 28 days
Renewal	The defendant may be further remanded for periods of up to 28 days, but only if it appears to the court, on the written or oral evidence of the approved clinician responsible for making the report, that this is necessary for completing the assessment of the defendant's mental condition
Maximum period	The total period of successive remands for report may not exceed a maximum of 12 weeks

Termination	The court may terminate the remand at any time
Notes	The power of further remanding the defendant may be exercised by the court in the defendant's absence if the defendant is legally represented and the legal representative is given the opportunity to be heard People remanded under this section are entitled to obtain a separate medical report from a doctor or approved clinician of their own choice and at their own expense, and to apply to the court on the basis of it for their remand to hospital to be terminated

Remand for treatment [section 36]

14.8 The Crown Court may order the remand to hospital of a defendant for treatment as set out figure 52.

Figure 52: Criteria for remand for report under section 36

Remand for treatment (section 36)	
May be exercised by	Crown Court only
in respect of a defendant who is	In custody awaiting trial before the court for an offence punishable with imprisonment (other than murder), or In custody at any stage of such a trial prior to sentence
If	The court is satisfied, on the written or oral evidence of two doctors, at least one of whom must be approved under section 12, that: • the defendant is suffering from mental disorder of a nature or degree which makes it appropriate for the defendant to be detained in a hospital for medical treatment, and • appropriate medical treatment is available
and	The court is satisfied, on the written or oral evidence of the approved clinician who would have overall responsibility for the defendant's case (and so be their 'responsible clinician'), or of some other person representing the managers of the relevant hospital, that arrangements have been made for the defendant to be admitted to that hospital within the 7 days starting with the day of the remand

14.9 As in section 35, for these purposes, mental disorder does not include learning disability, unless that learning disability is associated with abnormally aggressive or seriously irresponsible conduct on the part of the patient concerned.

14.10 Appropriate medical treatment means the same as it does in respect of applications for admission for treatment under part 2 of the Act (see paragraph 8.8).

14.11 As for section 35, the requirement that at least one of the doctors giving evidence about the defendant's mental disorder must be approved under section 12 is to be found in section 54(1).

14.12 If a remand for treatment is made, the arrangements in figure 53 apply.

Figure 53: Duration, renewal and termination of remand for report under section 36

Initial duration	Remand is in the first instance for the period specified by the court, which may be up to 28 days
Renewal	The defendant may be further remanded for periods of up to 28 days, but only if it appears to the court, on the written or oral evidence of the person's responsible clinician that a further remand is warranted
Maximum period	The total period of successive remands for treatment may not exceed a maximum of 12 weeks
Termination	The court may terminate the remand at any time
Notes	The power of further remanding the defendant may be exercised by the court in the defendant's absence if the defendant is legally represented and the legal representative is given the opportunity to be heard People remanded under this section are entitled to obtain a separate medical report from a doctor or approved clinician of their own choice and at their own expense, and to apply to the court on the basis of it for their remand to hospital to be terminated

14.13 For these purposes, the 'responsible clinician' means the approved clinician in overall charge of the patient's case in the hospital.

Courts' power to ask clinical commissioning groups for information about hospital places for defendants under 18 [section 39]

14.14 Clinical commissioning groups (CCGs) must respond to requests from courts in England and Wales for information about hospitals in their area, or elsewhere, with which arrangements could be made to admit a defendant aged under 18 whom the court is considering remanding to hospital under section 35 or 36.

14.15 CCGs must provide any relevant information they have, or could reasonably obtain. This includes information about the availability of accommodation or facilities in hospitals designed to be specially suitable for patients under aged 18. The same duty applies to local health boards in Wales and the Welsh Ministers.

Remands by virtue of other legislation

14.16 Remands under section 35 or 36 may also be made by courts by virtue of certain other pieces of legislation – see chapter 22.

Effect of remand under section 35 or 36 [sections 35(9), 35(10), 36(8) and 56]

Conveyance to hospital and return to court

14.17 The effect of the remand is, first, to direct a police officer, or other constable, or any other person directed by the court to do so, to convey the defendant to the hospital specified in the order within 7 days, including the day of remand, and, second, to entrust responsibility for the person's detention and reappearance in court to the managers of the hospital. Having agreed to do so before the remand was made, the hospital managers must admit and detain the patient.

Medical treatment

14.18 Patients remanded to hospital under section 35 are to be detained in the hospital, but the Act does not provide any authority to treat them for their mental disorder without their consent. They have the same rights to consent to and refuse treatment as patients who are not detained under the Act.

14.19 Patients remanded to hospital under section 36 may be treated for their mental disorder without their consent, in accordance with part 4 of the Act (see chapter 23).

Leave of absence, transfer and discharge

14.20 Patients remanded to hospital under section 35 or 36 may not be given leave of absence from the hospital. Nor may the hospital managers transfer them to another hospital. If necessary, an application may be made to the court for a new remand order or the court can order further remand under section 35(5).

14.21 Patients remanded under this section may not be discharged from detention in hospital by anyone except the courts while they remain subject to the remand.

Absconding

14.22 The rules about absence without leave which apply to most other detained patients do not apply to remanded patients. If a remanded patient absconds, either from the hospital in which they are detained or while being taken to or from the hospital, they may be arrested without warrant by any police officer, or other constable. They must then to be brought before the court that remanded them, which may (but need not) decide on some alternative approach to their case.

Effect on existing applications etc

14.23 A remand to hospital does not automatically affect any existing liability for detention for assessment or treatment on any other basis, nor bring a community treatment order (CTO) or guardianship to an end. But nor does it prevent them expiring or being discharged in the normal way.

Nearest relative

14.24 Patients remanded to hospital under section 35 or 36 do not have a nearest relative for the purposes of the Act.

Evidence to the courts on patients remanded to hospital under section 35 or 36 or given interim hospital orders [section 35(5), 36(4) and 38(5)] (actually 25.61-63)

14.25 A patient remanded to hospital for report under section 35 may only be further remanded after the first 28 days if the approved clinician responsible for making the report on the patient's mental condition gives written or oral evidence that further remand is necessary for completing the assessment.

14.26 Similarly, a patient remanded for treatment under section 36 may only be further remanded if the responsible clinician gives written or oral evidence that a further remand is warranted. And a court may only renew an interim hospital order (under section 38) if the responsible clinician gives evidence that the continuation of the order is warranted.

14.27 For further information on interim hospital orders, see chapter 18.

15: Hospital orders

Introduction

15.1 This chapter describes the provisions in part 3 of the Act which enable the courts to order offenders to be detained in hospital for treatment, rather than punishing them.

Hospital orders [section 37]

15.2 Courts may order the detention in hospital of mentally disordered offenders by making a hospital order as set out in figure 54.

Figure 54: Criteria for making hospital orders under section 37

Hospital order (section 37)		
May be made by	A magistrates' court or the Crown Court	
In respect of a defendant who is	*Where made by a magistrates' court:*	*Where made by the Crown Court:*
	Convicted by that court of an offence punishable on summary conviction with imprisonment, or Charged before that court with such an offence but who has not been convicted or whose case has not proceeded to trial, if the court is satisfied that the person did the act or made the omission charged	Convicted before that court for an offence punishable with imprisonment (other than murder)
If the court is satisfied	On the written or oral evidence of two doctors, at least one of whom must be approved under section 12, that • the offender is suffering from mental disorder of a nature or degree which makes it appropriate for the offender to be detained in a hospital for medical treatment, and • appropriate medical treatment is available.	

And the court is of the opinion	Having regard to all the circumstances, including the nature of the offence and the character and antecedents of the offender, and to the other available methods of dealing with the offender, that a hospital order is the most suitable method of dealing with the case
And it is also satisfied	On the written or oral evidence of the approved clinician who would have overall responsibility for the offender's case, or of some other person representing the managers of the relevant hospital, that arrangements have been made for the offender to be admitted to that hospital within the period of 28 days starting with the day of the order

15.3 For these purposes, mental disorder does not include learning disability, unless that learning disability is associated with abnormally aggressive or seriously irresponsible conduct on the part of the patient concerned.

15.4 Appropriate medical treatment means the same as it does in respect of applications for admission for treatment under part 2 of the Act (see paragraph 8.8 above).

15.5 Broadly speaking, 'antecedents' means the defendant's history, including any previous history of offending.

15.6 The requirement that at least one of the doctors giving evidence about the defendant's mental disorder must be approved under section 12 is to be found in section 54(1), rather than section 37 itself.

15.7 A hospital order is, essentially, an alternative to punishment. The court may not, at the same time as making a hospital order in respect of an offender, pass a sentence of imprisonment, impose a fine or make a community order, a youth rehabilitation order, or a referral order. Nor can the court make an order for a young offender's parent or guardian to enter into a recognizance to take proper care of and exercise proper control over the offender. The court may make any other order which it has the power to make, eg a compensation order.

15.8 To detain a patient in hospital as well as imposing a prison sentence, the Crown Court could, in certain circumstances, give hospital and limitation directions instead (see chapter 16). In very limited circumstances a hospital order may be made under section 51 of the Act in respect of patients who have been transferred under section 48 from custody to hospital while on remand (see paragraph 20.2 onward). A hospital order (including a hospital order with a restriction order under section 41) ceases to have effect if the offender is not admitted to the hospital named in the order within 28 days from the date of the making of the order.[76]

[76] R (DB) v Nottinghamshire Healthcare NHS Trust. 2008. EWCA Civ 1354. http://www.bailii.org/ew/cases/EWCA/Civ/2008/1354.html

15.9 Hospital orders under the Act may be made by virtue of several other pieces of legislation (see chapter 22).

Courts' power to ask for information about hospital **places** [section 39]

15.10 Clinical commissioning groups must respond to requests from courts in England and Wales for information about hospitals in their area, or elsewhere, with which arrangements could be made to admit a person in respect of whom the court is considering making a hospital order. Clinical commissioning groups must provide any relevant information they have, or could reasonably obtain. The same duty applies to local health boards in Wales and the Welsh Ministers.

15.11 If the person concerned is under 18, this includes information about the availability of accommodation or facilities in hospitals designed to be specially suitable for patients under 18 and the power also applies when the court is considering making an order for remand under section 35 or 36, or an order committing an offender under section 44.

Restriction orders [section 41]

15.12 A restriction order may be imposed alongside a hospital order by the Crown Court as set out in figure 55.

Figure 55: Criteria for imposing restriction orders

A restriction order may be imposed by the Crown Court if a hospital order has been made and:	
If	At least one of the doctors whose evidence is taken into account by the Court before deciding to give the hospital order has given evidence orally
And, having regard to	• the nature of the offence • the antecedents of the offender, and • the risk of the offender committing further offences if set at large
The Court thinks	It necessary for the protection of the public from serious harm for the person to be subject to the special restrictions which flow from a restriction order

15.13 It is not necessary for the registered medical practitioner whose evidence is taken orally to have recommended a restriction order.[77]

15.14 The effect of a restriction order is to impose a number of special restrictions on the patient. These are described in chapter 28.

[77] *R v Birch* (1989) 11 Cr. App. R(S). 202

15.15 If it imposes a restriction order, under section 47 of the Crime (Sentences) Act 1997[78] the court may specify a particular unit within a hospital as the place in which the patient is to be detained, rather than the hospital in general. In such cases, references in the legislation, and this Reference Guide, to hospitals have to be read as references to the specified hospital unit.

15.16 A restriction order lasts until it is lifted by the Secretary of State under section 42, or the patient is absolutely discharged from detention by the responsible clinician or hospital managers with the Secretary of State's consent under section 23 or by the Tribunal under section 73 – see chapters 6 and 21 respectively.

15.17 Some patients may nonetheless have restriction orders which are due to expire on a particular day, because:

- before 1 October 2007, courts could give restriction orders for a fixed period if they thought it appropriate, and
- patients transferred to England and Wales might be treated as if subject to a restriction order for only a fixed period, if the equivalent order to which they were previously subject in Scotland, Northern Ireland, the Isle of Man or any of the Channel Islands was only for a limited period (see chapter 34).

15.18 For the effect of the ending or lifting of a restriction order, see 21.17 onward. Unless the patient has been conditionally discharged, the hospital order does not end just because the restriction order does.

15.19 A magistrates' court may not impose a restriction order itself, but (subject to certain conditions) may commit a person in custody to the Crown Court with a view to the Crown Court doing so under section 43 – see chapter 17.

Interim hospital order [section 38]

15.20 Before deciding whether to make a hospital order, courts may, subject to certain conditions, make an interim hospital order instead for a period (in total) of no more than a year – see chapter 18.

Rights of appeal against conviction and sentence and associated duty on hospital managers [section 45 and various criminal justice measures]

15.21 Under the Criminal Appeal Act 1968,[79] a hospital order is a form of sentence and all patients admitted to hospital on the basis of a hospital order will have certain rights of appeal either to the Court of Appeal (Criminal Division) or to the Crown Court. This includes appeal against the conviction (or finding that

[78] Crime (Sentences) Act 1997. http://www.legislation.gov.uk/ukpga/1997/43
[79] Criminal Appeal Act 1968. http://www.legislation.gov.uk/ukpga/1968/19

the person had done the act in question) on which the order was based and against the order itself, including the restriction order, if there is one.

15.22 Section 45 of the Act itself specifically ensures that people given hospital orders by a magistrates' court under section 37(4) without being convicted have the same rights of appeal against the order as they would have if they had been convicted. The Crown Court hearing the appeal has the same powers it would have if the appeal were against conviction and sentence. Appeals in respect of children or young people given hospital orders by magistrates' courts without being convicted may be brought on their behalf by their parents or guardians. This applies to appeals against the order itself and against the finding that the child or young person had done the act in question.

15.23 In practice, the managers of the hospital in which patients are detained are responsible for ensuring that they are taken, with an escort, to court in connection with any appeal, as necessary. If any patient who is required to appear before the court is, in the opinion of the responsible clinician, unfit to appear, the Crown Court or the Registrar of Criminal Appeals, as the case may be, will need to be notified immediately.

Hospital order – authority to detain [section 40(1)]

15.24 The effect of a hospital order is, first, to confer authority on a police officer (or other constable), an approved mental health professional (AMHP), or any other person directed by the court to do so, to convey the patient to the hospital (or unit) specified in the order within 28 days and, second, to confer authority on the managers of the hospital to admit the patient within that period and to detain the patient.

Patients who abscond before being admitted under a hospital order [section 138]

15.25 If patients abscond between being given the hospital order and being admitted to the relevant hospital, they may be taken into custody and returned under section 138 of the Act (see chapter 20).

15.26 Patients without a restriction order ('unrestricted patients') may only be taken into custody during the six months starting with the date they went missing. There is no time limit where patients have been given a restriction order as well – restricted patients can be retaken at any time while their restrictions remain in force.

15.27 Any time during which patients are at large is ignored for the purposes of calculating the 28 day period during which they may be detained in a place of safety pending admission and during which they may be taken to and admitted to hospital. Time starts to run again when the patient returns or is taken into custody.

Effect of unrestricted hospital orders on patients once detained [section 40(4)]

15.28 Patients admitted to hospital under a hospital order without a restriction order are treated largely the same as patients detained on the basis of an application for admission for treatment under section 3. Like admission on that basis, the hospital order lasts for six months initially, but can be renewed.

15.29 The provisions of part 2 of the Act (and certain related provisions) which apply to unrestricted hospital order patients are set out in part I of schedule 1 to the Act. Some of them are applied with modifications, most of which are technical.

15.30 This is described in more detail in chapter 9, but there are three important differences worth noting in particular.

15.31 First, the initial six month maximum period of detention runs from the day that the hospital order is made by the court, not from the patient's admission to hospital, which could be several days later.

15.32 Second, hospital order patients' nearest relatives do not have the power to discharge them from hospital. These nearest relatives have rights to apply to the Tribunal instead (see chapter 6).

15.33 Third, patients admitted under a hospital order may not apply to the Tribunal until six months after the date of the making of the order (assuming the order is then renewed). This is because the initial decision to detain them has been made by an independent and impartial court. For the same reason, hospital managers are not required to refer the patient's cases to the Tribunal if the patient has not applied within the first six months of detention (see chapter 6).

Effect of restricted hospital order on patients once detained [section 41]

15.34 Patients admitted to hospital under a hospital order with a restriction order are also treated, in principle, like patients detained on the basis of an application for admission for treatment under part 2. However, there are many more differences in their case. These are summarised in chapter 21. One important difference is that, while the restriction order remains in force, the hospital order also remains in force and does not have to be renewed.

15.35 Part 1 of schedule 1 to the Act (described in paragraph 15.29) does not apply to restricted patients. Part 2 of that schedule applies instead.

Effect of a hospital order on existing authority to detain etc [section 40(5), 41(4) and section 55(4)]

15.36 When patients are admitted to hospital on the basis of a hospital order, any previous application for admission to hospital or application for guardianship under part 2 of the Act, and any previous unrestricted hospital order, unrestricted hospital direction, or unrestricted transfer direction or guardianship order under part 3 ceases to have effect. Restricted hospital orders do not end.

15.37 If the hospital order, or the conviction on which it is based, is quashed on appeal, any such previous application, order or direction will, in effect, be revived if it would still have been in force had the patient been in prison instead since the hospital order was made – see paragraph 25.54. In practice, a previous application or order will not still be in force if longer than six months has passed since the hospital order was given.

15.38 For a description of hospital directions, see chapter 16. For transfer directions, see chapters 19 and 20. For guardianship applications and orders, see chapter 28.

Written evidence [section 54]

15.39 Written evidence given by a doctor, or by someone representing the managers of a hospital, for the purpose of enabling the court to decide whether to make a hospital order may be received in evidence without further proof that it is, in fact, signed by the person in question or that that person has the necessary qualifications or authority to do so. The court may require the person concerned to give evidence orally.

15.40 In addition, if such evidence is submitted on the direction of the court by someone other than the defendant in question (or their representative), a copy has to be given to the defendant's legal representative (if they have one). If the defendant does not have a legal representative, then at least the substance of the report (if not the report itself) must be disclosed to the defendant, or if the defendant is a child or young person, to a parent or guardian who is present in court. Unless the report is only about arrangements for the defendant's admission to hospital, the defendant may have the person who signed the report called to give evidence orally and may call evidence to rebut the report.

Power of the Secretary of State to reduce the 28 day period for making a hospital order [section 54A]

15.41 The Secretary of State has the power to make an order to reduce the 28 day period:

- within which the court must be satisfied the defendant will be admitted to hospital, and

- during which patients may be detained in a place of safety pending that admission and during which the Secretary of State may direct that the patient be admitted to a different hospital (or unit, as the case may be) instead.

At the time of publication, no such order has been made.

16: Hospital and limitation directions

Introduction

16.1 This chapter describes the provisions in section 45A of the Act which allow the Crown Court to give hospital and limitation directions authorising the detention of offenders in hospital for treatment at the same time as passing a prison sentence.

Hospital and limitation directions [section 45A]

16.2 A hospital direction is a direction for a person's detention in hospital. A limitation direction is a direction that they be subject to the special restrictions in section 41 of the Act which also apply to people given restriction orders (see chapter 21).

16.3 A hospital direction may not be given without an accompanying limitation direction (although, as described below, a hospital direction may remain in force after the limitation direction has expired).

16.4 Courts may make hospital and limitation directions in the circumstances set out in figure 56.

Figure 56: Criteria for making hospital and limitation directions

Hospital and limitation directions (section 45A)	
May be given by	Crown Court
In respect of a person who is	Aged 21 or over and convicted before that court of an offence punishable with imprisonment (other than murder)
If the court is satisfied	On the written or oral evidence of two doctors, at least one of whom must be approved under section 12, and at least one of whom must have given evidence orally, that: • the offender is suffering from mental disorder of a nature or degree which makes it appropriate for the offender to be detained in a hospital for medical treatment, and • appropriate medical treatment is available
And the court	Has first considered making a hospital order under section 37, but has decided instead to impose a sentence of imprisonment

And it is also satisfied	On the written or oral evidence of the approved clinician who would have overall responsibility for the offender's case or of some other person representing the managers of the relevant hospital, that arrangements have been made for the offender to be admitted to that hospital within the 28 days starting with the day of the order.

16.5 As with the criteria for hospital orders:

- mental disorder here and throughout this chapter does not include learning disability, unless that learning disability is associated with abnormally aggressive or seriously irresponsible conduct on the part of the patient concerned
- appropriate medical treatment means the same as it does in respect of applications for admission for treatment under part 2 of the Act (see paragraph 8.8 above), and
- the requirement that at least one of the doctors giving evidence about the defendant's mental disorder must be approved under section 12 is to be found in section 54(1).

16.6 As with a restricted hospital order, on the making of a hospital and limitation direction, the court has the power to specify that the offender be admitted to a particular unit of the hospital in question. If so, references to hospitals are to be treated as if they were references to the particular unit in question.

16.7 Hospital and limitation directions may also be appealed and imposed on appeal by virtue of the Criminal Appeal Act 1968[80] (see chapter 20). An order under section 45A can only be made in respect of offenders aged 21 and over, because the court cannot decide to impose a sentence of imprisonment of offenders under 21.[81]

Provisions in respect of hospital orders which also apply to hospital and limitation directions

16.8 The following provisions described in chapter 4 also apply to hospital and limitation directions:

- courts' power under section 39 to ask clinical commissioning groups for information about hospital places (paragraph 14.14)
- courts' power to make an interim hospital order under section 38 before finally deciding how to deal with the offender (paragraph 18.2)

[80] Criminal Appeal Act 1968. http://www.legislation.gov.uk/ukpga/1968/19

[81] The Criminal Justice and Court Services Act (2000) contains provisions (which have not been brought into force) which would repeal the prohibition on 18-20s being sentenced to imprisonment. The Ministry of Justice has been keeping under review the question of whether to bring these provisions into force. Attorney General's Reference (No. 54 of 2011). 2011. EWCA Crim 2276. http://www.mentalhealthlaw.co.uk/AG%27s_ref_%28no_54_of_2011%29_%282011%29_EWCA_Crim_2276

- temporary detention in a place of safety pending admission to the hospital (or hospital unit) specified in the hospital direction, including the ability of the Secretary of State to direct that the offender be admitted to a different hospital (or unit) in exceptional circumstances (paragraph 18.3 to 18.16)
- rights of appeal against conviction and sentence and associated duty on hospital managers (paragraph 15.21)
- the effect on existing authority to detain etc (paragraph 19.26), and
- rules about written evidence (paragraph 19.39).

Hospital direction – authority to detain [section 45B(1)]

16.9 The effect of a hospital direction is, first, to confer authority on a police officer, or other constable, or on any other person directed by the court to do so, to convey the patient to the hospital, or unit, specified in the order within 28 days and, second, to confer authority on the managers of the hospital to admit the patient within that period and to detain the patient.

Patients who abscond before being admitted under a hospital order [section 138]

16.10 If patients abscond between being given the hospital and limitation direction and being admitted to the relevant hospital, they may be taken into custody and returned under section 138 of the Act (see chapter 11). Like patients subject to restricted hospital orders, there is no limit on the time during which that may be done.

16.11 Similarly, any time during which the patient is at large is ignored for the purposes of calculating the 28 day period during which they may be detained in a place of safety pending admission to hospital and during which they may be taken to and admitted to hospital. Time starts to run again when the patient returns or is taken into custody.

Effect of hospital and limitation directions on patients once detained [section 45B(2)]

16.12 For most purposes, patients subject to hospital and limitation directions are treated in the same way as patients subject to hospital orders and restriction orders.

16.13 This is because the Act says, in section 45B(2), that a hospital direction is to have effect in respect of any patient like a transfer direction and a limitation direction like a restriction direction. Section 47(3) then says that a transfer direction has effect like a hospital order, and section 49(2) says that a restriction direction has the same effect as a restriction order.

16.14 There are three important differences, set out below.

Limitation directions may be time-limited [section 50(2), (3) and (5)]

16.15 A limitation direction ends automatically on the patient's 'release date'.

16.16 The patient's release date is the day that the patient would have been entitled to be released from custody had the patient not be detained in hospital. Discretionary early release such as home detention curfew is not taken into account. For these purposes, any prison sentence which the patient was already serving when the hospital direction was given is taken into account as well as the sentence(s) passed at the same time as the direction was given. If the patient is serving a life sentence, or an indeterminate sentence, the release date is the date (if any) on which the person's release is ordered by the parole board.

16.17 Although the limitation direction ends on the release date, the hospital direction does not. So if patients are still detained in hospital on the basis of the hospital direction on their release date, they remain liable to be detained in hospital from then on like unrestricted hospital order patients (see chapter 15). This includes patients who are on leave of absence from hospital on their release date, but not those who have been conditionally discharged (see chapter 28) and who have not been recalled to hospital.

16.18 Hospital and limitation direction patients who are absent without leave, or are otherwise liable to be taken into custody, under the Act are also treated as being unlawfully at large from custody for the purposes of section 49(2) of the Prison Act 1952.[82] This may affect their release date.

While a limitation direction is in force, patients may be removed to prison [section 50(1) and (5)]

16.19 Unlike hospital order patients, hospital and limitation direction patients are detained primarily on the basis of a prison sentence. While the limitation direction remains in effect, the Secretary of State may direct that they be removed to prison (or equivalent) to serve the remainder of their sentence, or else release them on licence.

16.20 This is only possible where the Secretary of State is notified by the offender's responsible clinician, any other approved clinician, or by the Tribunal, that:

- the offender no longer requires treatment in hospital for mental disorder, or
- no effective treatment for the disorder can be given in the hospital in which the offender is detained.

16.21 When notified in this way by the responsible clinician, or any other approved clinician, the Secretary of State may:

- direct the offender's removal to a prison (or another penal institution) where the offender could have been detained if not in hospital, or

[82] Prison Act 1952. http://www.legislation.gov.uk/ukpga/Geo6and1Eliz2/15-16/52

- discharge the offender from the hospital on the same terms on which the offender could be released from prison.

See below for the procedure where the Tribunal is involved.

16.22 In practice, the Secretary of State expects clinical staff from the hospital and prison to meet to plan the patient's future care (a 'section 117 meeting') before directing the patient's removal to prison.

While a limitation direction is in force, discharge by the Tribunal requires the consent of the Secretary of State [section 74]

16.23 With one exception, if the Tribunal thinks that a patient subject to a restriction order would be entitled to be discharged, but the Secretary of State does not consent, the patient will be removed to prison. That is because the Tribunal has decided that the patient should not be detained in hospital, but the prison sentence remains in force until the patient's release date.

16.24 The patient will remain detained in hospital if the Tribunal thinks the patient would be entitled to conditional discharge, but recommends that the patient remain in hospital if the Secretary of State does not agree to a conditional discharge, (see paragraph 6.89 onwards).

Effect of removal to prison on hospital and limitation directions [section 50(1) and (5)]

16.25 If an offender is removed to custody, both the hospital direction and the limitation direction end when the offender arrives at the relevant prison or other institution.

17: Committal to Crown Court for restriction order

Introduction

17.1 This chapter describes the provisions under which magistrates' courts may commit offenders to the Crown Court if they think a restricted hospital order may be appropriate.

Committal to hospital [section 43(1)]

17.2 A magistrates' court has no power itself to make a restriction order, but it may commit an offender to the Crown Court for sentencing with a view to a restriction order being made in the circumstances set out in figure 57.

Figure 57: Criteria for committal to hospital

A magistrates' court may commit a person to the Crown Court with a view to a restriction order if	
The person	Is aged 14 or over, and
	Has been convicted by the court of an offence punishable on summary conviction by imprisonment
And	The court could make a hospital order under section 37
But having regard to	The nature of the offence The antecedents of the offender, and The risk of the offender committing further offences if set at large
The court thinks	That if a hospital order is made, a restriction order should also be made

Committal in custody [section 43]

17.3 The magistrates' court may commit the offender in custody (ie to prison or its equivalent).

Committal to hospital [section 44]

17.4 Alternatively, the court may direct that the patient be admitted to a hospital and be detained there until the Crown Court disposes of the case. The court may only do this if it is satisfied on written or oral evidence that arrangements have been made for the patient to be admitted to hospital.

17.5 That evidence must be given by the approved clinician who would have overall responsibility for the offender's case while in hospital or by someone else representing the managers of the hospital in question.

Effect of committal to hospital [section 44(3)]

17.6 The effect of the order is, first, to confer authority on a police officer (or other constable), an approved mental health professional (AMHP), or any other person directed by the court to do so, to convey the patient to the hospital specified in the order (there is no requirement to do so within 28 days) and, second, to confer authority on the managers of the hospital to admit and detain the patient there.

17.7 The court can also give any directions it thinks fit about the patient's transport from the hospital to the Crown Court. In practice, these directions will both authorise and require the managers of the relevant hospital to ensure that the patient is taken to the Crown Court as necessary.

Provisions in respect of hospital orders which also apply to committals to hospital [sections 44(3) and 51(4)]

17.8 The following provisions described in chapter 15 in relation to hospital orders also apply in these cases:

- temporary detention in a place of safety pending admission to the specified hospital, including the ability of the Secretary of State to direct that the offender be admitted to a different hospital in exceptional circumstances (see paragraphs 15.22 to 15.28), and
- rules about written evidence (see paragraph 15.39).

17.9 Apart from the fact that they do not have to be conveyed to hospital within 28 days, patients committed to hospital are treated as if subject to a restricted hospital order (see chapter 21).

Action for the Crown Court [section 43(2) and (3), 51(7)]

17.10 The Crown Court is required to inquire into the circumstances of the patient's case and either:

- make a hospital order (with or without a restriction order), as if the offender had been convicted before the Crown Court, rather than by the magistrates' court, or
- deal with the offender in some other way the magistrates' court would have been able to originally.

17.11 Under section 51(7), if it is impracticable or inappropriate to bring the patient before the court, the court may also make a hospital order in the patient's absence under section 51(5), as if the patient were subject to a restricted transfer direction. But it may only do this if the criteria for making such an order (described in paragraph 20.22) are met.

17.12 Before making a decision on how to deal with the patient, the Crown Court has the power to remand the patient to hospital under section 35 or 36 (see chapter 14) or make an interim hospital order under section 38 (see chapter 18).

18: Interim hospital orders

Introduction

18.1 This chapter describes the provisions under which courts may detain offenders in hospital for treatment under an interim hospital order before finally deciding how to dispose of their cases.

Interim hospital orders [section 38]

18.2 Before deciding whether to give an offender a hospital order, hospital and limitation directions, a prison sentence, or some other criminal justice disposal, a court may make an interim hospital order, detaining the patient in hospital for a maximum (in total) of 12 months, as set out in figure 58.

Figure 58: Criteria for making interim hospital orders

Interim hospital order (section 38)		
May be made by	A magistrates' court or the Crown Court	
In respect of a person who is	*Where made by the magistrates' court*	*Where made by the Crown Court*
	Convicted by that court of an offence punishable on summary conviction with imprisonment	Convicted by that Court of an offence punishable with imprisonment (other than murder)
If the court is satisfied	On the written or oral evidence of two doctors, at least one of whom must be approved under section 12 and at least one of whom is employed at the hospital which is to be specified in the order, that: • the offender is suffering from mental disorder, and • there is reason to suppose that the mental disorder is such that it may be appropriate for a hospital order to be made	
And it is also satisfied	On the written or oral evidence of the approved clinician who would have overall responsibility for the offender's case or of some other person representing the managers of the relevant hospital, that arrangements have been made for the offender to be admitted to that hospital within the 28 days starting with the day of the order	

18.3 As with hospital orders, the requirement that at least one of the doctors giving evidence about the defendant's mental disorder must be approved under section 12 is to be found in section 54(1).

18.4 Unlike hospital orders, one of the doctors giving evidence about the patient's mental disorder must be employed at the hospital in which the patient is to be detained.

18.5 Interim hospital orders may also be given under certain other pieces of legislation – see chapter 22.

Duration and renewal of interim hospital orders [sections 38(2), (5) and (6) and 45A(8)]

18.6 An interim order lasts for the period specified by the court, which cannot be more than 12 weeks. It may be renewed for further periods of no more than 28 days at a time, and it cannot remain in force for more than 12 months in total.

18.7 The interim hospital order may be made by the court or renewed by the court without the patient being present, provided the patient is legally represented and the legal representative is given an opportunity to be heard. The same applies if the court decides to make a hospital order in place of the interim hospital order (but not if the Crown Court decides to give hospital and limitation directions instead).

18.8 The court must end the interim hospital order if it makes a hospital order or deals with the patient in some other way, eg by imposing a fine or a prison sentence, or (if the Crown Court) by imposing a prison sentence and giving hospital and limitation directions at the same time.

18.9 Because interim hospital orders (like hospital orders, hospital and limitation directions and guardianship orders) are a form of sentence, patients can appeal against them in the same way they may appeal against other sentences. Under section 11(5) of the Criminal Appeal Act 1968,[83] a court that has imposed an interim hospital order may end it and make its final sentencing decision, even though an appeal against the order is still outstanding.

Provisions in respect of hospital orders which also apply to interim hospital orders [section 40]

18.10 The following provisions described in chapter 15 in relation to hospital orders also apply to interim hospital orders:

- courts' power under section 39 to ask clinical commissioning groups for information about hospital places (see paragraph 14.14)
- rights of appeal against conviction and sentence and the associated obligations of hospital managers (see paragraph 15.21)
- rules about written evidence under section 54 (see paragraph 15.39), and

[83] Criminal Appeal Act 1968. http://www.legislation.gov.uk/ukpga/1968/19

- the Secretary of State's power under section 54A to reduce the time period within which patients must be admitted to hospital (see paragraph 15.41).

Interim hospital order – authority to detain [section 40(1) and (3)]

18.11 The effect of an interim hospital order is, first, to require a police officer (or other constable) or any other person directed by the court to do so, to convey the patient to the hospital specified in the order within 28 days starting with the day of the order and, second, to require the managers of that hospital to admit the patient within that period and to detain the patient in accordance with the Act.

Absconding while subject to an interim hospital [section 38(7)]

18.12 Patients subject to interim hospital orders who abscond from hospital or while being conveyed to or from hospital may be arrested without a warrant by any police officer, or other constable. Once arrested, they are to be brought before the court which imposed the interim hospital order as soon as practicable. The court may, if it wishes, then terminate the order and deal with the person in question in any other way it could have dealt with them originally had the order never been made.

Effect of interim hospital orders on patients once detained [section 38, 40 and 56]

18.13 A patient subject to an interim hospital order is detained in accordance with the provisions of section 38 and is in a different position to hospital order patients.

18.14 Patients subject to interim hospital orders cannot be discharged or given leave of absence from hospital by their responsible clinician, nor discharged or transferred to another hospital or to guardianship by the hospital managers, or discharged by the Tribunal. The court may, in effect, discharge them by ending the interim hospital order and deciding to deal with them without making a hospital order or hospital and limitation direction.

18.15 Patients subject to interim hospital orders may be treated without consent under part 4 of the Act (see chapter 23). In principle, this applies even when detained in a place of safety pending admission to hospital.

18.16 Patients subject to interim hospital orders do not have a nearest relative for the purposes of the Act.

19: Transfer of sentenced prisoners to hospital

Introduction

19.1 This chapter describes the provisions under which the Secretary of State may transfer sentenced prisoners from prison to detention in hospital for treatment.

Transfer to hospital of sentenced prisoners [sections 47]

19.2 The Secretary of State may make a transfer direction in the circumstances set out in figure 59. A transfer direction is a warrant directing that a patient be taken to and detained in the hospital specified in the warrant.

Figure 59: Criteria for transfer directions in respect of sentenced prisoners

Transfer directions for sentenced prisoners (section 47)	
May be given in respect of a person who is serving a sentence of imprisonment which includes a person who is:	Detained in pursuance of any sentence or order for detention made by a court in criminal proceedings, or
	Detained in pursuance of any sentence or order for detention made by a court in armed forces disciplinary proceedings (except a sentence of service detention), or
	Committed to custody under section 115(3) of the Magistrates' Courts Act 1980 (which relates to persons who fail to comply with an order to enter into recognizances to keep the peace or be of good behaviour), or
	Committed by a court to a prison or other institution to which the Prison Act 1952 applies in default of payment of any sum adjudged to be paid on conviction

If the Secretary of State	Is satisfied, by reports from at least two doctors, at least one of whom must be approved under section 12, that: • the prisoner is suffering from mental disorder • the mental disorder is of a nature or degree which makes it appropriate for the prisoner to be detained in a hospital for medical treatment, and • appropriate medical treatment is available
And	The Secretary of State is of the opinion, having regard to the public interest and all the circumstances, that it is expedient to direct the prisoner's transfer
If a transfer direction is given	The Secretary of State may (but need not) also give a restriction direction under section 49

19.3 A decision to transfer a prisoner at the end of their sentence requires heightened scrutiny to be applied by the Secretary of State as to the evidence on which the decision is based and whether the necessary criteria are met.[84] If transfer is not appropriate or possible, consideration may need to be given to the use of a civil section if admission to hospital is necessary.

19.4 The reference to persons detained in pursuance of any sentence or order for detention made by a court in criminal proceedings covers people under 18 and under 21 who cannot be sentenced to imprisonment.[85]

19.5 As with the criteria for hospital orders:

- mental disorder here and throughout this chapter does not include learning disability, unless that learning disability is associated with abnormally aggressive or seriously irresponsible conduct on the part of the patient concerned
- appropriate medical treatment means the same as it does in respect of applications for admission for treatment under part 2 of the Act (see paragraph 8.8), and
- the requirement that at least one of the doctors giving evidence about the defendant's mental disorder must be approved under section 12 is to be found in section 54(1).

[84] R (TF) v Secretary of State for Justice. 2008. EWCA Civ 1457. http://www.bailii.org/ew/cases/EWCA/Civ/2008/1457.html

[85] The Criminal Justice and Court Services Act (2000) http://www.legislation.gov.uk/ukpga/2000/43 contains provisions (which have not been brought into force) which would repeal the prohibition on 18-20s being sentenced to imprisonment. The Ministry of Justice has been keeping under review the question of whether to bring these provisions into force.

Restriction directions [section 49]

19.6 The Secretary of State may also issue a warrant directing that the transferred patient be subject to the special restrictions under section 41 which apply to patients given restricted hospital orders. Such directions are referred to in the Act as 'restriction directions'.

19.7 If the Secretary of State also makes a restriction direction, under section 47 Crime (Sentences) Act 1997 the transfer direction can specify that the patient is to be admitted to a particular unit of the hospital in question. In such cases, references to hospitals are to be treated as references to the particular hospital unit in question.

Patient to be transferred to hospital within 14 days [section 47(2)]

19.8 The transfer direction ceases to have effect if the patient has not been admitted to the hospital, or unit, in question by the end of the 14 days starting with the day it is given. The hospital, or unit, specified in the transfer direction must take every reasonable step to admit the patient within the 14 days for which the warrant is valid. In practice, a further transfer direction could be given if necessary.

Effect of an unrestricted transfer direction [section 47(3)]

19.9 Patients given transfer directions without restriction directions are treated for almost all purposes in exactly the same way as patients given unrestricted hospital orders. The main exception is that they may apply to the Tribunal for discharge during the first six months following the transfer direction – see chapter 6.

19.10 That in turn means they are treated, for most purposes, as if they had been admitted to hospital on the basis of an application for admission for treatment under part 2 of the Act (see chapter 23 for fuller details). The transfer direction lasts for six months initially, but may be renewed.

19.11 Unrestricted transfer direction patients cannot be returned from hospital to prison to complete their sentences in the same way as restricted direction patients, even if they no longer require treatment. Their sentences and the power to impose licence conditions (and to recall the offender following any breach of licence conditions) continue to run notwithstanding that there has been a transfer to hospital.[86]

Effect of a restricted transfer direction [section 47(3) and 49]

19.12 Sentenced prisoners given transfer directions and restriction directions are treated for most purposes in the same way as patients given restricted hospital orders (see chapters 15 and 21). One effect of this is that, while a

[86] R (Miah) v Secretary of State for the Home Department. 2004. EWHC 2569 (Admin). http://www.bailii.org/ew/cases/EWHC/Admin/2004/2569.html

restriction direction is in force, the transfer direction also remains in force and does not need to be renewed.

19.13 Special arrangements apply to the discharge of restricted transfer direction patients from hospital, because they are detained primarily on the basis of a prison sentence and are liable to be returned to prison to complete their sentence(s) if they no longer need to be in the hospital. These arrangements, which are described later in this chapter, are like those for patients given hospital and limitation directions (except that, by definition, transferred prisoners will already have been in prison at some point).

Automatic expiry of restriction directions [section 50(2), (3) and (4)]

19.14 Like a limitation direction, a restriction direction ends automatically on the patient's 'release date'.

19.15 The patient's release date is the day on which the patient would have been entitled to be released from custody had the transfer direction not been given. If the patient is serving a life sentence, or an indeterminate sentence, the release date is the date (if any) on which the person's release is ordered by the parole board.

19.16 Although the restriction direction ends on the release date, the transfer direction does not. If patients are still detained in hospital on their release date on the basis of a transfer direction, they remain liable from then on to be detained in hospital as unrestricted patients. This includes patients who are on leave of absence from hospital on their release date, but not those who have been conditionally discharged (see chapter 21) and who have not subsequently been recalled to hospital.

19.17 As with hospital and limitation direction patients, going absent without leave from hospital, or otherwise absconding, under the Act may affect the release date of a patient transferred to hospital under a restricted transfer direction (see paragraph 16.18).

Return to prison [section 50(1)]

19.18 Restricted transfer direction patients may be returned to custody by the Secretary of State to serve the remainder of their sentence, or the Secretary of State may exercise any power of releasing them on licence or discharging them under supervision which would have been exercisable had the patient been so returned to custody.

19.19 As with the removal of hospital and limitation direction patients to prison, this is only possible where the Secretary of State is notified by the offender's responsible clinician, any other approved clinician, or by the Tribunal, that:

- the offender no longer requires treatment in hospital for mental disorder, or

- no effective treatment for the disorder can be given in the hospital in which the offender is detained.

19.20 When notified in this way by the responsible clinician, or any other approved clinician, the Secretary of State may:

- direct the offender's removal to a prison (or other establishment) where the offender could have been detained if not in hospital, or
- discharge or release the offender from the hospital as the Secretary of State could have done if the offender had been removed to custody.

See below for the procedure where the Tribunal is involved.

19.21 In practice, the Secretary of State expects clinical staff from the hospital and prison to meet to plan the patient's future care (a 'section 117 meeting') before directing the patient's return to prison.

Discharge of restricted transfer direction patients by the Tribunal [section 74]

19.22 Like hospital and limitation direction patients, restricted transfer direction patients can only be discharged by the Tribunal if the Secretary of State agrees.

19.23 With one exception, if the Tribunal thinks that a patient would be entitled to be discharged if subject to a restriction order, but the Secretary of State does not consent, the patient will be removed to prison. This is because the Tribunal has decided that the patient should not be detained in hospital, but the prison sentence remains in force and the patient has yet to reach their release date.

19.24 The patient will remain detained in hospital if the Tribunal thinks the patient would be entitled to conditional discharge, but recommends that the patient remain in hospital if the Secretary of State does not agree to that conditional discharge. This is described more fully in chapter 6.

Effect of removal to prison on transfer direction and restriction direction [section 50(1)]

19.25 If an offender is returned to custody, both the transfer direction and the restriction direction end when the offender arrives at the relevant prison or other institution.

Effect of a transfer direction on existing authority to detain etc [section 40(5), 47(3) and 55(4)]

19.26 Like patients detained as a result of a hospital order, when patients are admitted to hospital on the basis of a transfer direction, any previous application for admission, application for guardianship, unrestricted hospital order, or guardianship order ceases to have effect. A previous restricted hospital order does not end.

19.27 If the prison sentence the patient would otherwise be serving, or the conviction on which it is based, is quashed on appeal, the transfer direction would fall and any such previous application, order or direction will, in effect, be revived if it would still be in force had the patient remained in prison instead of being transferred to hospital – see paragraph 25.54.

20: Transfer of unsentenced prisoners to hospital

Introduction

20.1 This chapter describes the provisions under which the Secretary of State may transfer unsentenced prisoners from prison, or other forms of custody, eg immigration removal centre, to hospital for treatment where that is urgently needed.

Transfer to hospital of unsentenced prisoners [section 48]

20.2 A transfer direction is a warrant directing that a patient be taken to and detained in the hospital specified in the warrant.

20.3 The Secretary of State may make a transfer direction in respect of an unsentenced prisoner only in the circumstances set out in figure 60. The key difference between this and arrangements for sentenced patients is that an unsentenced prisoner must be in urgent need of treatment if a transfer direction is to be given.

Figure 60: Criteria for transfer directions in respect of unsentenced prisoners

Transfer directions for unsentenced patients (section 48)	
May be exercised in respect of	People remanded in custody by a magistrates' court ('magistrates' remand prisoners'). This does not cover under-18s remanded to local authority accommodation under sections 91 and 92 Legal Aid, Sentencing and Punishment of Offenders Act 2012[87]
	Civil prisoners, ie persons committed by a court to prison for a limited term, but who are not sentenced prisoners (as described in chapter 8) ('civil prisoners')
	People detained under the Immigration Act 1971[88] or under section 62 of the Nationality, Immigration and Asylum Act 2002[89] ('immigration detainees')
	People detained in a prison, but not serving a sentence of imprisonment or falling within the above categories– usually people remanded by the Crown Court ('other remand prisoners')

[87] Legal Aid, Sentencing and Punishment of Offenders Act 2012. http://www.legislation.gov.uk/ukpga/2012

[88] Immigration Act 1971. http://www.legislation.gov.uk/ukpga/1971/77

[89] Nationality, Immigration and Asylum Act 2002. http://www.legislation.gov.uk/ukpga/2002/41

If the Secretary of State	Is satisfied, by reports from at least two doctors, at least one of whom must be approved under section 12, that: • the person is suffering from mental disorder of a nature or degree which makes it appropriate for the person to be detained in a hospital for medical treatment • the person is in urgent need of such treatment, and • appropriate medical treatment is available
And	The Secretary of State is of the opinion, having regard to the public interest and all the circumstances, that it is expedient to direct the person's transfer

20.4 As with transfer directions for sentenced prisoners:

- mental disorder here and throughout this chapter does not include learning disability, unless that learning disability is associated with abnormally aggressive or seriously irresponsible conduct on the part of the patient concerned
- appropriate medical treatment means the same as it does in respect of applications for admission for treatment under part 2 of the Act (see paragraph 8.8 above), and
- the requirement that at least one of the doctors giving evidence about the defendant's mental disorder must be approved under section 12 is to be found in section 54(1).

Restriction directions [section 49]

20.5 In certain cases, the Secretary of State must also give a restriction direction, and in other cases may do so, as follows:

Figure 61: Secretary of State restriction direction

Magistrates' or other remand prisoner	Civil prisoner or an immigration detainee
Secretary of State must also give a restriction direction under section 49	Secretary of State may also give a restriction direction under section 49

20.6 As with sentenced patients, if the Secretary of State also makes a restriction direction, under section 47 Crime (Sentences) Act 1997 the transfer direction can specify that the patient is to be admitted to a particular unit of the hospital in question. In such cases, references to hospitals are to be treated as references to the particular hospital unit in question.

Effect of a transfer direction in respect of an unsentenced patient [section 48(3)]

20.7 Transfer directions and restriction directions for unsentenced patients have the same effect as they do for sentenced patients. So:

- the hospital, or unit, specified in the transfer direction must admit the patient, but the direction ceases to have effect if that does not happen within the 14 days starting with the day the direction is given
- patients given transfer directions without restriction directions (unrestricted transfer direction patients) are treated for most purposes in the same way as patients given unrestricted hospital orders and cannot be returned to custody from hospital
- patients given transfer directions and restriction directions (restricted transfer order patients) are treated for most purposes in the same way as patients given restricted hospital orders, but can be returned to custody from hospital
- if a restricted patient is returned to custody, both the transfer direction and the restriction direction expire on the patient's arrival there, and
- any previous application for admission, application for guardianship, unrestricted hospital order, unrestricted hospital direction or guardianship order (but not a restricted hospital order) ceases to have effect when the transfer direction is given.

20.8 Unlike sentenced prisoners, unsentenced patients do not have a 'release date' on which restriction directions end. Instead, there comes a point at which transfer directions themselves (as well as restriction directions, if relevant) automatically expire, as described below.

20.9 There are also differences in the circumstances in how, if at all, patients may be returned to custody.

Automatic expiry of transfer directions for unsentenced prisoners [sections 51(1), 52(1) and 53(1)]

20.10 Transfer directions automatically end in the circumstances set out in figure 62.

Figure 62: Automatic expiry of transfer directions for unsentenced prisoners

Class of detainee (see paragraph 20.3 above)	Transfer direction expires
Magistrates' remand prisoners (section 52(2))	At the end of the period of remand (or further remand), unless the patient is sent in custody to the Crown Court for trial or to be dealt with in some other way (in which case the transfer direction expires when the court disposes of the case), or unless the court directs the transfer direction should expire earlier
Other remand prisoners (section 51(2))	When the person's case is disposed of by the relevant court or the person is remitted to custody or released on bail
Civil prisoners and immigration detainees (section 53(1))	At the end of the period during which the person would, but for their transfer to hospital, be liable to be detained in the prison or other institution from which they were transferred to hospital, or when the person is remitted to custody

Discharge by the Tribunal [section 74]

20.11 Unsentenced prisoners subject to transfer directions under section 48 have the right to apply to the Tribunal for their discharge from detention in hospital – see chapters 6.

20.12 If the Tribunal orders the discharge of a patient who is not also subject to a restriction direction, the patient will be free to leave hospital and will not be returned to custody.

20.13 Different arrangements apply to restricted patients. Where the Tribunal decides that such a patient would be entitled to be discharged either absolutely or conditionally if they were subject to a restricted hospital order (rather than transfer direction), it must inform the Secretary of State. If the patient would be entitled to conditional discharge, the Tribunal may recommend that, if not so discharged, the patient continue to be detained in hospital (rather than being returned to custody).

20.14 Unless the Tribunal has recommended that such a restricted patient continue to be detained in hospital, the Secretary of State must then issue a warrant directing the patient's return to prison, or any other place of detention in which the patient could have been detained but for being in hospital. If the Tribunal has decided that the patient would be entitled to be conditionally discharged, but has made a recommendation for the patient's continued detention in hospital if not so discharged, the patient remains detained and subject to the restricted transfer direction as before.

Magistrates' remand prisoners – further remands etc [section 52(2) to (7)]

20.15 Where a transfer direction has been given in respect of a defendant remanded in custody by a magistrates' court, the court may exercise its normal power of further remand in custody without the defendant being brought to court from hospital, provided the defendant has appeared before the court within the previous six months.

20.16 If defendants are further remanded in custody, they remain in hospital – the Secretary of State does not have to issue a new transfer direction.

20.17 If the court sends the defendant to the Crown Court, the transfer direction remains in force, but the patient is then treated for most purposes like an 'other remand prisoner' instead (see paragraph 20.22 onward below).

20.18 The court may send patients subject to transfer directions to the Crown Court for trial (under sections 51 or 51A of the Crime and Disorder Act 1998) in their absence. It may only do so if the patient in question is legally represented and the court is satisfied on the written or oral evidence of the patient's responsible clinician that the patient is unfit to take part in the proceedings.

Magistrates' remand prisoners – return to prison etc [section 52(5)]

20.19 A magistrates' court may direct that a magistrates' remand prisoner's transfer direction is to cease to have effect before the current period of remand has ended. It may also direct that a transfer direction is to end even though the patient has already been sent in custody to the Crown Court and is therefore no longer treated, for most purposes, as a magistrates' remand prisoner (see paragraph 201.7).

20.20 In either case, the court may only do so if it is satisfied, on the written or oral evidence of the patient's responsible clinician, that:

- the patient no longer requires treatment in hospital for mental disorder, or
- no effective treatment for his disorder can be given in the hospital to which the patient has been transferred.

20.21 When ending a transfer direction like this, the court may remand the prisoner in some other way.

Other remand prisoners – hospital orders in the defendant's absence [section 51(5)]

20.22 While a remand prisoner (other than a magistrates' remand prisoner) remains subject to a transfer direction, the relevant court can make a hospital order (either with or without a restriction order) in the patient's absence and (if the person is awaiting trial) without convicting the patient if the three criteria described in the figure 63 are met.

Figure 63: Criteria for making a hospital order under section 51

<table>
<tr><td rowspan="3">To make a hospital order in the patient's absence under section 51(5), the relevant court must</td><td>Think it is impracticable or inappropriate to bring the patient before the court, and</td></tr>
<tr><td>Be satisfied, on the written or oral evidence of at least two doctors, at least one of whom is approved under section 12, that:
• the patient is suffering from mental disorder of a nature or degree which makes it appropriate for the patient to be detained in a hospital for medical treatment, and
• appropriate medical treatment is available</td></tr>
<tr><td>And be of the opinion, after considering any depositions or other documents it requires, that it is proper to make such an order</td></tr>
</table>

20.23 Under section 51(7), this also applies to patients committed to hospital under section 44 (see chapter 17) and section 43.

20.24 A hospital order made in these circumstances has the same effect as any other hospital order made in the normal way under section 37 (see chapter 15).

Other remand prisoners – return to prison etc [section 51(3) and (4)]

20.25 Both the relevant court and the Secretary of State may, in certain circumstances, return remand prisoners to custody, as set out in figure 64. The court, but not the Secretary of State, may also release the patient on bail.

20.26 Neither of these powers apply to magistrates' remand prisoners, unless they have been sent to the Crown Court (see section 52).

Figure 64: Release and return to prison of other remand prisoners

<table>
<tr><td colspan="3">Other remand prisoner [section 51]</td></tr>
<tr><td>While the transfer direction is in force</td><td>If the Secretary of State is notified by the patient's responsible clinician, any other approved clinician or by the Tribunal that:</td><td>If the relevant court is satisfied on the written or oral evidence of the patient's responsible clinician that</td></tr>
</table>

	The patient no longer requires treatment in hospital for mental disorder, or no effective treatment for his disorder can be given in the hospital to which the patient has been transferred	
Then	The Secretary of State may direct the patient's return to any place where the patient could have been detained if not in hospital	If the Secretary of State has not remitted the patient to prison or equivalent already, the relevant court may do so, or, if it could otherwise do so, release the prisoner on bail

20.27 If a patient is released on bail by the court, both the transfer direction and the accompanying restriction direction come to an end, just as it would if the patient had been returned to prison.

Civil prisoners and immigration detainees – return to custody [section 53]

20.28 Civil prisoners and immigration detainees given unrestricted transfer directions may not be returned to custody.

20.29 But if they are subject to restricted transfer directions then the Secretary of State may issue a warrant directing that they be remitted to any place they at which they could have been detained if not in hospital.

20.30 The Secretary of State may only do this if notified by the patient's responsible clinician, any other approved clinician, or by the Tribunal that:

- the patient no longer requires treatment in hospital for mental disorder, or
- no effective treatment for the disorder can be given in the hospital to which the patient has been transferred.

20.31 In those cases, both the transfer direction and the restriction direction cease to have effect when the person arrives at the prison or other place of detention.

21: Restricted patients

Introduction

21.1 This chapter summarises the effect of restriction orders, limitation directions and restriction directions on patients who are, or have been, detained under part 3 of the Act. These patients are collectively known as 'restricted patients' as defined in section 79(1).

21.2 For a description of when these orders and directions may be imposed, see the previous chapters.

Effect of restrictions [sections 41 and 42 and part 2 of schedule 1 in particular]

21.3 Restricted patients are subject to various special restrictions compared to other patients ('unrestricted patients') detained in hospital by order of the courts or transferred by the Secretary of State from prison (or other places of detention) to hospital.

21.4 In summary, the main differences are as set out in figure 65.

Figure 65: Summary of main differences in application of provisions to restricted and unrestricted patients

Provision	Application to restricted patients
Leave of absence (section 17)	Responsible clinicians may only grant restricted patients leave of absence from hospital with the consent of the Secretary of State
Recall from leave of absence (section 17)	The Secretary of State may recall patients from leave of absence at any time. This is in addition to the power of responsible clinicians to recall patients from leave (although the responsible clinician cannot recall after 12 months beginning with the first day of leave)
Community treatment order (CTO) (section 17A)	Does not apply. Restricted patients may not be discharged onto CTO, but may be conditionally discharged – see paragraph 21.11 onward
Absence without leave (section 18)	There is no time limit after which the patient may no longer be taken into custody and returned to hospital or any other place they ought to be

Provision	Application to restricted patients
Transfer from one hospital to another (section 19)	Hospital managers may only transfer patients from one hospital to another with the consent of the Secretary of State (even if both hospitals are under the same management)
Transfer to guardianship (section 19)	Does not apply. Restricted patients may not be transferred to guardianship
Renewal of authority to detain (section 20)	Does not apply. The authority to detain does not expire, so no renewal is required
Confirmation of authority to detain after absence without leave (section 21B)	Does not apply. The authority to detain does not expire however long the patient is absent without leave
Ending of authority to detain after six months imprisonment (section 22)	Authority to detain does not expire however long the imprisonment
Discharge by responsible clinicians and hospital managers (section 23)	The responsible clinician and hospital managers may only discharge patients with the consent of the Secretary of State
Nearest relatives (section 26)	Does not apply. Restricted patients do not have a nearest relative for the purposes of the Act
Applications to the Tribunal (sections 66 and 69)	Does not apply. The rules on when patients may apply are a little different to other patients, largely because there is no renewal of authority to detain – see chapter 6
Applications to the Tribunal by nearest relatives (sections 66 and 69)	Does not apply. Restricted patients do not have a nearest relative for the purposes of the Act
Hospital managers' duty to refer to the Tribunal (section 68)	Does not apply, but under section 71(2) the Secretary of State has a duty to refer patients if they have not had a hearing for 3 years (1 year if under 18) – see chapter 6 for further details
Tribunal's general discretion to discharge (section 72)	Does not apply The relevant powers of the Tribunal in relation to restricted patients are in section 73 and 74

21.5 In addition, there are a number of special arrangements which are unique to restricted patients, summarised in figure 66.

Figure 66: Summary of special arrangements which only apply to restricted patients

Provision	Effect
Specification of units within hospitals (section 47 of the Crime (Sentences) Act 1997)	Hospital orders, hospital directions and transfer directions for restricted patients may specify a particular unit within a hospital as the place in which a patient is to be detained Rules on leave of absence, transfer, etc apply accordingly. So, for example, hospital managers require the consent of the Secretary of State to transfer a patient between units – or to allow a patient to visit a different unit – within the same hospital, if the patient's order or direction specifies a particular unit
Discharge by Secretary of State (section 42)	All restricted patients may be discharged by the Secretary of State
Conditional discharge (sections 42 and 73)	The Secretary of State may discharge restricted patients conditionally rather than absolutely – in which case they remain liable to be recalled to hospital The Tribunal must discharge restricted patients conditionally rather than absolutely unless satisfied that it is not appropriate to do so. This does not apply to patients subject to a restriction direction or limitation direction Conditional discharge is described more fully in chapter 27

Provision	Effect
Return or removal to prison (sections 50 to 53)	Patients transferred to hospital from prison may only be returned to prison if they are subject to a restriction direction. In some circumstances, unsentenced prisoners transferred to hospital must be returned to custody – see chapters 19 and 20 Patients subject to hospital and limitation directions can be removed to prison in certain circumstances to serve the remainder of the prison sentence(s) imposed at the same time as the directions – see chapter 15 Patients subject to restriction orders cannot be removed to prison under the Act – although, in practice, they would be removed to prison if subsequently they were to receive a prison sentence or were remanded in custody and not transferred or remanded back to hospital under the Act
Tribunal discharge of hospital and limitation direction and restricted transfer direction patients (section 74)	Because they are subject to a prison sentence, the Tribunal cannot discharge patients subject to hospital and limitation directions or sentenced prisoners subject to restricted transfer directions without the Secretary of State's consent If the Secretary of State does not consent to the discharge, patients are removed to prison instead, unless the Tribunal has recommended that a patient who would be entitled to conditional discharge should remain in hospital Similar arrangements apply to unsentenced patients subject to restricted transfer directions, except that unless the Tribunal recommends that they remain in hospital, the Secretary of State must return the patient to custody See chapter 6
Reports to Secretary of State (section 41(6))	Responsible clinicians must examine restricted patients and send a report to the Secretary of State at intervals decided by the Secretary of State (which must not be more than one year)
Attendance in the interests of justice etc (section 42(6))	The Secretary of State can direct that a restricted patient be taken to any place in Great Britain (but not Northern Ireland) if it is desirable in the interests of justice or for a public inquiry (see paragraphs 21.25 and 21.26)

21.6 In practice, one important consequence of restrictions is that patients remain subject to ongoing case-management by the Mental Health Casework Section of the Ministry of Justice, on behalf of the Secretary of State. See also Code of Practice paragraphs 22.53 and 22.86.

Absolute discharge – ending of restrictions and the associated authority for detention [section 42(1) and 73]

21.7 The Secretary of State may discharge restricted patients absolutely at any time by issuing a warrant to that effect.

21.8 The Secretary of State may also consent to the discharge of restricted patients by the responsible clinician, or the hospital managers under section 23 (as modified by schedule 1).

21.9 Restricted patients may also be discharged absolutely by the Tribunal in certain circumstances, although not patients subject to a limitation direction or restriction direction, see chapter 6.

21.10 Absolute discharge by the Tribunal or by (or with the consent of) the Secretary of State, automatically brings to an end the special restrictions and the underlying hospital order, hospital direction or transfer direction. The patient therefore ceases to be liable to be detained.

Conditional discharge [section 41(6), 42, 73 and 75]

21.11 In certain circumstances, restricted patients must be conditionally, rather than absolutely, discharged by the Tribunal, see chapter 6.

21.12 In addition, the Secretary of State may conditionally discharge restricted patients at any time, by issuing a warrant to that effect.

21.13 Conditionally discharged patients may be recalled to hospital by the Secretary of State at any time where it is necessary to protect the public from the actual or potential risk posed by that patient (or to protect the patient themselves) and that risk is linked to the patient's mental disorder. Patients recalled to hospital become detained patients again.

21.14 See chapter 27 for a description of the effect of conditional discharge.

Expiry of restrictions while associated authority for detention remains in force [section 41(4), 50(2) and (5)]

21.15 As described in earlier chapters, there are circumstances in which restriction orders, limitation directions and restriction directions will expire while the associated hospital order, hospital direction or transfer direction remains in force. Those circumstances are described in the figure 67.

Figure 67: Expiry of restrictions while authority for detention remains in place

Patient subject to	Restrictions end automatically at	Notes
Hospital order and restriction order	The end of period for which the restriction order was imposed	This will only happen where the restriction order was given in England or Wales before 1 October 2007 and the court chose to give a restriction order for a fixed period, or where the patient is treated as subject to a restriction order of limited duration on transfer from an equivalent order imposed outside England or Wales
Hospital and limitation direction	On the patient's 'release date'	The release date is the date (if any) on which patients would have been entitled to be released from custody had they not been detained in hospital instead (see paragraph 16.16) or when the Parole Board direct the release of the individual
Restricted transfer direction (sentenced prisoner)		

21.16 In practice, the same effect will sometimes result from an appeal against sentence. It is possible for a restriction order to be quashed without the associated hospital order also being quashed, and for a hospital and limitation direction to be replaced with an unrestricted hospital order.

Secretary of State's power to lift restrictions while patients remain detained [section 42(1)]

21.17 The Secretary of State has the discretion to lift a restriction order, limitation direction or restriction direction without at the same time discharging the associated hospital order, hospital direction or transfer direction. The Secretary of State may do this if satisfied that the restrictions are no longer necessary for the protection of the public from serious harm.

21.18 Only the Secretary of State has the power to lift restrictions in this way without discharging the underlying authority to detain, although, as explained above, the same effect may result from an appeal against sentence.

Effect of expiry or lifting of restrictions on detained patients [section 41(4) and 55(4)]

21.19 If restrictions expire or are lifted while they remain detained, patients are treated as if they were subject to an unrestricted hospital order, hospital direction or transfer direction, as the case may be, given on the day the restrictions ended.

21.20 In other words, patients are treated as if they had newly been made subject to an unrestricted order or direction, except that all such patients are able to apply to the Tribunal within the first six months of their new status, even if they are subject to hospital orders – see chapter 6.

21.21 The Secretary of State no longer has a role in their continuing detention.

21.22 If sentenced prisoners subject to transfer directions, or patients subject to hospital directions, were to have their restrictions lifted before their release date, the effect is that they cannot be removed to custody even though their sentence is still in force. In practice, this is unlikely to happen.

21.23 If the Secretary of State were to lift restrictions from an unsentenced transfer direction patient, the patient's transfer direction would still expire automatically at the normal time (see paragraph 20.10). During that period the patient could no longer be returned to custody.

21.24 If patients have already been conditionally discharged when their restrictions expire or are lifted (and have not been recalled to hospital), they are treated as having been absolutely discharged. As a result, they can no longer be recalled to hospital – see chapter 27.

Secretary of State's power to direct restricted patients to be taken to any place in Great Britain in the interests of justice etc [section 42(6)]

21.25 The Secretary of State may direct people to transport a restricted patient to anywhere in England, Wales or Scotland, if satisfied that the patient's attendance there is desirable in the interests of justice or for the purposes of any public inquiry.

21.26 Unless the Secretary of State says otherwise, the patient is to be kept in custody on the journey to the destination, while there and on the journey back to the hospital (or unit) in which the patient is detained.

Related material

- Ministry of Justice Mental Health Casework Section. First Floor, Grenadier House, 99-105 Horseferry Road, London SW1P 2DD
  Ministry of Justice Switchboard: 020 3334 3555
  General: enquiry.mhu@noms.gsi.gov.uk

22: Other legislation under which part 3 remands, orders and directions may be made

Introduction

22.1 This chapter summarises various provisions in other legislation which allow the courts or the Secretary of State to make remands, orders and directions under part 3 of the Act, or their equivalent. It summarises the main effects, including the more important special arrangements that would not normally apply under part 3, but does not attempt to deal comprehensively with all the small differences in the way the Act applies to such patients.

Defendants who are not fit to stand trial or who have been found not guilty by reason of insanity

22.2 Under section 5 of the Criminal Procedure (Insanity) Act 1964,[90] where a person is found unfit to plead, but to have done the act or made the omission of which they were accused, the court may make a hospital order under section 37 of the Act. It may also do so if the defendant is found not guilty by reason of insanity.

22.3 Prior to amendments made by the Domestic Violence, Crime and Victims Act 2004 (DVCVA),[91] different arrangements applied to people arraigned before 31 March 2005. Until then, the courts could not make a hospital order under the Act itself, but would make an 'admission order' which, for the most part, had the same effect as a hospital order. Courts could also make guardianship orders under the Act. Some admission orders may still be in force.

22.4 To make a hospital order, the courts must have the evidence required by the Act. In other words, they require the same medical evidence as they do when making a hospital order after a conviction. They do not formally require evidence from the hospital managers that a hospital place is available – if an order is made, the hospital specified in it is under a duty to admit the patient.

22.5 Following either finding, the hospital order may be given with or without a restriction order. If the offence charged is murder, and a hospital order is given, the court must always make a restriction order, whether or not the normal criteria for making a restriction order are met.

---

90 Criminal Procedure (Insanity) Act 1964. http://www.legislation.gov.uk/ukpga/1964/84
91 Domestic Violence, Crime and Victims Act 2004 . http://www.legislation.gov.uk/ukpga/2004/28

22.6 Pending a decision as to whether to make a hospital order, the court may make a remand under section 35 or 36 of the Act or an interim hospital order under section 38. For these purposes, the court may do this even if the defendant was charged with murder.

22.7 When patients are given a hospital order for these reasons, the managers of the hospital named in the order are under an obligation to admit them immediately. Unlike normal hospital orders, it is not possible for patients to be detained temporarily in a place of safety while arrangements are made for their admission to the hospital.

22.8 Patients admitted to hospital when found unfit to be tried have not received a full criminal trial, and may be sent back for trial by the prosecuting authority if that authority is satisfied, after consulting their responsible clinician, that they can now properly be tried. The Secretary of State may also do this, if the patient concerned is still subject to a restriction order and still detained in hospital. This includes patients on leave of absence from hospital, but not those who have been conditionally discharged and not recalled to hospital. Before doing so, the Secretary of State must consult the patient's responsible clinician.

22.9 The general principle observed by the Secretary of State is that people who have been accused of an offence ought, if possible, to be brought to trial so that they may have an opportunity of having their guilt or innocence determined by a court. In practice, the Secretary of State will consult the responsible clinician about a relevant patient's fitness for trial during the first six months of their detention and regularly thereafter.

22.10 If sending patients back for trial, the Secretary of State may remit them either directly to the court or to prison to await trial. The patient's hospital order (and restriction order) ceases to apply on their arrival at the court or prison.

22.11 Equivalent arrangements apply under the section 169 of and schedule 4 to the Armed Forces Act 2006,[92] which contain similar provisions.

Appeals and retrials

22.12 Under various provisions of the Criminal Appeal Act 1968,[93] the Court of Appeal may make hospital or guardianship orders under section 37 and hospital or limitation directions under section 45A in the case of convicted offenders in the same way as the court which originally heard the case. Under sections 6 and 14 of the same Act, the Court of Appeal may also make hospital orders in the case of people it finds should originally have been found unfit to be tried or to be not guilty by reason of insanity, in essentially the same way as a lower court (see paragraphs 22.2 to 22.11).

[92] Armed Forces Act 2006. http://www.legislation.gov.uk/ukpga/2006/52
[93] Criminal Appeal Act 1968. http://www.legislation.gov.uk/ukpga/1968/19

22.13 The Court of Appeal may also make remands under sections 35 and 36 and interim hospital orders under section 38. If it makes an interim hospital order, the responsibility for deciding when to renew or end the order falls to the lower court. It is also the lower court which must decide what sentence to impose at the end of the interim hospital order, which might – but need not – be a hospital order or hospital and limitation directions.

22.14 Under section 8 of that Act, where a conviction is quashed and someone who is liable to be detained under an order or direction under part 3 of the Act (except a remand under sections 35, 36 or an interim hospital order under section 38) is ordered to be retried, the order or direction in question continues in force pending the retrial, unless it ends or the patient is discharged from it in the normal way. Likewise, where a conviction is quashed and someone who has been discharged from an order or direction under part 3 onto is ordered to be retried, the person remains a community treatment order (CTO) patient pending the retrial – and the patient can be discharged, or the order can be revoked or otherwise come to an end, in the normal way.

22.15 Where a retrial is ordered in the case of someone who is liable to be detained under a remand under section 36 or an interim hospital order under section 38, the Court of Appeal may make an order for that person's continued detention, in which case part 3 applies as if the patient were subject to a restricted transfer direction. That means, amongst other things, that the patient can be given leave of absence and discharged with the consent of the Secretary of State without the case having to be referred back to the court. The same applies where the Court of Appeal makes an order for the continued detention in hospital pending trial of someone whose appeal against a finding of unfitness to be tried it has upheld.

22.16 Similarly, under section 16 of the Courts-Martial (Appeals) Act 1968,[94] the Appeal Court may (like courts-martial) make a hospital order under section 37 where it finds a defendant unfit to stand trial or not guilty by reason of insanity, and may also make remands under section 35 and 36, and interim hospital orders under section 38.

22.17 Under the same Act, if the Appeal Court quashes a conviction and orders the retrial of a person who is detained under part 3 of the Act (or who was detained under part 3 but has since been discharged onto CTO), the person's detention or CTO continues, in the normal way, pending the retrial. The same applies where the court quashes a finding that a person was unfit to be tried and the person is therefore to be tried.

---

[94] These and related provisions of the Courts-Martial (Appeals) Act 1968 http://www.legislation.gov.uk/ukpga/1968/20 are amended by the Armed Forces Act 2008. At the time of publication, those amendments were not yet in force.

Prosecution appeals against decisions of certain appeal courts

22.18 Under sections 5 and 5A respectively of the Administration of Justice Act 1960, and sections 37 and 37A of the Criminal Appeal Act 1968,[95] the relevant appeal court may make an order continuing a patient's detention or CTO under the Act, where the prosecution is granted, or gives notice of its intention to apply for, permission to appeal against a decision made on appeal. The court may only do this if the patient would be detained under the Act or a CTO patient but for its own decision made on appeal.

22.19 If the patient would, but for the decision of the court, have been detained under an interim hospital order under section 38 of the Act, the effect of any such order authorising continued detention is that part 3 applies as if the patient were subject to a restricted transfer direction. That means that the limit on the maximum duration of an interim hospital order does not apply, and that the patient acquires the right to apply to the Tribunal for discharge.

22.20 Similarly, under sections 43 and 43A respectively of the Courts-Martial (Appeals) Act 1968, the Appeal Court may make an order authorising the defendant's continued detention or CTO under the Act, if the Director of Service Prosecutions is granted, or gives notice of its intention to apply for, leave to appeal to the House of Lords, and the defendant would, but for the Court's decision, be liable to be detained under the Act or a CTO patient, as applicable.

Contempt of court

22.21 Under section 14 of the Contempt of Court Act 1981, instead of committing a person to prison for contempt of court, superior courts have the same power to remand a person for report under section 35 of the Act as the Crown Court has in respect of a person on trial before it. Similarly, these courts can make a hospital order, interim hospital order or guardianship order under the Act in the same way that the Crown Court could in respect of a person convicted of an offence.

22.22 The relevant court requires the same medical and other evidence that the Crown Court would normally need, and must apply the same criteria. For these purposes 'superior court' includes the county court, but not a magistrates' court.

Other powers of the courts

22.23 In certain circumstances relating to breaches of orders and injunctions under section 51 of the Family Law Act 1996,[96] magistrates' courts may make a hospital or guardianship order under section 37 of the Act. In similar circumstances, the power to remand for report under section 35 of the Act

---

[95] Criminal Appeal Act 1968. http://www.legislation.gov.uk/ukpga/1968/19

[96] Family Law Act 1996. http://www.legislation.gov.uk/ukpga/1996/27

may be exercised by the courts under sections 48 and 63L of the same Family Law Act 1996 and under section 156 of the Housing Act 1996.[97]

Offenders transferred from overseas

22.24 Under the Colonial Prisoners Removal Act 1884,[98] certain mentally disordered offenders may be transferred from detention in a British overseas territory to detention in a hospital in England or Wales. Where this is to happen in the case of a patient who was found unfit to be tried, or not guilty by reason of insanity, the Secretary of State will issue a warrant directing the patient's detention in a specified hospital. That warrant has the same effect as a restricted hospital order under section 37 (and 41) of the Act. In any other case, the Secretary of State will make a transfer direction (with or without a restriction direction) under section 47 (and 49). A patient who was originally found unfit to be tried, but who recovers sufficiently, may be returned to the overseas territory to be tried.

22.25 It is also possible for mentally disordered offenders detained abroad to be transferred to detention in the UK under the Repatriation of Prisoners Act 1984,[99] where the UK has a relevant agreement with the country in question. If such a person is to be detained in a hospital in England, the Secretary of State will issue a warrant which will, in effect, make the person subject to an appropriate order or direction made under part 3 of the Act on the day the warrant takes effect.

22.26 Patients are then treated for most purposes as if they were subject to the appropriate order or direction given under the Act in the normal way. However, if the warrant effectively makes a patient subject to a hospital order, with or without a restriction order, the patient can apply to the Tribunal during the first six months of the order.

[97] Housing Act 1996. http://www.legislation.gov.uk/ukpga/1996/52
[98] Colonial Prisoners Removal Act 1884. http://www.legislation.gov.uk/ukpga/Vict/47-48/31
[99] Repatriation of Prisoners Act 1984. http://www.legislation.gov.uk/ukpga/1984/47

Care, support and treatment in hospital

These chapters describe the provisions of the Act dealing with medical treatment for mental disorder. These provisions primarily apply to people who are liable to be detained in hospital or who are community treatment order (CTO) patients. Some provisions apply to all mental health patients, regardless of whether they are, or could be, detained under the Act.

23: Medical treatment

Introduction

23.1 This chapter describes the provisions in part 4 of the Act which deal with medical treatment for mental disorder. Part 4 primarily applies to people who are liable to be detained in hospital and to patients on a community treatment order (CTO) who have been recalled to hospital. But some provisions apply to all mental health patients, regardless of whether they are (or could be) detained under the Act.

Patients to whom part 4 applies ('detained patients') [section 56]

23.2 Except for those which apply to all patients, the provisions described in this chapter only apply to the patients set out in figure 68. This chapter refers to them as 'detained patients'.

Figure 68: Patients who are detained patients for the purposes of this chapter

Detained patients in this chapter includes those who are	Detained patients in this chapter does not include those who are
Liable to be detained on the basis of an application for admission for assessment or treatment under part 2 (sections 2 and 3)	Liable to be detained on the basis of an emergency application (section 4) unless or until the second medical recommendation is received
Remanded to hospital for treatment under section 36	Remanded to hospital for a report under section 35
Subject to a hospital order, interim hospital order, hospital direction, transfer direction or committed to hospital under part 3 (except as noted in the second column)	Detained in a place of safety in accordance with directions under section 37(4) or 45A(5) pending admission to hospital, on the basis of a hospital order or hospital and limitation directions
CTO patients recalled to hospital	CTO patients not recalled to hospital
	Conditionally discharged restricted patients
	Detained under the 'holding powers' in section 5
	Detained in a place of safety under section 135 or 136

Meaning of medical treatment for mental disorder [section 145]

23.3 The meaning of medical treatment is described in paragraphs 1.17 onward. It is not limited to what might be considered 'medical' treatment – it includes nursing, psychological therapies, and specialist mental health habilitation, rehabilitation and care.

23.4 Medical treatment for mental disorder means treatment for the purpose of alleviating, or preventing a worsening of, a patient's mental disorder, or one or more of its symptoms or manifestations.

23.5 'Symptoms' and 'manifestations' include the way a disorder is experienced by the individual concerned and the way in which the disorder manifests itself in the person's thoughts, emotions, behaviour and actions.

23.6 Medical treatment includes treatment of physical health problems only to such extent that such treatment is part of, or ancillary to, treatment for mental disorder, eg treating wounds self-inflicted as a result of mental disorder. Otherwise the Act does not regulate medical treatment for physical health problems.[100] The Code of Practice provides guidance in relation to physical healthcare. See for example Code of Practice paragraphs 24.57-24.62. Other guidance is included in relation to supporting people with long term conditions and disabilities, including reasonable adjustments.

Section 57, 58 and 58A treatments

23.7 Part 4 applies to all forms of medical treatment for mental disorder. Certain types of treatment are subject to special rules set out in sections 57, 58 and 58A. The treatments covered by these sections are summarised in figure 69.

23.8 The special rules concerned are explained more fully later in this chapter, and are summarised in figure 73 at the end of the chapter.

Figure 69: Summary of types of treatment to which the special rules in sections 57, 58 and 58A apply

Section	Types of treatments	For
Section 57	Neurosurgery for mental disorder Surgical implantation of hormones to reduce male sex drive Other treatments specified in regulations (none at time of publication)	All patients

[100] The Code of Practice provides guidance on promoting good physical health. See, for example paragraphs 24.57- 24.62.

Section	Types of treatments	For
Section 58	Treatments specified in regulations (none at the time of publication) Medication (not otherwise subject to special rules) after three months of medication first being administered except medication administered as part of electro-convulsive therapy (ECT)	Detained patients as described in figure 68
Section 58A	ECT Medication administered as part of ECT Other treatments specified in regulations (none at the time of publication)	Detained patients as described in figure 68 All other children and young people under 18

Approved clinician or person in charge of the treatment

23.9 Part 4 refers in several places to the approved clinician, or to the person, in charge of the treatment. That means the clinician in charge of the particular treatment in question for the patient.

23.10 The clinician in charge of treatment must be an approved clinician, if the treatment is being given:

- without the patient's consent
- with the patient's consent, but on the basis of a certificate issued under section 58 or in relation to a patient over 18 a certificate issued under 58A by that clinician – see paragraphs 23.31 and 23.43, or
- pending compliance with section 58 and with the consent of a CTO patient who has been recalled to hospital, in order to avoid serious suffering – see paragraph 24.42.

23.11 Where a patient has a responsible clinician in overall charge of their case, the responsible clinician need not be in charge of any particular form of treatment. There may be different clinicians in charge of different forms of treatment.

Second opinion appointed doctors [sections 57, 58, 58A and 119(2)]

23.12 In this chapter, a 'second opinion appointed doctor' (SOAD) means a registered medical practitioner (a doctor) appointed by the Care Quality Commission (CQC). SOADs provide an independent medical view on whether it is appropriate for certain treatments to be given to individual patients. They can be members of the CQC itself, but do not have to be.

23.13 In order to carry out their functions under part 4 of the Act, SOADs may:

- visit, interview and examine any detained patient, in private, in any hospital in which patients may be detained under the Act, and
- require the production of and inspect any records relating to the treatment of the patient in that hospital.

Other people appointed by CQC to provide an independent opinion on a patient's capacity to consent to treatment under section 57 (see paragraph 23.16 onward) have the same power to visit and interview (but not examine) patients and to inspect records. Anyone who obstructed access to patients or their records without reasonable cause would be guilty of the offence of obstruction under section 129 of the Act (see chapter 33)

23.14 The approved clinician, or other person, in charge of the treatment in question cannot also act as the patient's SOAD, nor can the patient's responsible clinician, if they have one.

The meaning of 'appropriate' [section 64(3)]

23.15 In several cases, SOADs must decide if it is appropriate for a particular treatment to be given to a patient. This means they must decide if the treatment is 'appropriate' in the patient's case taking into account the nature and degree of the mental disorder from which the patient is suffering and all other circumstances of the case. (See also Code of Practice paragraphs 24.6-24.7.)

Medical treatment of detained patients without consent [section 63]

23.16 Unless the special rules in sections 57, 58 or 58A apply, detained patients may be given medical treatment for the mental disorder from which they are suffering without their consent, provided the treatment is given by or under the direction of the approved clinician in charge of the treatment in question, who need not be the patient's responsible clinician.

Treatment requiring consent and second opinion [section 57 and regulation 27]

23.17 Section 57 applies to any surgical operation for destroying brain tissue or the functioning of brain tissue. In other words, neurosurgery for mental disorder, sometimes called 'psychosurgery'.

23.18 It is applies to any other forms of treatment set out in regulations. At the time of publication, the only treatment included in regulations is surgical implantation of hormones for the purpose of reducing male sex drive.

23.19 This Reference Guide refers to treatments to which section 57 applies as 'section 57 treatments'.

23.20 No-one, whether or not a detained patient, may be given a section 57 treatment for mental disorder unless all three of the following requirements are met:

- they consent to it
- a SOAD and two other people appointed by CQC have certified in writing that the patient is capable of understanding the nature, purpose and likely effects of the treatment in question and has consented to it, and
- the SOAD also certifies in writing that it is appropriate for the treatment to be given to the patient (see paragraph 23.14).

23.21 Before deciding whether to certify that the treatment is appropriate, the SOAD must consult a nurse and one other person who have both been professionally concerned with the patient's treatment. The second person consulted must not be either a doctor or a nurse. In practice, the second person will typically be a psychologist, social worker, occupational or other therapist. Consultation with these two professionals must be in addition to any consultation with the person in charge of the proposed treatment, or the patient's responsible clinician, if they have one.

23.22 Certificates authorising section 57 treatment must be given using form T1 (the equivalent Welsh form will have been used if the patient was a Welsh patient at the time). The effect of section 59 is that a certificate may either relate to a one-off administration of a section 57 treatment (or treatments), or to a plan under which the patient would be given section 57 treatments on more than one occasion. The certificate may limit treatment under a plan to only a specific period, after which a new certificate would be needed if further treatment was required.

23.23 If the patient subsequently withdraws consent to a treatment specified in the certificate, section 60 means the certificate no longer authorises that treatment. The same applies if the patient ceases to be capable of understanding the nature, purpose and likely effect of a treatment, in other words, where patients no longer have the capacity to decide for themselves whether to go ahead or continue with the treatment.

23.24 Section 64(1A) means that the clinician in charge of a section 57 treatment does not have to be an approved clinician.

Treatment requiring consent or second opinion [section 58 and 62A(2) and regulation 27]

23.25 Unlike section 57, section 58 applies only to detained patients (as described in figure 68).

23.26 The treatments to which section 58 applies ('section 58 treatments') are:

- treatments specified in regulations under section 58(1)(a) – none at the time of publication, and
- medication for mental disorder (unless included in the first category, or a

section 57 or 58A treatment) if three months or more have elapsed since medication was first given to the patient during an unbroken period of compulsion ('medication after three months').

23.27 An unbroken period of compulsion means a period during which the patient has been continuously been a detained patient (as defined above) or a CTO patient.

23.28 For example, the period is not broken because patients move directly from detention under section 2 to detention under section 3. Nor is it broken where patients become CTO patients, then have their CTO revoked and so became detained patients again, nor by a withdrawal of consent by the patient to the treatment.

23.29 The period would be broken if the patient had at any time been discharged from detention without becoming a CTO patient, if the patient is placed on guardianship or, in the case of restricted patients, if the patient had at any point been conditionally discharged.

23.30 The three month period runs from the first administration of any medication for mental disorder, not only the medication in question. It does not matter whether that medication was given with the patient's consent or by using the powers in the Act to give treatment without consent. The three month period does not run from the date of the start of patient's detention (and, by definition, cannot start before the patient was first detained).

23.31 At the time of publication, no treatments are specified in regulations, so only medication after three months is covered by section 58. If, in due course, any type of medication were to be specified in regulations, section 58 would apply to that type of medication at all times. There would be no exception for the first three month period. Medication specifically for the purposes of ECT is covered by section 58A, not section 58.

23.32 A detained patient may not be given a section 58 treatment unless one of the three sets of conditions set out in figure 70 is met.

Figure 70: Conditions for giving treatment under section 58

Section 58 treatment may be given if:	
either	the patient has consented to the treatment, and either the approved clinician in charge of it, or a SOAD, has certified that the patient is capable of understanding the nature, purpose and likely effects of the treatment and has consented to it

or	a SOAD has certified in writing that • the patient is capable of understanding the nature, purpose and likely effects of the treatment, but has not consented to it, and • it is appropriate for the treatment to be given
or	a SOAD has certified in writing that: • the patient is not capable of understanding the nature, purpose and likely effects of the treatment, and • it is appropriate for the treatment to be given

23.33 The effect is that a section 58 treatment may not be given to a patient who cannot, or will not, consent to it, unless it is approved by a SOAD.

23.34 As with section 57, before deciding whether to certify that treatment is appropriate, the SOAD must consult a nurse and one other person (not a nurse or doctor), who have both been professionally concerned with the patient's treatment. Again, this must be in addition to any consultation with the approved clinician in charge of the proposed treatment, or the patient's responsible clinician, if different.

23.35 Like a section 57 certificate, a certificate under section 58 may relate to more than one type of treatment and may authorise both one-off administration or a course of treatment, either on a open-ended basis, or only for a specific period.

23.36 The clinician in charge of a section 58 treatment must be an approved clinician, unless the treatment is being given with the patient's consent and on the basis of section 58 certificate issued by a SOAD. It is section 61, rather than section 58 itself, which says that the clinician in charge of section 58 treatment without the patient's consent must be an approved clinician.

23.37 A section 58 certificate ceases to apply to a treatment if the premise on which it was given no longer applies. In other words:

- a certificate given on the basis that the patient consents no longer applies to any treatment to which the patient withdraws consent, or if the patient loses the capacity to consent to it
- a treatment approved by a SOAD on the basis that a patient cannot consent to it, ceases to be approved if the patient gains (or regains) the capacity to consent to it, or
- a treatment approved by a SOAD on the basis that the patient is refusing to consent to it, ceases to be approved if the patient loses the capacity to consent to it, and therefore refuse it.

23.38 The certificate could continue to apply to any other treatments, eg if the patient has only withdrawn consent to one of the types of treatment specified in the certificate.

23.39 The combined effect of sections 60 and 62(3) is that in the first two cases described in paragraph 23.36 treatment, or a course of treatment, that has already been started may be continued pending re-compliance with section 58, if the approved clinician in charge of the treatment considers that discontinuing it would cause serious suffering to the patient. In other words, it may be continued for as long as it takes to issue or obtain a new certificate, or for it to be decided that a new certificate should not be issued.

23.40 Certificates by approved clinicians or SOADs saying that patients have consented to section 58 treatment are to be given on form T2. SOAD certificates saying that section 58 treatment is appropriate even though the patient either cannot or will not consent are to be given on form T3. The equivalent Welsh form will have been used by a SOAD if the patient was detained in Wales at the time the certificate was originally given.

Treatment requiring consent and/or a second opinion [section 58A and regulation 27]

23.41 Section 58A applies to detained patients (as described in figure 70) and to all other patients aged under 18 (whether or not they are detained).

23.42 The treatments to which section 58A applies ('section 58A treatments') are:

- electro-convulsive therapy (ECT), and
- treatments specified in regulations under section 58A(1)(b).

23.43 At the time of publication, the only treatments specified in regulations are medication administered as part of ECT.

23.44 A detained patient aged 18 or over may only be given a section 58A treatment if one of the two sets of conditions set out in figure 71 is met.

Figure 71: Conditions for giving treatment under section 58A to detained patients aged 18 or over

Section 58A treatment may be given to a detained patient aged 18 or over if:	
either	the patient has consented to the treatment, and the approved clinician in charge of it, or a SOAD, has certified that the patient is capable of understanding the nature, purpose and likely effects of the treatment and has consented to it
or	a SOAD has certified in writing that: • the patient is not capable of understanding the nature,

	purpose and likely effects of the treatment, but • it is appropriate for the treatment to be given, and • giving the treatment would not conflict with an advance decision or a decision made by a donee or deputy or by the Court of Protection in accordance with the Mental Capacity Act 2005 (MCA)[101]

23.45 The effect is that section 58A cannot be used to treat patients who have the capacity to consent to treatment, but who have not done so.

23.46 In the conditions described above, and in the figure below, an advance decision means an advance decision by the patient to refuse the treatment in question, which the SOAD is satisfied is valid and applicable to the treatment, as those terms are defined in sections 24 to 26 of the MCA. In other words, an advance decision to refuse treatment which a clinician would have to respect in any other circumstances.

23.47 A donee (more often termed an 'attorney') means a donee of a lasting power of attorney (as defined by section 9 of the MCA) created by the patient. A deputy means a deputy appointed for the patient by the Court of Protection under section 16 of the MCA. In both cases a decision means a decision which that person takes on behalf of the patient within the scope of their authority and in accordance with the MCA. In other words, a decision which would be effective in any other circumstances.

23.48 Patients aged under 18 may not be given a section 58A treatment unless one of the two sets of conditions set out in figure 72 is met.

Figure 72: Conditions for giving treatment under section 58A to patients aged under 18

Section 58A treatment may be given to a patient under 18 if:	
either	the child or young person has consented to the treatment, and a SOAD has certified that: • the child or young person is capable of understanding the nature, purpose and likely effects of the treatment and has consented to it, and • it is appropriate for the treatment to be given.
or	a SOAD has certified in writing that: • the child or young person is not capable of understanding the nature, purpose and likely effects of the treatment, but

[101] Mental Capacity Act 2005. http://www.legislation.gov.uk/ukpga/2005/9/contents

	• it is appropriate for the treatment to be given, and • (if the patient is 16 or 17 years old) giving the treatment would not conflict with decision made by a deputy or by the Court of Protection in accordance with the MCA.

23.49 In other words, no child or young person under 18 may be given a section 58A treatment for mental disorder unless it is approved by a SOAD.

23.50 If the second set of conditions applies and the child or young person is a detained patient, no further legal authority is needed to give the treatment. If the child or young person is not a detained patient, then as well as the certificate, it is still necessary to have the normal legal authority to treat the patient which would be required if section 58A did not exist. Depending on the circumstances, that might, eg come from a court order, or, in the case of a young person aged 16 or 17, the provisions of the MCA.

23.51 Before deciding to give a certificate in the case of a patient, of any age, who is not capable of understanding the nature, purpose or likely effects of the proposed treatment, the SOAD must consult a nurse and one other person, not a nurse or doctor, who have both been professionally concerned with the patient's treatment. This must be in addition to any consultation with the approved clinician, or other person, in charge of the proposed treatment, or with the patient's responsible clinician, if they have one.

23.52 Like other certificates under part 4, certificates under section 58A may relate to more than one type of treatment and may authorise both one-off administration or a course of treatment, either on a open-ended basis, or only for a specific period.

23.53 The combined effect of section 58A itself and sections 61 and 64(1B) is that the clinician in charge of a section 58A treatment must be an approved clinician, unless the treatment is being given:

- to a child or young person under 18 who is not a detained patient, or
- in any other case, with the patient's consent and on the basis of section 58A certificate issued by a SOAD.

23.54 Like a certificate under section 58, a section 58A certificate ceases to apply to a treatment if the premise on which it was given no longer applies (see paragraph 23.36). If it has ceased to apply because a patient who had consented has now lost capacity to consent, or a patient who lacked capacity to consent has now gained it, the effect of sections 60 and 62(3) is that the treatment in question may be continued if the clinician in charge of the treatment considers that discontinuing it would cause serious suffering to the patient. Because treatment may only be continued 'pending compliance with section 58A', this does not allow treatment to be continued against the wishes of a patient who has the capacity to refuse it.

23.55 A new section 58A certificate is not required just because a young person reaches the age of 18.

23.56 Certificates by approved clinicians or SOADs saying that patients aged 18 or over have consented to section 58A treatment are to be given on form T4. A SOAD certificate saying that section 58A treatment is appropriate for a patient aged under 18 who has consented is to be given on form T5. A SOAD certificate saying that section 58A treatment is appropriate even though the patient (of any age) either cannot or will not consent is to be given on form T6. The equivalent Welsh form will have been used by a SOAD if the patient was a Welsh patient at the time the certificate was originally given.

Cases of urgency where sections 57, 58 and 58A do not apply – immediately necessary treatment [section 62]

23.57 Sections 57 and 58 do not apply if the treatment in question is:

a) immediately necessary to save the patient's life
b) a treatment which is not irreversible, but which is immediately necessary to prevent a serious deterioration of the patient's condition
c) a treatment which is not irreversible or hazardous, but which is immediately necessary to alleviate serious suffering by the patient, or
d) treatment which is not irreversible or hazardous, but which is immediately necessary to prevent the patient from behaving violently or being a danger to himself or to others and represents the minimum interference necessary to do so.

23.58 Section 58A does not apply to ECT if the ECT falls with a) or b) in paragraph 23.57 above. Regulations about other section 58A treatments can say which of the categories of immediately necessity above apply in each case. At time of publication only categories a) and b) apply.

23.59 A treatment is irreversible if it has irreversible physical or psychological consequences which are unfavourable to the patient. A treatment is not irreversible merely because it has irreversible consequences which are of benefit to the patient. A treatment is hazardous if it entails 'significant physical hazard to the patient'.

23.60 The fact that sections 57, 58 or 58A are disapplied does not mean that the treatment can automatically be given. All it means is that the particular requirements of those sections do not apply. There would still need to be a lawful basis on which to give the treatment in question.

23.61 For detained patients, the required authority might be found in section 63, as described in paragraph 23.15, provided the treatment is given by or under the direction of an approved clinician. Otherwise, the treatment could only be given with the patient's consent, or where, under the MCA or any other law, treatment is given in the patient's best interests in the absence of the patient's consent.

Disapplication of sections 58 and 58A in respect of CTO patients recalled to hospital [section 62A]

23.62 In certain circumstances, sections 58 and 58A do not apply to CTO patients who have been recalled to hospital, including those patients whose CTOs are then revoked. Typically, this is where the treatment in question has already been certified as appropriate by a SOAD in a 'part 4A certificate', although that is not the only case), (see chapter 29).

Reporting to CQC on treatments approved by SOADs [section 61]

23.63 Where a SOAD has certified that a treatment is appropriate and that treatment has, in fact, been given to the patient, reports on the treatment and the patient's condition must be to be sent to CQC. This does not apply to certificates given by SOADs on forms T2 or T4, or the Welsh equivalents, because in those cases the SOAD is only certifying the patient's consent, not the appropriateness of the treatment.

23.64 Reports must be submitted to CQC whenever CQC requests. For detained patients, or CTO patients who were recalled to hospital and detained there at the time of the treatment, they must automatically be made:

- on the next occasion on which the patient's responsible clinician sends a report to the hospital managers under section 20 in order to renew detention (see paragraphs 25.29 to 29.34), section 20A to extend a CTO (see paragraphs 26.72 to 26.79), or section 21B to confirm the detention or CTO of a patient who had been absent without leave for more than 28 days (see paragraphs 25.42 to 25.49 and 26.85 to 226.90 respectively), or
- for restricted patients, at the end of six months starting with the day of the patient's hospital order, hospital direction or transfer direction, or (for treatment after those first six months) on the next occasion that the responsible clinician makes a report on the patient to the Secretary of State for Justice (see paragraph 25.59).

23.65 The reports must be made by the approved clinician in charge of the treatment in question. In some cases, this may mean that more than one person may have to report on the same patient at the same time.

23.66 For section 57 treatments and section 58A treatments for patients aged under 18 who are not detained patients, section 64 says that 'approved clinician in charge of the treatment' means the person in charge of the treatment in question, whether or not that person is an approved clinician.

CQC's power to withdraw certificates [section 61(3) and 62(3)]

23.67 Under section 61(3), CQC may at any time notify the person in charge of a particular treatment that a SOAD certificate, other than one merely confirming a patient's consent, will no longer apply to that treatment from a specified date. The certificate may continue to apply to other types of treatments.

23.68 If so, the treatment must be stopped unless or until a new certificate is obtained, or a certificate is no longer needed because, for example, the patient is now consenting. As result of section 62(3) a treatment or a course of treatment which is already in progress may continue if the clinician in charge of it considers that discontinuing it would cause serious suffering to the patient, pending (re-)compliance with section 57, 58 or 58A, as applicable. For detained patients, the person in charge of the treatment must be an approved clinician, unless it is a section 57 treatment.

Summary of the requirements of sections 57, 58 and 58A

23.69 Figure 73 gives a summary of the requirements of sections 57, 58 and 58A.

Figure 73: Summary of requirements of sections 57, 58 and 58A

Section	Detained patient who can consent	Detained patient who cannot consent	Other patient	Section does not apply if treatment is
57	Consent and second opinions	Not permitted	Consent and second opinions	Immediately necessary under section 62 in the view of the clinician in charge
58	Consent or second opinion	Second opinion		Immediately necessary under section 62 in the view of the approved clinician in charge, or authorised by section 62A instead (recalled CTO patients only)
58A	Consent (and, if under 18, second opinion)	No contrary advance decision or decision of attorney, deputy or Court of Protection and second opinion.	Under 18s only: second opinion (in addition to normal authority to treat)	Immediately necessary under section 62 in the view of the approved clinician in charge[102] but only to save patient's life or prevent serious deterioration[103] Authorised by section 62A instead (recalled CTO patients only)

These requirements and decisions are represented as figures 94, 95 and 96 in Annex D together with a written explanation of each figure.

[102] The clinician in charge does not need to be an approved clinician if the patient is under 18 and neither detained nor a CTO patient.

[103] What counts as 'immediately necessary' under section 62 may be different for any further forms of treatment added to section 58A by regulations in due course.

24: Medical treatment of CTO patients (part 4a)

Introduction

24.1 This chapter describes the provisions of part 4A of the Act which apply to patients on a community treatment order (CTO), except when they have been recalled to hospital. It also describes the special provisions in part 4 which apply to CTO patients when they have been recalled to hospital.

Definitions

24.2 Definitions of 'medical treatment', 'approved clinician in charge of the patient's treatment', ''second opinion appointed doctor' (SOAD), 'appropriate', 'donee' (or 'attorney'), 'deputy', 'section 57 treatment', 'section 58 treatment' and 'section 58A treatment' in chapter 23 also apply in this chapter.

Key requirements of part 4A [sections 64A and 64B]

24.3 Medical treatment for mental disorder may not be given, by anyone, in any circumstances, to CTO patients who have not been recalled to hospital, unless the requirements of part 4A of the Act are met. The only exception is treatment given in accordance with section 57, (see paragraph 23.17 onwards).

24.4 The requirements of part 4A are of two types – authority and certification:

- in all cases, the person giving the treatment must have the authority to do so
- in most cases, if the treatment is a section 58 or 58A type treatment, at present, medication and electro-convulsive therapy (ECT), the certificate requirement must also be met.

24.5 A treatment is a 'section 58 type treatment' if it would be a section 58 treatment if the patient were detained (see paragraphs 23.25 – 23.40). Likewise, a 'section 58A type treatment' is a treatment to which would be a section 58A treatment if the patient were detained (see paragraphs 23.40 – 23.56).

Authority to treat – patients aged 16 or over [section 64C(2), 64D, 64G, 64J and 64K and regulation 28]

24.6 Whether or not the certificate requirement also applies, there must always be authority to give the treatment.

24.7 If the patient has the capacity to consent to the treatment in question, the patient's own consent provides the authority for giving it.

24.8 Patients aged 16 or over have capacity to consent unless they lack capacity to make the decision, as defined in the Mental Capacity Act 2005 (MCA).

24.9 If someone else is empowered under the MCA to consent on the patient's behalf when the patient lacks capacity to consent themselves, then that other person's consent to the treatment would provide the necessary authority. That other person could be an attorney (donee), a deputy or the Court of Protection itself, (see also Code of Practice chapter 7).

24.10 In any other case, there will only be authority to give treatment to a CTO patient aged 16 or over if the following conditions are met:

- first, the person giving the treatment has taken reasonable steps to establish whether the patient does or does not have capacity to consent to it
- second, having taken those steps, the person giving the treatment reasonably believes, when giving the treatment, that the patient lacks capacity to consent to it
- third, either the person giving the treatment has no reason to believe that the patient objects to the treatment, or the person giving the treatment does have reason to believe that the patient objects, but it is not necessary to use any force against the patient in order to give the treatment
- fourth, the person giving the treatment is either the approved clinician who is in charge of the treatment in question, or someone acting under that approved clinician's direction
- fifth, giving the treatment does not conflict with an advance decision made by the patient which the person giving the treatment is satisfied is both valid and applicable to the treatment in question, and
- sixth, giving the treatment does not conflict with a decision lawfully made by an attorney, a deputy or the Court of Protection.

24.11 In deciding whether a patient objects to treatment, the person concerned must consider all the reasonably ascertainable evidence. This includes what can be ascertained about the patient's behaviour, wishes, feelings, views, beliefs and values, both past and present. Evidence from the past should only be considered where it remains appropriate to do so. In other words, it should not be considered where it is no longer relevant because, for example, it is undisputed that the patient's views or beliefs have since changed.

24.12 The third, fourth, fifth and sixth conditions above do not apply if the treatment is immediately necessary and:

- either it is not necessary to use force against the patient, or

- the treatment needs to be given in order to prevent harm to the patient and the force used is a proportionate response to the likelihood of the patient suffering harm and the seriousness of that harm.

24.13 In addition, a certificate is not required for any form of treatment if it is:

- immediately necessary to save the patient's life
- a treatment which is not irreversible, but which is immediately necessary to prevent a serious deterioration of the patient's condition
- a treatment which is not irreversible or hazardous, but which is immediately necessary to alleviate serious suffering by the patient, or
- treatment which is not irreversible or hazardous, but which is immediately necessary to prevent the patient from behaving violently or being a danger to himself or to others and represents the minimum interference necessary to do so.

If the treatment is ECT, only the first or the second categories apply.

24.14 In summary, the effect of this is that:

- unless the person giving the treatment reasonably believes that the patient lacks capacity to consent, they cannot treat the patient unless the patient consents. If the patient does not consent, the treatment cannot be given unless the patient is recalled to hospital
- if the person giving the treatment reasonably believes that the patient lacks capacity to consent, then treatment can be given, but only if the strict criteria set out above are met. Amongst other things, this means that, except in an emergency, physical force cannot be used in order to give the treatment against the patient's objections (unless the patient's attorney or deputy, or the Court of Protection, has consented to it on their behalf), and
- where patients have an attorney or deputy who can consent to the treatment on their behalf, that person's lawful consent provides authority to give the treatment. Conversely, except in emergencies, treatment cannot be given if it goes against a lawful decision of such an attorney or deputy

Similarly, treatment can be given if it is authorised by a decision of the Court of Protection and, except in emergencies, it cannot be given if it goes against a decision of the Court, and except in emergencies, treatment cannot be given contrary to a valid and applicable advance decision by the patient to refuse the treatment.

24.15 By definition, decisions of attorneys, deputies and the Court of Protection will only be relevant where patients lack capacity to take the relevant decisions for themselves.

Authority to treat – patients under 16 [section 64E(6), 64F, 64G 64J and 64K)]

24.16 For children and young people under 18 the issues of competence and capacity are different. For details of competence for under 16 year olds and capacity of 16 and 17 year olds, see Code of Practice paragraphs 19.24 – 19.37.

24.17 If the child has the competence to consent to the treatment in question, the patient's own consent provides the necessary authority for giving it.

24.18 In any other case, there will only be authority to give the treatment if the following conditions are met:

- first, the person giving the treatment has taken reasonable steps to establish whether the child is or is not competent to consent to it
- second, having taken those steps, the person giving the treatment reasonably believes that the child is not competent to consent
- third, either the person giving the treatment has no reason to believe that the patient objects to the treatment, or the person giving the treatment does have reason to believe that the patient objects, but it is not necessary to use any force against the patient in order to give the treatment, and
- fourth, the person giving the treatment must either be the approved clinician who is in charge of the treatment in question, or someone acting under that approved clinician's direction.

24.19 As with older patients, the third and fourth conditions above do not apply if:

- the treatment is immediately necessary, and
- if it is necessary to use force against the patient, the treatment needs to be given in order to prevent harm to the patient and the use of such force is a proportionate response to the likelihood of the patient suffering harm and the seriousness of that harm.

24.20 The term 'immediately necessary' has the same meaning as for older patients (see paragraph 24.13 above), and clinicians must take the same factors into account in deciding whether a child is objecting (see paragraph 24.11).

24.21 A parent, or another person with parental responsibility, cannot consent to treatment for mental disorder on behalf of a child or young person who is a CTO patient. Nor can they refuse such treatment on such a patient's behalf.

Certificate requirement – CTO patients of any age [sections 64B, 64C, 64E and 64H and regulation 28]

24.22 If the treatment in question is a section 58 or 58A type treatment, then as well as there being authority to give the treatment, it is normally necessary for the treatment in question to have been approved by a 'part 4A certificate'. The exceptions to this rule are set out below.

24.23 A part 4A certificate is a certificate given by a SOAD certifying that it is appropriate for one or more forms of section 58 or section 58A type treatments to be given to a CTO patient.

24.24 The SOAD must specify on the certificate the forms of treatment to which it applies and any conditions to which the approval of any or all of those forms of treatment is subject. The SOAD may also specify which (if any) of the treatments approved on the certificate may be given to the patient on recall to hospital without the need for a separate certificate under part 4 of the Act (see paragraph 24.33 onward).

24.25 Before issuing the certificate, the SOAD must consult two other people who have been professionally concerned with the patient's medical treatment. Only one of those two people may be a doctor and neither may be the patient's responsible clinician or the approved clinician in charge of any of the treatments that are to be specified on the certificate.

24.26 As a result, the certificate would not authorise any treatment if, at the time it is proposed to give the treatment, the person who is now the patient's responsible clinician or the approved clinician in charge of the treatment in question happens to be one of the two people who were originally consulted by the SOAD before giving the certificate.

24.27 Part 4A certificates are to be given by SOADs using form CTO11 (but a patient in England may have a part 4A certificate on the equivalent Welsh form, if it was originally given in accordance with the Welsh regulations instead). Where a community patient has capacity to consent, or if under 16 is competent to consent, to treatment and has done so, then form CTO12 should be completed. For these purposes, SOADs may at any reasonable time visit and interview CTO patients in a hospital, another establishment as defined in the Care Standards Act 2000 (eg a care home or a children's home) or any other place to which they are given access. They may also require the production of and inspect records relating to the patient's treatment there. Anyone who obstructed their access to patients or their records without reasonable cause would be guilty of the offence of obstruction under section 129 of the Act (see chapter 34).

Exceptions to the certification requirement [sections 64B(3), 64C(4) to (9), 64E(3) to (5) and 64G]

24.28 A certificate is not required for any medication which is a section 58 type treatment:

- during the period of one month starting with the day on which the patient became (or last became) a CTO patient, or

- if less than three months has passed since the patient was first administered medication during an unbroken period of detention and CTO, or an unbroken succession of periods of detention and CTO.

24.29 In other words, as well as the equivalent of the three month rule in section 58 (see paragraphs 23.26 to 23.30), there is also no requirement for a certificate for section 58 type treatment during the first month of any period of a CTO. But both of these exceptions only apply to medication, and neither applies to medication used as part of ECT because it is a section 58A treatment. Nor would these exceptions apply to any type of medication that was specified in regulations under section 58(1)(a) of the Act in due course. At the time of publication, no such regulations had been made.

24.30 In addition, a certificate is not required for any form of treatment if it is:

- immediately necessary to save the patient's life, or
- a treatment which is not irreversible, but which is immediately necessary to prevent a serious deterioration of the patient's condition,

or (unless it is a section 58A treatment)

- a treatment which is not irreversible or hazardous, but which is immediately necessary to alleviate serious suffering by the patient a treatment which is not irreversible or hazardous, but which is immediately necessary to prevent the patient from behaving violently or being a danger to himself or to others, and represents the minimum interference necessary to do so. (See paragraph 23.57 for further explanation).

24.31 But even if a certificate is not necessary, for whichever reason, there must still be authority to give the treatment, as described earlier in this chapter.

CTO patients recalled to hospital [section 62A]

24.32 Part 4A does not apply to the treatment of CTO patients who have been recalled to hospital, unless or until they are released from the resulting detention in hospital (see paragraph 8.71 to 8.85).

24.33 Part 4 applies to such patients instead, but with four differences.

24.34 First, treatment which would otherwise require a certificate under section 58 or 58A can be given without such a certificate if it is expressly approved instead by the patient's part 4A certificate (if the patient has one).

24.35 For these purposes, a treatment is only expressly approved by a part 4A certificate if the SOAD who gave the certificate explicitly states in it that the treatment in question may be given to a patient who has been recalled.

24.36 Such approval may be subject to conditions which must be followed. The conditions could be different from those which apply when the patient has not been recalled. A SOAD might, for example, specify that treatment on recall may only be given if a patient who has the capacity to consent to it does so.

24.37 A part 4A certificate cannot authorise treatment under section 58A for which there would be no authority under part 4A itself, if the patient had not been recalled. In particular, it cannot authorise treatment without the consent of a person who has the capacity (or, in the case of a patient under 16, the competence) to consent to the ECT (or other treatment) in question. Nor can it authorise section 58A treatment contrary to a valid and applicable advance decision, or the decision of an attorney, deputy or the Court of Protection.

24.38 Second, medication which would otherwise require a certificate under section 58 can be given without such a certificate if the certificate requirement in part 4A would not yet apply to the treatment because less than one month has passed since the making of the patient's CTO (see paragraph 24.30).

24.39 In other words, no certificate is required for the administration of most medication to a patient who has been a CTO patient for less than a month.

24.40 Third, treatment that was already in progress on the basis of a part 4A certificate before the patient was recalled can be continued temporarily without a certificate, even if the part 4A certificate does not expressly approve it, if the approved clinician in charge of the treatment in question considers that withdrawing the treatment would cause serious suffering to the patient. This also applies if treatment was already being continued after the withdrawal of a part 4A certificate – see paragraph 24.46.

24.41 This exception only applies pending compliance with section 58 or 58A. In other words, it applies only for the time it takes to obtain the certificate that would normally be required, or for a SOAD to decide that it is not appropriate to issue such a certificate.

24.42 These exemptions to the requirements for certificates under part 4 also apply to patients whose CTOs have been revoked. For section 58 type treatments, the first and second exemptions, described in paragraphs 24.35 and 24.39 respectively, apply only pending compliance with section 58 itself.

24.43 Figure 74 summarises the circumstances in which the requirement to have a certificate under sections 58 or 58A of part 4 does not apply to CTO patients recalled to hospital, or whose CTOs have been revoked.

Figure 74: Summary of exemptions from part 4 certificate requirements for CTO and former CTO patients

A section 58 or 58A certificate is not required for a CTO patient who has been recalled to hospital, or for a patient whose CTO has just been revoked, if:	
Medication which needs a certificate after 3 months under section 58	***ECT and other section 58 and 58A treatments***
It is specifically authorised in the part 4A certificate for use on recall;† or	It is specifically authorised in the part 4A certificate for use on recall;[104] or
Before the patient was recalled, it was properly being provided on the basis of a part 4A certificate (including one which had been withdrawn) and is only being continued to avoid serious suffering to the patient and pending a new certificate, or	Before the patient was recalled, it was properly being provided on the basis of a part 4A certificate (including one which had been withdrawn) and is only being continued to avoid serious suffering to the patient and pending a new certificate, or
It is permitted under part 4 anyway without a certificate because it is immediately necessary, or	It is permitted under part 4 anyway without a certificate because it is immediately necessary.
It is less than one month since the patient became a CTO patient.	

CTO patients in hospital without having been recalled

24.44 Part 4A continues to apply to CTO patients who are in hospital, either voluntarily or when complying with a condition of their CTOs without having been recalled.

Withdrawal of part 4A certificates [section 64H]

24.45 Care Quality Commission (CQC) may at any time notify the person in charge of the treatment in question that a part 4A certificate will cease to apply from a certain date.

24.46 Once the certificate ceases to apply, it can no longer be used to comply with whatever certificate requirement needs to be met. Treatment which cannot be given without a certificate must either be stopped completely, or suspended while a new certificate is sought.

[104] Once the patient's CTO is revoked, these exemptions only apply to section 58 type treatments pending compliance with section 58.

24.47 Pending compliance with the relevant requirement for a certificate, treatment may be continued temporarily if the person in charge of the treatment in question considers that withdrawing the treatment would cause serious suffering to the patient. This continues to apply even if the patient is recalled to hospital.

Reports to CQC on treatment given in accordance with a part 4A certificate [section 64H(4) and 61(1)]

24.48 Where treatment has been given on the basis of a part 4A certificate, the person in charge of the treatment must send CQC a report under section 64H on the treatment and the patient's condition when requested to do so by CQC.

24.49 In addition, a report must be given automatically to CQC under section 61 if treatment is given on the basis of a part A certificate to a CTO patient who has been recalled to hospital, including one whose CTO is then revoked, in lieu of a SOAD certificate under section 58 or 58A (see paragraphs 24.32 to 24.43). This will only apply to treatment to which the patient either did not, or could not consent.

24.50 In such cases, a report must be submitted by the approved clinician in charge of the treatment at the same time it would have to be given if the treatment had, in fact, been given on the basis of section 58 or 58A SOAD certificate (see paragraphs 23.63 – 23.65). This means the approved clinician must make a report to CQC on the next occasion that the responsible clinician submits a report under section 20 to renew the patient's detention, under section 20A to extend the patient's CTO, or under section 21B to confirm the patient's detention or CTO after absence without leave for more than 28 days.

Leaving hospital

Patients who leave hospital may be fully discharged or allowed on leave temporarily under section 17 of the Act, placed under guardianship or be discharged onto a community treatment order (CTO). Patients on section 17 leave remain liable to be detained under the Act and patients subject to a CTO may be recalled to hospital for further medical treatment if necessary.

The Secretary of State for Justice may conditionally discharge a restricted patient at any time, by issuing a warrant to that effect and in certain circumstances restricted patients may be conditionally discharged by the Tribunal.

Where patients are placed under guardianship the guardian may be a local authority or a private individual.

The Act requires clinical commissioning groups and local authorities to arrange after-care for certain patients who have been detained for treatment under the Act to help their further recovery and re-integration into the community. This after-care must meet a need arising from or related to the person's mental disorder and have the purpose of reducing the risk of a deterioration of the person's mental condition.

25: Leaving hospital (planned discharge and absence without leave)

Introduction

25.1 This chapter describes the main provisions of the Act which apply to patients leaving hospital.

Leave of absence from hospital [section 17 and regulation 19]

25.2 Responsible clinicians may give part 2 and unrestricted part 3 patients leave to be absent from the hospital in which they are detained, subject to any conditions they think are necessary in the interests of the patient, or for the protection of other people. Responsible clinicians may not delegate this power to anyone else.

25.3 Leave of absence can be given either for a temporary absence, after which the patient is expected to return to hospital, or as a period of trial leave to assess the patient's suitability for discharge. It can also be given for a series of temporary absences. Leave of absence can be extended without the patient having to return to hospital.

25.4 If responsible clinicians think it is necessary in the interests of the patient or for the protection of other persons, they can direct that the patient remains in custody during leave. This is commonly termed 'escorted leave'.

25.5 Patients on escorted leave may be kept in the custody of an officer on the staff of the hospital or of any other person authorised in writing by the hospital managers (or by someone authorised by the hospital managers to give that authorisation on their behalf). If the leave was granted on condition that they stay in another hospital, then patients can also be kept in the custody of any officer on the staff of that other hospital.

25.6 Escorted leave arrangements can be used, for example, to allow detained patients to be escorted on outings, to attend other hospitals for treatment, or to have home visits on compassionate grounds.

25.7 Escorted leave to Scotland, Northern Ireland, the Channel Islands or the Isle of Man can only be granted if the law in the jurisdiction in question allows the patient to be kept in custody once there. At the time of publication, this applies only in Scotland.[105] For escorted leave from another jurisdiction to England or Wales, see paragraph 11.21.

Leave for Court Proceedings – restricted patients

25.8 Where a court directs the attendance of a patient, the Secretary of State for Justice will rarely refuse consent. Consent must still be sought and details with regard to dates, location, reasons for attendance and security measures will need to be provided. Those patients detained under section 48 of the Act will be given a general permission on transfer on the assumption that legal proceedings will inevitably need to be completed.

25.9 Secretary of State for Justice's consent is required for restricted patients attending court for legal proceedings other than criminal.

Leave for emergency medical treatment – restricted patients

25.10 Aside from routine medical appointments and/or treatment when the Secretary of State for Justice's consent is required, the responsible clinician may use their discretion if presented with an acute situation in which the restricted patient requires emergency hospital treatment. Examples of such conditions are heart attack, stroke, and penetrative wounds and burns. Emergency or urgent treatment may also be needed for non-life threatening but urgent conditions such as fractures. The Ministry of Justice should be notified as soon as practicable of the circumstances of the treatment, including arrangements to manage any risks and when the patient in returned to the secure hospital.

25.11 Leave may not be granted by responsible clinicians to patients detained under section 5, remanded under sections 35 or 36, detained in hospital as a place of safety, or subject to an interim hospital order under section 38.

25.12 Patients who are detained for treatment may be entitled to after-care provided by (or for) clinical commissioning groups (CCGs) and local authorities under section 117 of the Act while they are on leave of absence – see chapter 24.

Duty to consider community treatment order before granting longer term leave [section 17(2A) and (2B)]

25.13 Responsible clinicians may not grant longer term leave to part 2 patients or to unrestricted part 3 patients without first considering whether the patient should instead go onto a community treatment order (CTO) – see Code of Practice paragraphs xx.

---

[105] The law in Scotland gives powers to restrain or retake a patient on escorted leave from England who is in Scotland: the Mental Health (Cross-border Visits)(Scotland) Regulations 2008.SSI. 2008/181 http://www.legislation.gov.uk/ssi/2008/181 .made under section 309A of the Mental Health (Care and Treatment) (Scotland) Act 2003 apply sections 301 to 303 of that Act. http://www.legislation.gov.uk/asp/2003/13

25.14 Granting longer term leave means granting leave indefinitely or for a period of more than seven consecutive days, or extending existing leave so that in total it would last for more than seven consecutive days.

25.15 This is not relevant to restricted patients, because they cannot become CTO patients. In practice, and for the same reason, it is not relevant to patients detained for assessment under section 2.

Recall from leave [section 17(4)]

25.16 Responsible clinicians may recall patients from leave if they think it is necessary to do so in the interests of the patient's health or safety or for the protection of other persons.

25.17 A patient can only be recalled if, in the opinion of the responsible clinician, the patient's condition makes it necessary for the patient to become an in-patient again.[106] Except in an emergency, patients should not be recalled from leave of absence without up-to-date clinical evidence that they remain mentally disordered.[107]

25.18 To recall a patient, the responsible clinician must issue a notice in writing of the recall to be given to the patient or to the person, if there is one, in charge of the patient during their leave. The reasons for recall should be fully explained to the patient and a record of the explanation included in the patient's notes.

25.19 Restricted patients may also be recalled at any time by the Secretary of State for Justice. They could not be recalled by their responsible clinician in the unlikely circumstances that they had already been absent on leave for more than 12 months.

25.20 Patients cannot be recalled after they have been discharged or after the authority for their detention has expired.

Absence without leave [sections 18 and 21B and regulation 19]

25.21 Where part 2 or part 3 patients:

- are absent from hospital without having been given leave to be absent
- do not go to, or absent themselves without permission from, any place at which they are required to reside as a condition of leave, or
- fail to return from leave either at the end of a period of leave or when recalled

they are treated as absent without leave (AWOL) under the Act. The same applies to patients detained under the 'holding powers' in section 5 who go absent from the hospital.

[106] R v Hallstrom, ex p. W (No. 2); R v Gardner, ex p. L. 1986. 2 All ER 306.
[107] Kay v United Kingdom. 1998. 40 BMLR 20.

25.22 For patients AWOL from a CTO, see paragraphs 26.67 to 26.71. For patients who abscond in other circumstances, see chapter 11.

25.23 Patients who are AWOL may be taken into custody in England or Wales under section 18 and be returned or taken, as the case may be, to the hospital or place in question by the following people:

- any staff of the hospital
- any approved mental health professional (AMHP) acting on behalf of a local authority, or an approved social worker in Northern Ireland
- any police officer (or other constable), or
- any person authorised in writing by the managers of the hospital in which the person is liable to be detained or of another hospital where the patient is required to reside as a condition of leave, which includes someone authorised in writing on behalf the managers by someone authorised by the managers to do so.

For patients who go AWOL to Scotland, the Isle of Man or any of the Channel Islands, see chapter 31.

25.24 If patients do not go to, or go absent without permission from, a hospital at which they are required to reside as a condition of leave, they may also be taken into custody and returned or taken to that hospital by any staff of that hospital or any person authorised by its managers.

25.25 Patients, other than restricted patients, cannot be taken into custody under section 18 after whichever is the later date below:

- the end of their current period of detention, ignoring any extra time that would be allowed if the patient were to return or be taken into custody right at the end of that period – see paragraph 25.38, or
- if the patient is detained on the basis of an application for admission for treatment under section 3, or is a part 3 patient, the end of the six months starting on the first day of the absence without leave.

25.26 For these purposes, the fact that the responsible clinician has already made a report renewing the patient's detention (see paragraph 25.30) is irrelevant unless the renewed period of detention has already started when the patient goes absent.

25.27 There is no such time limit for restricted patients. They may be retaken for as long as they remain subject to restrictions.

Examples

Patient detained under section 5(4)

Mr A was an informal patient who was detained under section 5(4) at noon on 1 January when he tried to leave the hospital. He then went absent before the approved clinician in charge of his treatment could attend and make a report under section 5(2). He can only be retaken until 6pm the same day (six hours after his detention), ie at the end of the period for which he could have been detained under section 5(4).

Patient detained under section 5(2)

Mrs P was also an informal patient who was detained at noon on 1 January. She went absent at the same time as Mr A. But because she was detained under section 5(2), rather than 5(4), she can be retaken until noon on 4 January (72 hours after her detention).

Patient detained under section 2

Mr C was admitted to hospital at noon 1 January, on the basis of an application for assessment under section 2. He went absent later that day. He can be retaken until his detention under section 2 would normally expire at the end of 28 January (28 days from his detention date).

Patient detained under section 4

Miss B was also admitted for assessment at the same time as Mr C and also went absent. But she was admitted on the basis of an emergency application under section 4. So, unless the second medical recommendation is received in the interim, she can only be retaken until the end of 72 hours from her admission, ie noon on 4 January.

Patients detained under section 3

Mr O was already detained in hospital under section 3 when he went absent without leave in the evening of 1 January. Section 3 patients can be retaken until the end of their current period of detention, or six months starting with the day they went absent, whichever is later. Mr O's current period of detention is due to expire at the end of 7 January. Therefore, six months from when he went absent (starting that day) is later than when his current detention expires, so he can be retaken until the end of 30 June.

The responsible clinician had already made a report to renew Mr O's detention for another six months to 7 July before he went absent, but because his current period of detention had not yet expired when he went absent, that renewal is not taken into account.

Mrs Y was also detained under section 3 when she went absent at the same time as Mr O on 1 January. Unlike Mr O, her current period of detention is not due to expire until 15 October. Because that date is later than six months from when she went absent, the end of 15 October is also the latest time by which she may be retaken.

25.28 If patients are taken into custody, or come voluntarily to the place they ought to be, after being AWOL for more than 28 days, eg on or after 29 January in the examples above, their detention expires automatically at the end of the week starting with the day of their return to the relevant hospital, or other place), unless their responsible clinician renews the authority for their detention. See paragraphs 25.21 and 25.42 onward.

Expiry and renewal of authority for detention [section 20 and regulations 13 and 26]

25.29 Patients detained for treatment, rather than assessment, under part 2 and unrestricted part 3 patients may be detained initially for a maximum of six months. The authority for their detention can then be renewed for a further six months, and subsequently for a year at a time. This does not apply to restricted patients, as the authority for their detention does not have to be renewed.

> **Example**
>
> Mr K is admitted on the basis of an application for admission for treatment under section 3 on the evening of 1 January 2016. Therefore:
>
> - his initial maximum period of detention lasts until the end of 30 June 2016
> - if renewed, his second period would last until the end of 31 December 2016
> - if renewed again, his third period would last until the end of 31 December 2017, and so on.

25.30 At some point during the final two months of the first and each subsequent period of detention, responsible clinicians must examine patients in order to decide whether they meet the criteria for renewal.

25.31 The criteria for renewal are that:

- the patient is suffering from mental disorder of a nature or degree which makes it appropriate for the patient to receive medical treatment in hospital
- it is necessary for the health or safety of the patient, or for the protection of others, that the patient should receive this treatment
- such treatment cannot be provided unless the patient continues to be detained, and
- appropriate medical treatment is available for the patient.

Mental disorder and appropriate medical treatment mean the same for these purposes as they do in the criteria under which patients were initially detained.

25.32 If responsible clinicians think the criteria are met, they must make a report to that effect to the hospital managers under section 20. Responsible clinicians:

- must first consult at least one other person who has been professionally concerned with the patient's treatment, and
- may not make the report unless another person who has been professionally concerned with the patient's treatment, but who belongs to a different profession, states in writing that they agree that the renewal conditions are met.

25.33 The report, and the statement of agreement by the second professional who is from a different profession must be made using form H5 and sent to the hospital managers, who must record their receipt of it in part 3 of the form.

25.34 Unless the managers decide to discharge the patient (see paragraph 25.45 onward below), they must arrange for the patient to be told about the renewal. They must also take whatever steps are reasonably practicable to arrange for the person they think is the nearest relative to be informed, unless the patient has requested otherwise, or the patient does not have a nearest relative. They must do this as soon as practicable after the decision is made not to discharge the patient. Information given to nearest relatives must be in writing, but may be communicated by electronic means (eg email) if the nearest relative agrees.

25.35 The effect of the report is to renew the authority for detention (ie the relevant application, order or direction) for a further six months or a year (as applicable) from the date it would otherwise expire, not the date of the report itself.

Patients absent without leave as deadline for renewal report approaches [section 21 and 21A and regulation 26]

25.36 Special arrangements apply if patients are AWOL at any point during the week which ends on the day that their current period of detention is due to expire, and a renewal report has yet to be made.

25.37 If patients have not been taken into custody, or do not come voluntarily, to the hospital or place where they are required to reside before the end of the period during which they can be taken into custody under section 18 (as described in paragraph 25.23), their period of detention expires, and no renewal report can be made.

25.38 If they are taken into custody under section 18, or come voluntarily to the relevant hospital or place, during the period allowed by that section, the period of detention is treated as not expiring until the end of the week starting with the day the patient arrives back at the hospital or other place, as the case may be.

25.39 Responsible clinicians therefore have a week from the day of the patient's return to examine the patient and send the report to renew the authority for detention to the hospital managers. So, if the patient returns on Monday, the responsible clinician has until the end of the following Sunday to submit the report.

25.40 If patients are taken into custody, or come voluntarily to the relevant hospital or place, within the 28 days starting with the day they went AWOL (ie before the end of 28 January if they went absent on 1 January), the renewal report is to be made under section 20 in the normal way. Any such report would therefore have to be agreed by a second professional – see paragraph 25.32.

25.41 If patients are taken into custody, or come voluntarily to the relevant hospital or place, after more than 28 days, it is not normally necessary to make a report under section 20. That is because the patient's detention has anyway to be confirmed by a report under section 21B, and that report can also serve as a renewal report in place of a report under section 20 (see paragraph 25.42 to 25.49).

Example – return from AWOL within 28 days

Mr G and Miss Q were both detained under section 3 on 1 January. Their current period of detention is therefore due to expire at the end of 30 June.

They both went absent on 27 June before their responsible clinicians, who had left it very late, were able finally to decide whether they should make renewal reports.

Mr G is found and returned to the hospital on Friday 28 June. The deadline for making the renewal report is extended for one week from his return, to the end of Thursday 4 July. If his responsible clinician sends a renewal report on form H5 to the managers before then, Mr G's period of detention will be renewed until 31 December.

Miss Q decides to come back to the hospital herself, but not until Wednesday 24 July. The deadline in her case is therefore extended for one week from her return, to the end of Tuesday 30 July. If a report is made by then, her detention will be renewed until 31 December as well.

Confirmation of detention of patients who have been absent without leave for more than 28 days [section 21B and regulations 14 and 26]

25.42 Where part 2 patients or unrestricted part 3 patients are taken into custody, or come voluntarily to the relevant hospital or other place, after being AWOL for more than 28 days, their responsible clinician must examine them and, if appropriate, submit a report using form H6 to the hospital managers confirming that the criteria for continued detention are met. This must be done however long remains until the patient's detention next needs to be renewed.

25.43 The criteria for continued detention are the same as the criteria for renewing detention (described at paragraph 25.31).

25.44 Unless such a report is submitted to the managers, the patient's detention expires automatically at the end of the week starting with the day on which the patient arrives at the relevant hospital or place, as the case may be. So if the patient arrives on Monday, the report must be submitted by the end of the following Sunday.

25.45 Responsible clinicians must submit a report during this period, if they think that the criteria are met. But they must first consult one or more other people who have been professionally concerned with the patient's treatment and an AMHP acting on behalf of a local authority. There is no requirement in this case to obtain a statement of agreement from a second professional from a different profession.

25.46 The managers must record their receipt of the report in part 2 of the same form H6.

25.47 A report made under this procedure will renew the patient's detention if it would already have expired if the patient had not gone AWOL, or if it would expire on the day the report is submitted (see paragraph 25.50).

25.48 In addition, if the patient's detention is due to expire in the period of two months starting with the day on which the report is submitted to the managers, the responsible clinician may, but need not, indicate on the form that it is to act as any renewal report which would otherwise have to be made under section 20 during that period.

25.49 Unless the managers decide to discharge the patient, they should arrange for the patient and, where relevant, the nearest relative to be informed of any report under section 21B in the same way as if it were a report under section 20 itself (see paragraph 25.34). They must also take whatever steps are reasonably practicable to arrange for the person they think is the nearest relative to be informed, unless the patient has requested otherwise, or does not have a nearest relative.

Patients who return from absence without leave and whose detention would otherwise have expired [section 21A and 21B and regulation 26]

25.50 In some cases, the responsible clinician's report under section 20 or 21B renewing the detention of a patient who has been AWOL will be made on or after the day the old period of detention was originally due to expire. If so, that report is treated as having retrospectively renewed the detention from the end of the old period of detention in the normal way.

25.51 In the rare circumstances where the patient's detention would otherwise have expired has expired twice since they went AWOL, the responsible clinician's report under section 21B is treated as having renewed the detention on both occasions.

25.52 If a patient's detention is renewed retrospectively, either once or twice in this way, the hospital managers must take whatever steps are reasonably practicable to arrange for the patient to be told about the renewal. They must also take such steps to arrange for the person they think is the nearest relative to be informed, unless the patient has requested otherwise, or does not have a nearest relative.

25.53 The patient must be told of the retrospective renewal both orally and in writing. Information given to nearest relatives must be in writing, but may be communicated by electronic means (eg email) if the nearest relative agrees.

Patients who are imprisoned etc [section 22 read with sections 18, 21 and 21A]

25.54 Special rules apply to patients detained on the basis of an application for admission for treatment under section 3 and unrestricted part 3 patients, if they are imprisoned, remanded or otherwise detained in custody by any court in the UK while liable to be detained in hospital.

25.55 Such patients automatically cease to be liable to be detained on the basis of the relevant application, order or direction if they remain in custody for longer than six months in total. Until then, they remain formally liable to be detained in hospital, unless discharged in the interim.

25.56 If they are released during that six month period, they are treated as if they had gone AWOL from the hospital on the day of their release, except that they may be retaken only during the 28 days starting with that day.

25.57 Because they are treated as AWOL, if the authority for their detention would otherwise have expired, or is about to expire, it will not in fact expire until the end of the week starting with the day of the patient's return to hospital, provided that the patient is taken into custody or returns during the 28 day period allowed (see paragraph 25.38).

25.58 As a result, if the patient's current period of detention is otherwise due to expire, responsible clinicians will always have at least a week in which to examine the patient and submit a report renewing the patient's detention under section 20 (see paragraph 25.30 onward). Because patients cease to be liable to detention if they have not returned to hospital within the permitted 28 days, it will never be necessary to make a report confirming their detention under section 21B.

Example – return from AWOL after more than 28 days

Mrs J was also detained under section 3 on 1 January 2016 and her current period of detention is therefore due to expire at the end of six months on 30 June 2016.

Mrs J went absent on 24 June before her responsible clinician had examined her to decide whether to make a report under section 20 renewing her detention from 1 July for a further six months.

Mrs J is found some distance away and taken into custody on Sunday 9 October. She is brought back to the hospital on Monday 10 October.

Because she has been absent for more than 28 days, her responsible clinician must confirm her detention by making a report on form H6 under section 21B. Unless this is done before the end of Sunday 16 October, she will no longer be detained.

Having examined Mrs J, the responsible clinician makes the report on Tuesday 15 November, confirming that she meets the criteria for continuing detention.

Because her last period of detention expired while she was absent, this report automatically renews her detention retrospectively from 1 July 2016, which means her detention is now due to expire on 31 December 2016.

Because that is less than two months away, the responsible clinician has the option of indicating on the form H6 that it is also to serve as a report renewing Mrs J's detention again from 1 January 2017.

The responsible clinician decides to do that. Mrs J's detention is therefore renewed for one year from 1 January 2017 without the responsible clinician needing to make a separate report on form H5 under section 20.

Reports to the Secretary of State for Justice on restricted patients [section 41(6) and 45A(3)]

25.59 Responsible clinicians must examine restricted patients and send a report to the Secretary of State for Justice at intervals decided by the Secretary of State, which must not be more than one year.

25.60 Responsible clinicians should also inform the Secretary of State for Justice if a patient subject to hospital and limitation directions, or a restricted transfer direction, no longer requires treatment for mental disorder, or if no effective treatment can be given in the hospital. The Secretary of State will then consider whether the patient should be removed to prison, or equivalent (see chapters 5, 8 and 9). In the case of restricted transfer patients who were remanded in custody by a magistrates' court before being transferred ('magistrates' remand prisoners'), it is the magistrates' court that should be informed – see paragraph 20.17).

Evidence to the courts on patients remanded to hospital under section 35 or 36 or given interim hospital orders [section 35(5), 36(4) and 38(5)]

25.61 A patient remanded to hospital for report under section 35 may only be further remanded after the first 28 days if the approved clinician responsible for making the report on the patient's mental condition gives written or oral evidence that further remand is necessary for completing the assessment.

25.62 Similarly, a patient remanded for treatment under section 36 may only be further remanded if the responsible clinician gives written or oral evidence that a further remand is warranted. And a court may only renew an interim hospital order (under section 38) if the responsible clinician gives evidence that the continuation of the order is warranted.

25.63 For further information on remands to hospital and interim hospital orders, see chapters 14 and 18 respectively.

26: Community treatment orders

Introduction

26.1 This chapter describes the provisions in the Act (principally sections 17A to 17G) which deal with community treatment orders (CTOs). Certain patients can be discharged from detention by means of a CTO, while remaining liable to recall to hospital for further medical treatment if necessary.

Definitions

26.2 Patients who are subject to a CTO are described in the Act as 'community patients'. This Reference Guide refers to them as 'CTO patients' to avoid confusion with people receiving treatment in the community without being subject to the Act.

26.3 A 'part 2 CTO patient' is one who was detained on the basis of an application for admission for treatment (section 3) immediately before becoming a CTO patient.

26.4 A 'part 3 CTO patient' is one who was detained on the basis of an unrestricted hospital order, hospital direction or transfer direction immediately before becoming a CTO patient.

26.5 'Responsible clinician' means the same as it does in relation to a detained patient, namely the approved clinician in overall charge of the patient's case.

26.6 'Responsible hospital' means the hospital whose managers have responsibilities in relation to the CTO patient in question. Initially, at least, this will be the hospital in which the patient was liable to be detained immediately before becoming a CTO patient. Responsibility can subsequently be assigned to another hospital using the procedure described in paragraphs 26.126 to 26.130.

Delegation of hospital managers' functions in relation to CTO patients [sections 32(3) and 142B and regulations 3, 19 and 26]

26.7 The provisions described in this chapter include various duties on hospital managers. The meaning of hospital managers is described in paragraph 1.22.

26.8 As hospital managers are, in most cases, an organisation, they do not have to perform their functions personally. The same general rules which apply to delegation of hospital managers' functions in relation to detention also apply to CTO (see paragraphs 31.7 to 31.17).

Eligible patients [section 17A and Schedule 1]

26.9 CTOs may be made only in respect of patients who are liable to be detained in hospital for treatment on the basis of one of the orders and directions set out in figure 75. CTOs may not be made in respect of patients detained in hospital on the basis of an application for admission for assessment under section 2 or 4, nor restricted patients.

Figure 75: Patients who may become CTO patients

Patients may become CTO patients if they are detained on the basis of	Section
An application for admission for treatment	section 3
A hospital order (without a restriction order)	section 37 or 51
A hospital direction (but no longer a limitation direction)	section 45A
A transfer direction (without a restriction direction)	section 47 or 48
or If they are treated as being subject to one of the above, eg as a result of transfer from guardianship or from outside England or Wales	

Criteria for CTO [section 17A]

26.10 The criteria for making a CTO are that:

- the patient is suffering from mental disorder of a nature or degree which makes it appropriate for the patient to receive medical treatment
- it is necessary for the patient's health or safety or for the protection of other persons that the patient should receive such treatment
- subject to the patient being liable to be recalled as mentioned below, such treatment can be provided without the patient continuing to be detained in a hospital
- it is necessary that the responsible clinician should be able to exercise the power under section 17E(1) to recall the patient to hospital (see paragraphs 26.31 onward), and
- appropriate medical treatment is available for the patient.

26.11 'Mental disorder' and 'appropriate medical treatment' mean the same in relation to CTOs as they do in the criteria for detention for treatment under section 3 (see paragraphs 8.7 and 8.8). This means that 'mental disorder' does not include learning disabilities, unless the learning disability is associated with abnormally aggressive or seriously irresponsible conduct on the part of the patient concerned (see paragraphs 1.12 to 1.14).

Procedure for making a CTO [section 17A and regulation 6]

26.12 Responsible clinicians may make a CTO if they are satisfied that the relevant criteria are met.

26.13 In determining whether it is necessary that they should be able to exercise the power of recall under section 17E, the factors that responsible clinicians must consider include what risk there would be of a deterioration of the patient's condition if the patient were not detained in a hospital, for example, as a result of refusing or neglecting to receive the medical treatment required for the mental disorder. In doing so, responsible clinicians must have regard to the patient's history of mental disorder and any other relevant factors.

26.14 Before a CTO may be made, an approved mental health professional (AMHP), acting on behalf of a local authority, must agree with the responsible clinician's opinion that all the criteria are met and agree that it is appropriate for the patient to become a CTO patient.

26.15 The CTO, and the AMHP's agreement to it, must be put in writing using form CTO1. That form is then to be sent to the managers of the hospital in which the patient was liable to be detained as soon as reasonably practicable.

Conditions to be included in a CTO [section 17B and regulation 6]

26.16 CTOs must specify conditions which the CTO patient will be expected to comply with.

26.17 All CTOs must include conditions ('mandatory conditions') requiring patients to make themselves available for examination so that:

- the responsible clinician can decide whether to make a report extending the CTO under section 20A (see paragraph 27.71 below), and
- a second opinion doctor (SOAD) can decide whether to give a certificate ('a part 4A certificate') authorising certain kinds of treatments for the patient (see chapter 24).

26.18 The CTO may include other conditions which the responsible clinician (with the AMHP's agreement) thinks are necessary or appropriate for one or more of the following reasons:

- ensuring that the patient receives medical treatment
- preventing risk of harm to the patient's health or safety, or
- protecting other people.

26.19 The conditions, with the exception of the mandatory conditions are not directly enforceable. If a patient fails to comply with any condition, the responsible clinician may take that failure into account when considering whether it is necessary to use the power to recall the patient to hospital (see paragraphs 26.31 onwards).

26.20 The conditions of a CTO must not deprive a person of their liberty. The precise scope of the term 'deprivation of liberty' is not fixed. In its 19 March 2014 judgment (Cheshire West)[108] the Supreme Court clarified that there is a deprivation of liberty in circumstances where a person is under continuous control and supervision, is not free to leave and lacks capacity to consent to these arrangements. The Supreme Court noted that factors which are not relevant in determining whether there is a deprivation of liberty include the person's compliance or lack of objection and the reason or purpose behind a particular placement. The relative normality of the placement, whatever the comparison made, is not relevant. A deprivation of liberty in relation to a person who lacks capacity may be authorised by an authorisation under Schedule A1 to the Mental Capacity Act 2005 or a Court of Protection order.

Variation and suspension of conditions [section 17B(4) and (5), and regulation 6]

26.21 The responsible clinician may subsequently vary the conditions, or temporarily suspend any of them, at any time. The agreement of an AMHP is not required. The responsible clinician must record any variation on form CTO2 and send that form to the managers of the responsible hospital as soon as reasonably practicable.

Effect of a CTO [section 17D]

26.22 A CTO is an order for the patient's discharge from detention in hospital, subject to the possibility of the patient being recalled to hospital for further medical treatment, if necessary. As with any other discharge from detention, the patient does not necessarily have to leave hospital immediately, or may already have done so on leave of absence.

26.23 While a CTO is in force, the application for admission for treatment, or the order or direction under part 3, on the basis of which the patient was detained immediately before being made subject to the CTO remains in force, but the hospital managers' authority to detain the patient is suspended.

26.24 The authority to detain the patient does not need to be renewed while it is suspended, and so will not expire while the patient remains a CTO patient. An order or direction under part 3 may come to an end for another reason, eg if the patient's conviction is quashed on appeal, in which case so too will the CTO.

26.25 When a patient's CTO ends the patient will be discharged absolutely both from the CTO and the underlying authority for detention. This does not apply if the reason for the CTO ending is its revocation by the responsible clinician following the patient's recall to hospital. Where the CTO is revoked, the underlying authority for detention is, in effect, revived (see paragraph 26.57 to 26.59).

---

[108] P v Cheshire West and Chester Council and another and P and Q v Surrey County Council. 2014. WLR 2. https://www.supremecourt.uk/decided-cases/docs/UKSC_2012_0068_Judgment.pdf

26.26 Where the Act refers to patients who are 'detained' or 'liable to be detained' this does not include CTO patients. References in other legislation to patients detained or liable to be detained under the Act do not include CTO patients.

Duty to inform nearest relatives about discharge onto CTOs [section 133]

26.27 Hospital managers have a duty under section 133 to take whatever steps are practicable to inform the person they think is the nearest relative that a detained patient is to be discharged from hospital, unless the patient or the relative has asked that such information should not be given, or there is no nearest relative. This duty applies equally where patients are to be discharged from hospital by means of a CTO. If practicable, the information should be given at least seven days before the date of discharge.

Information for patients and nearest relatives about CTO [section 132A]

26.28 Section 132A requires the managers of the responsible hospital to take whatever steps are practicable to ensure that CTO patients understand:

- the effect of the provisions of the Act which apply to them as CTO patients, and
- their rights to apply to the Tribunal.

This action must be taken as soon as practicable after the patient becomes a CTO patient, and must include providing the necessary information both orally and in writing. For hospital managers' additional duty to give information to CTO patients on recall to hospital, see paragraphs 26.45 to 26.46.

26.29 The hospital managers must also take whatever steps are practicable to give or send a copy of the written information to the person they think is the patient's nearest relative, unless the patient requests otherwise, or does not have a nearest relative. This must be done either at the same time, or within a reasonable time afterwards.

Information about independent mental health advocates for CTO patients [section 130D]

26.30 The managers of the responsible hospital must take steps to give CTO patients information about the availability of independent mental health advocates (IMHA). Unless the patient requests otherwise, or does not have a nearest relative, the managers must also take whatever steps are practicable to give this information to the person they think is the patient's nearest relative. This must be done as soon as practicable after the CTO is made (see chapter 4).

Recall of patients to hospital [section 17E and regulation 6]

26.31 CTO patients may be recalled to hospital if their responsible clinician decides that they need to receive medical treatment for their mental disorder in a hospital and that, if they were not recalled to hospital to receive that treatment, there would be a risk of harm to the patient's health or safety, or to other people.

26.32 There is also a power to recall patients to hospital if they fail to comply with one of the mandatory conditions to attend for examination described in paragraph 26.18.

26.33 Unless the patient's responsible hospital is in Wales, responsible clinicians must recall patients by giving them written notice of recall using form CTO3. For patients in Wales see paragraph 26.40.

26.34 The notice in form CTO3 may only be served on the patient in one of the three ways set out in figure 76. The time at which it is deemed to have been served – in other words, when the patient is deemed to have received the notice – depends on the way in which it is served, again as set out in the figure.

Figure 76: Service of notices recalling CTO patients to hospital

Method of serving the recall notice	Notice deemed to have been served
Delivering the notice by hand to the patient	As soon as it is given to the patient.
Delivering the notice by hand to the patient's usual or last known address	At the start of day which follows the day on which it is delivered to that address. For example, if it is delivered at noon (even on a weekend or bank holiday), it is deemed to have been served immediately after midnight that night.
Sending it by pre-paid first class post (or its equivalent) to the patient at the patient's usual or last known address	On the second business day after it is posted. For example if it is posted on Monday, it is deemed to have been delivered on Wednesday. But if it is posted on Friday, it is deemed to have been delivered on Tuesday. Weekends and public holidays do not count as business days.

26.35 The responsible clinician must send a copy of the form to the managers of the hospital to which the patient is recalled as soon as reasonably practicable. If that is not the responsible hospital, the responsible clinician must also tell those managers the name and address of the responsible hospital.

26.36 Patients may be recalled to any hospital, not just their responsible hospital. In practice, patients should not be recalled to any hospital unless it has been established that the hospital can accept them – hospital managers are not obliged to accept patients just because a responsible clinician has issued a recall notice.

26.37 Patients recalled to hospital do not have to be admitted as in-patients, eg they could be recalled for out-patient treatment instead.

26.38 Patients may be recalled even if they are already in hospital at the time. This could happen, for example, if a patient attends hospital either voluntarily or to comply with a condition of the CTO, but then refuses to accept the treatment the responsible clinician thinks is needed. If the patient, or someone else, would be at risk if the patient does not have that treatment, the patient could be formally recalled to allow the treatment to be given without the patient's consent.

26.39 If the patient's responsible hospital is in Wales, recall must be done in accordance with the equivalent Welsh regulations, even if the patient is to be recalled to a hospital in England. That will involve using a Welsh statutory form, rather than CTO3, to give the patient notice of the recall.

Effect of recall to hospital [section 17E(6), 17F(6) and regulation 6]

26.40 The issue of a recall notice gives the managers of the relevant hospital the power to detain the patient at the hospital specified in the recall notice for up to 72 hours from the time at which the patient is first detained there as a result of the recall. The 72 hour period does not run from the time the recall notice was issued, unless the patient was already in the hospital at the time and was immediately detained as a result.

26.41 The start of the patient's detention must be recorded by the managers of the hospital in question, or an officer authorised by them in writing, using form CTO4.

26.42 If patients who are recalled to hospital do not come to the hospital as required, or go absent from the hospital once there, they are considered absent without leave (AWOL), and may be taken into custody and brought,(or returned, to the hospital, in accordance with the rules described in paragraphs 26.67 to 26.75).

26.43 While detained in hospital on recall, CTO patients are subject, with certain exceptions to the same rules on medical treatment as other patients detained in hospital (see chapter 23). They are not subject to any of the other provisions about detained patients described in chapter 25, or elsewhere in this Reference Guide, because they are not considered to be 'liable to be detained' in the terms of the Act.

Duty to give information to patients recalled to hospital [regulation 6(7)]

26.44 As soon as practicable, the managers of the hospital to which a patient is recalled must take whatever steps are reasonably practicable to arrange for the patient to be informed, orally and in writing, of the provisions of the Act under which the patient has been recalled and the effect of those provisions, eg that the patient may be detained for up to 72 hours. Wherever possible the responsible clinician should give the patient, or arrange for the patient to be given, oral reasons for the recall before it happens, taking into account any risks arising from giving notice of the recall.

26.45 The responsible clinician must take whatever steps are reasonably practicable to ensure that that patient understands the provisions of part 4 of the Act to the extent that they are relevant to the patient's case. Part 4 of the Act deals with treatment for mental disorder, especially treatment without consent (see chapter 23). There are certain differences in the way it applies to CTO patients who are recalled to hospital – see paragraph 24.32 onward.

Transfer of recalled patients to another hospital [section 17F(2) and regulations 9 and 12]

26.46 While patients are being detained in hospital on recall, the managers of the hospital in question may authorise their transfer to another hospital. The maximum 72 hour period of detention in hospital on recall continues to run from the original time that the patient was detained, despite the transfer.

26.47 No particular procedure need be followed if the patient is to be transferred to a hospital under the management of the same hospital managers.

26.48 To authorise transfer from a hospital in England to a hospital under different management, whether in England or Wales, the hospital managers of the first hospital must use form CTO6. They may not authorise the transfer unless they are satisfied that arrangements have been made for the patient's admission to the new hospital.

26.49 The hospital managers of the hospital from which the patient is to be transferred must give the managers of the new hospital a copy of the record of the time the patient was detained as a result of being recalled to hospital (ie form CTO4). This must be done before, or at the time, that the patient is transferred.

26.50 The hospital managers of the new hospital must record the time of the patient's admission there using the same form CTO6 on which the transfer was originally authorised.

26.51 If an NHS patient is recalled to an independent hospital, an officer authorised by the relevant NHS body may also authorise the patient's transfer to another hospital under different management. The relevant NHS body is the one which has contracted with the independent hospital to act as the responsible hospital.

26.52 A transfer between hospitals while a patient is recalled does not change the responsible hospital. There is a separate procedure for changing the responsible hospital (see paragraphs 26.127 to 26.134).

26.53 Hospital managers may authorise officers to authorise transfers and make any necessary records on their behalf.

26.54 Patients whose transfer has been authorised may be conveyed to the new hospital by an officer of the managers of either hospital or by any person authorised by the managers of the hospital to which to patient is being transferred. This may only be done during the 72 hour period for which the patient may be detained on the basis of the recall.

26.55 Transfers from hospitals in Wales to hospitals in England must be done in accordance with the equivalent Welsh regulations. That will involve using a Welsh statutory form, rather than form CT06, to authorise the transfer and to record the patient's admission to the new hospital.

Revocation of CTOs [section 17F(3) and (4) and regulation 6(8)]

26.56 If the responsible clinician decides that a patient meets the Act's criteria for admission to hospital for treatment (see paragraph 8.8) the clinician may revoke the patient's CTO, subject to the agreement of an AMHP acting on behalf of a local authority. The AMHP must agree not only that the criteria are met but also that revocation is appropriate.

26.57 A CTO may only be revoked while the patient is detained in hospital as a result of being recalled.

26.58 An order revoking a CTO – and the AMHP's agreement to it – must be made using form CTO5. The form must then be sent to the hospital managers of the hospital to which the patient was recalled, who must in turn send a copy of it to the managers of the hospital which was, until then, the responsible hospital, if they are different.

26.59 Revocation of a CTO revives the hospital managers' authority to detain the patient, which was suspended when the CTO was first made (see paragraph 26.23). In other words, patients become liable to be detained again on the basis of the application for admission, or the order or direction, which authorised their detention immediately before they became CTO patients.[109]

[109] As a result of transitional arrangements for patients subject to after-care under supervision (ACUS) immediately before 3 November 2008, some ACUS patients may become CTO patients without being detained again in the interim. If such patients have their CTOs revoked, they are treated as if they are liable to be detained on the basis of an application for admission for assessment under section 3, regardless of the actual authority under which they were detained before becoming ACUS patients. The Department of Health has issued separate guidance on these and other transitional arrangements relating to the abolition of ACUS. The transitional provisions themselves are to be found in the Mental Health Act 2007 (Commencement No. 6 and After-care under Supervision: Savings, Modifications and Transitional Provisions) Order. 2008. SI 2008/1210. http://www.legislation.gov.uk/uksi/2008/1210

26.60 The Act then applies to them as it would if they had never been on CTO. The only differences are that, for the purposes of expiry and renewal of the authority to detain, patients are treated as if they had first been detained on the day the CTO is revoked.

> **Example**
>
> Mr B was first detained on the basis of an application for treatment on 1 January 2015. His detention was renewed under section 20 for six months with effect from 1 July 2015 and then again from 1 January 2016 for one year. It is therefore due to expire again on 31 December 2016 unless renewed once more.
>
> In fact, he was discharged onto a CTO on 1 April 2015. He was recalled to hospital on 2 June and unfortunately the CTO had to be revoked on 4 June.
>
> Mr B's detention is therefore revived from 4 June 2015 and will be due to expire at the end of six months on 3 December 2015, unless renewed under section 20. If it is renewed, it will be initially renewed for six months to expire on 3 June 2016, and then, if necessary, for one year at a time.

26.61 If a patient has been recalled to a hospital which is not their responsible hospital, the application, order or direction is treated as if it referred to the new hospital instead.

26.62 The hospital managers of the hospital in which the patient is now detained must refer the patient's case to the Tribunal as soon as practicable after the revocation of the CTO – see chapter 6. For patients' own rights to apply to the Tribunal when their CTO is revoked, see chapter 6.

26.63 There is nothing to prevent a patient whose CTO has been revoked subsequently becoming a CTO patient again by being given a new CTO.

Release from recall [section 17F(5) to (7) and 5(6)]

26.64 A recalled patient may only be detained for a maximum of 72 hours unless the CTO is revoked. Otherwise, the patient is automatically released at the end of that period, and must be allowed to leave the hospital. The 'holding powers' in section 5 may not be used to keep the patient in hospital after the end of the 72 hours (Code of Practice chapter 18).

26.65 The responsible clinician may release a recalled patient from detention at any time before the end of the 72 hour period.

26.66 On release, the patient continues to be a CTO patient and so remains subject to the CTO and its conditions as before, unless those conditions have been varied (or suspended) in the normal way while the patient was recalled to hospital.

Recalled CTO patients who are absent without leave [section 18 and 21(4)]

26.67 Where CTO patients are at any time absent from the hospital to which they have been recalled, or to which they have been transferred while recalled, they are considered to be AWOL. They may be taken into custody under section 18 and taken to the hospital by any AMHP, police officer, or other constable, any officer on the staff of the hospital in question, or by any person authorised in writing by the responsible clinician or the hospital managers of that hospital.

26.68 This may only be done during the period before:

- the CTO expires, ignoring any extra time that would be allowed if the patient were to return or be taken into custody right at the end of that period (see paragraph 26.81), or
- the end of the six months starting with the first day of the absence without leave, if that is later.

26.69 For these purposes, the fact that the responsible clinician has already made a report extending the patient's CTO (see paragraph 26.74) is irrelevant unless the extended period has already started when the patient goes absent.

26.70 If patients are taken into custody, or come to the hospital voluntarily, before the end of the period during which they could be taken into custody, the 72 hours for which they can be detained effectively starts again on their arrival at the hospital. In other words, they can be detained for a further 72 hours, even if they had already been detained for part of that period before they went AWOL.

26.71 If patients are taken into custody, or come to the hospital voluntarily, after being absent for more than 28 days (ie on or after 29 January if they went absent on 1 January), their CTO expires at the end of the week starting with the day of their arrival at the hospital unless it is confirmed by the responsible clinician (see paragraphs 26.81 and onwards).

Expiry and extension of CTOs [section 20A and 20B and regulations 13 and 26]

26.72 Unless extended, a CTO expires at the end of the six months starting with the day on which it is made. So, if it is made on 1 January, it expires at the end of 30 June. If is not extended and the CTO expires, the patient the underlying authority for detention (whether it is an application for admission for treatment under part 2 or an order or direction under part 3) also cease to have effect.

26.73 A CTO can be extended for a further six months, and then for a year at a time. At some point during the final two months of the first and each subsequent period for which the CTO is in force, the responsible clinician must examine the patient in order to decide whether the patient meets the conditions for extension. The responsible clinician may recall the patient to hospital for this purpose, because being available for this examination is one of the mandatory conditions to be included in all CTOs (see paragraph 26.17).

26.74 The conditions for extension, which mirror the criteria for making a CTO in the first place, are that:

- the patient is suffering from mental disorder of a nature or degree which makes it appropriate for the patient to receive medical treatment
- it is necessary for the patient's health or safety or for the protection of other persons that the patient should receive such treatment
- subject to the patient continuing to be liable to be recalled as mentioned below, such treatment can be provided without the patient being detained in a hospital
- it is necessary that the responsible clinician should continue to be able to exercise the power of recall under section 17E(1) to recall the patient to hospital, and
- appropriate medical treatment is available for the patient.

26.75 In determining whether the fourth criterion, power of recall, above is met, the factors which responsible clinicians must consider include the same factors they are required always to consider when making CTOs initially (see paragraph 26.13).

26.76 If responsible clinicians think the criteria are met, they must make a report to that effect to the hospital managers under section 20A. Responsible clinicians:

- must first consult one or more other people who have been professionally concerned with the patient's medical treatment, and
- may not make the report unless an AMHP acting on behalf of a local authority confirms in writing that the criteria are met and that it is appropriate to extend the CTO.

26.77 The report, and the AMHP's statement of agreement, must be made using form CTO7 and sent to the managers of the responsible hospital, who must record their receipt of it in part 4 of the form.

26.78 The effect of the report is to extend the CTO for a further six months or a year, as applicable, from the date it would otherwise expire, not the date of the report itself.

26.79 Unless the hospital managers decide to discharge the patient (see paragraph 26.117), they must arrange for the patient to be told about the extension. They must also take whatever steps are reasonably practicable to arrange for the person they think is the patient's nearest relative to be informed as soon as practicable after their decision, unless the patient has requested otherwise, or does not have a nearest relative. Information given to nearest relatives must be in writing, but may be communicated by electronic means (eg email) if the nearest relative agrees. For information about the nearest relative, see chapter 2.

Patients absent without leave as deadline for extension report approaches [section 21 and 21A and regulations 14 and 26]

26.80 Special arrangements apply if patients are AWOL at any point during the week which ends on the day their CTO is due to expire, and an extension report has yet to be made. These arrangements are equivalent to those for part 2 detained patients described in chapter 27.

26.81 If patients have not been taken into custody, or do not attend the hospital voluntarily, before the end of the period during which they can be taken into custody under section 18, their CTOs expire and no extension report can be made.

26.82 If patients are taken into custody, or attend the hospital voluntarily, during that period, their CTOs are treated as not expiring until the end of the week starting with the day they arrive at the hospital.

26.83 Responsible clinicians therefore have a week from the day of the patient's arrival at the hospital to submit the extension report. If the patient arrives on Monday, the responsible clinician has until the end of the following Sunday to submit the report.

26.84 If patients are taken into custody, or attend the hospital voluntarily, during the 28 days starting with the day they went AWOL, ie before the end of 28 January, if they went AWOL on 1 January, the extension report is to be made in the normal way – and must therefore be agreed by an AMHP acting on behalf of a local authority.

26.85 If patients are taken into custody, or attend the hospital voluntarily after more than 28 days, it is not normally necessary to make an extension report under section 20A. That is because the patient's CTO has anyway to be confirmed by a report under section 21B, and that report can also serve as an extension report in place of a report under section 20A (see paragraph 26.87 and onwards).

Confirmation of CTOs for patients who have been absent without leave for more than 28 days [section 21B and regulations 14(3) and 26)]

26.86 Where recalled CTO patients are taken into custody, or attend the relevant hospital voluntarily, after being AWOL for more than 28 days, their responsible clinician must examine them and, if appropriate, submit a report using form CTO8 to the managers of the responsible hospital confirming that the conditions for the CTO are met. This is equivalent to the procedures for detained part 2 patients.

26.87 The criteria for continuing the CTO are the same as the criteria for extending it, described at paragraph 26.75 above.

26.88 Unless such a report is submitted, a patient's CTO expires automatically at the end of the week starting with the day on which they arrive at the hospital.

26.89 Responsible clinicians must make a report during this period if they think that the conditions are met. The responsible clinician must first consult one or more other people who have been professionally concerned with the patient's medical treatment and an AMHP who is acting on behalf of a local authority. There is no requirement in this case to obtain a statement of agreement from the AMHP.

26.90 The managers of the responsible hospital must record their receipt of the report in part 2 of the same form CTO8.

26.91 As described in paragraph 26.95, a report submitted under this procedure will extend the patient's CTO if it would otherwise already have expired, or if it would expire on the day the report is submitted to the managers). If so, the hospital managers must take the steps described there to arrange for the patient and, where relevant, the nearest relative to be informed.

26.92 In addition, if the patient's CTO is due to expire during the period of two months starting with the day on which the report is given to the managers, the responsible clinician may, but need not, indicate on the form that it is also to act as an extension report which would otherwise have to be made during that period under section 20A.

26.93 In that case, unless they decide to discharge the patient (see paragraph 26.117), the managers must take steps to arrange for the patient and, where relevant, the nearest relative to be informed of the report in the same way as if it were a report under section 20A itself.

Patients who return from absence without leave and whose CTO would otherwise have expired [sections 21, 21A and 21B and regulation 26]

26.94 In some cases, the responsible clinician's report under section 20A or 21B extending the CTO of a patient who has been AWOL will be made on or after the day the CTO was originally due to expire because the period for which the CTO is in force has been extended by section 21. If so, that report is treated as having retrospectively extended the CTO from when it would otherwise have expired in the normal way.

26.95 In the rare circumstances where the patient's CTO would otherwise have expired twice since they went AWOL, the responsible clinician's report under section 21B is treated as having extended the CTO on both occasions.

26.96 If a patient's CTO is extended retrospectively, either once or twice, in this way, the hospital managers must take whatever steps are reasonably practicable to arrange for the patient to be told about the extension. They must also take such steps to arrange for the person they think is the nearest relative to be informed, unless the patient has requested otherwise, or does not have a nearest relative.

26.97 The patient must be told of the retrospective extension both orally and in writing. Information given to nearest relatives must be in writing, but may be communicated by electronic means (eg email) if the nearest relative agrees.

Patients who are imprisoned etc [section 22, read with sections 18, 21 and 21A]

26.98 Special rules apply to CTO patients who are imprisoned, remanded or otherwise detained in custody by any court in the UK. These are similar to those for part 2 detained patients.

26.99 Such patients automatically cease to be CTO patients if they remain in custody for longer than six months in total.

26.100 Until then, they formally remain CTO patients, unless discharged from their CTO in the interim. If they are released from custody during that six month period, they are treated as if they had gone AWOL on the day of their release.

26.101 Because patients in this situation are treated as being AWOL, if such a patient's CTO would otherwise have expired, or is about to expire, it will not in fact expire until the end of the week starting with the day of the patient's return to hospital (if the patient had already been recalled to hospital when first imprisoned) or (if not) the date of the patient's release from custody.

26.102 The effect of this is that, if the patient's CTO is otherwise due to expire, responsible clinicians will always have at least a week in which to examine the patient and submit a report extending the CTO, if appropriate, under section 20A.

26.103 Although CTO patients released from custody after less than six months are treated as having gone AWOL, they may only automatically be taken into custody and returned to a hospital if they had already been recalled to that hospital when they were first imprisoned. Even then, that can only be done during the 28 day period starting with the date of their release.

26.104 The normal rules about recalling patients to hospital apply to patients released from custody during whatever period remains of their CTO (including the one week extension, where relevant). They can, if necessary, be recalled to hospital in order to be examined with a view to making a report extending their CTOs (see paragraph 26.33). If they failed to attend, they would be considered AWOL in the normal way, and could therefore be taken into custody at any time during the six months starting with the day they failed to attend, as described in paragraphs 26.68 onward.

Discharge of part 2 CTO patients by their nearest relatives [sections 23 and 25 and regulations 3 and 25]

26.105 Nearest relatives may discharge part 2 CTO patients from CTOs – and therefore from the underlying application for admission for treatment as well – in the same way as they can discharge patients detained in hospital on the basis of an application for admission for treatment under section 3.

26.106 Nearest relatives must give a written discharge order. Before doing so, they must give the managers of the responsible hospital not less than 72 hours notice in writing of their intention to discharge the patient. The notice does not have to be given in any particular form.

26.107 Like a notice of discharge from detention, the notice, and the order for discharge itself, must either be delivered to an officer of the managers of the responsible hospital authorised by them to receive it, be sent by prepaid post to those managers at that hospital, or, if the managers agree, be sent using the managers' internal mail system. The 72 hour period starts to run from the time: when the notice is received by the authorised person; when it is sent by pre-paid post, then when it is received at the hospital to which it is addressed, or otherwise the second business day (if first class post) or fourth business day (if second class post) following the day of posting (unless the contrary is shown), or when it is put into the internal mail system, as the case may be.

26.108 If responsible clinicians consider that, if discharged from CTOs, patients are likely to act in a manner dangerous to other persons or themselves, they may make a report to that effect using form M2 and send it to the managers of the responsible hospital before the end of the 72 hour notice period.

26.109 Unlike other statutory forms used in connection with the Act, a notice given on form M2 may be formally served on the managers, if they agree, by faxing it to them, or by emailing, or otherwise sending them, a scanned version, or other electronic reproduction, of the completed and signed form. It may not be signed electronically.

26.110 The effect of such a report is to veto the nearest relative's decision to discharge the patient. It also prevents the nearest relative from discharging the patient from the CTO at any time in the six months following the date of the report.

26.111 If the responsible clinician issues this report, the managers must arrange for the nearest relative to be informed in writing without delay. The nearest relative may then apply to the Tribunal for the patient's discharge instead – see chapter 6.

26.112 If the responsible clinician does not make a report within the 72 hour notice period, the patient must be discharged from the CTO in accordance with the nearest relative's order. If the patient happened to be recalled to hospital at the time, they would have to be released from the hospital, because the authority to detain them on recall would no longer exist.

26.113 Nearest relatives cannot order patients to be released from detention in hospital on recall without also discharging them from the CTO.

26.114 Nearest relatives cannot order the discharge of part 3 CTO patients, but can apply to the Tribunal instead in certain circumstances (see chapter 7).

Discharge of CTO patients by their responsible clinicians [section 23 and regulation 18]

26.115 Responsible clinicians may discharge CTO patients (including part 3 CTO patients) at any time, by making a written order. The order must be sent to the managers of the responsible hospital as soon as practicable after it is made, but it is effective even before it is submitted to the managers.

Discharge of CTO patients by the hospital managers [section 23]

26.116 The managers of the responsible hospital may also discharge CTO patients at any time by making a written order. They must always consider doing so when the responsible clinician makes a report extending the CTO, as described in paragraph 26.77 onward.

26.117 Where the managers are an NHS trust, NHS foundation trust, special health authority or local health board, or another body of persons (eg a company), they may only delegate the discharge function to the same three or more people to whom they can delegate decisions about discharging detained patients (see paragraph 26.117). As with detention, the three people to whom the discharge function is delegated must be unanimous in their decision to discharge. If the decision is taken by more than three people, as well as a majority in favour, that majority must be made up of at least three people in favour of discharge before a decision to discharge can be made.

26.118 Like nearest relatives, the managers cannot order patients to be released from recall to hospital, except by discharging them from the CTO itself.

Discharge of CTO patients by the Tribunal [part 5]

26.119 CTO patients may also be discharged from CTO by the First-tier Tribunal (or Upper Tribunal on appeal). For information on this, and an explanation of the rights of patients and their nearest relatives to apply for discharge, see chapter 6.

26.120 In certain circumstances, the managers of the responsible hospital have a duty to refer CTO patients' cases to the Tribunal, including when a patient's CTO is revoked. The Secretary of State for Health may also refer cases to the Tribunal at any time. See chapter 6 for further information on these powers and duties.

26.121 The Tribunal cannot release patients from periods of recall to hospital (except by discharging them from the CTO itself). Nor can it discharge patients onto CTOs in the first place, although it may recommend that the responsible clinician consider doing so – see paragraphs 6.73 and 6.74.

Duty of managers to inform nearest relative of discharge of CTO patient [section 133]

26.122 Where a CTO patient is to be discharged, the managers of the responsible hospital must take whatever steps are practicable to inform the person they think is the patient's nearest relative, unless the patient or the nearest relative has asked that such information should not be given, or the patient does not have a nearest relative. If practicable, the information should be given at least 7 days before the date of discharge. The obligation to inform the nearest relative does not apply where the patient is being discharged on the nearest relative's own order (see paragraph 26.105).

Visiting and examination of patients in relation to use of powers of discharge [section 24)]

26.123 As with discharge from detention, any doctor or approved clinician may be authorised by or on behalf of a nearest relative to visit and examine a patient. Authorised people have a right to inspect records relating to the patient's detention or treatment in any hospital or any after-care services provided for the patient under section 117, in order to advise on the use of the nearest relative's power of discharge.

Discharge from a CTO – general points

26.124 Discharge from a CTO means discharge from the CTO and the underlying authority for detention, whether it is an application for admission for treatment under part 2 or an order or direction under part 3.

26.125 The effect is that the patient can no longer be recalled to hospital or required to stay in hospital.

Reassignment of responsibility for CTO patients [section 19A and regulations 17 and 26]

26.126 Responsibility for a CTO patient may be transferred from the managers of one hospital to another, by reassigning responsibility for the patient in accordance with regulations made under section 19A.

26.127 The managers of the responsible hospital may authorise this using form CTO10 if the new responsible hospital is not under the same management as the responsible hospital and is in England. They may only do so if the managers of the new hospital agree to the assignment and specify a date on which it is to take place.

26.128 If responsibility is to be assigned to a hospital in Wales, the procedures in the equivalent Welsh regulations apply instead, and the equivalent Welsh form must be used.

26.129 Once responsibility is assigned, the new hospital becomes the responsible hospital. The underlying authority for the patient's detention is treated as if it had always specified the new responsible hospital as the one in which the patient was detained when first discharged onto the CTO.

26.130 A change of responsible hospital does not change the date on which the CTO is due to expire, nor the period for which it could, if appropriate, be extended.

26.131 The managers of the hospital to which responsibility for a patient is to be, or has been, assigned must notify the patient of the reassignment of responsibility either before or as soon as practicable afterward. Unless the patient has requested otherwise, or does not have a nearest relative, those managers must also take whatever steps are reasonably practicable to have the person they think is the patient's nearest relative informed, again either before or as soon as practicable after the reassignment. Information given to nearest relatives must be in writing, but may be communicated by electronic means (eg email) if the nearest relative agrees.

26.132 Hospital managers may authorise any officer to exercise their functions in relation to assignment on their behalf.

26.133 If an independent hospital is the responsible hospital for an NHS patient, an officer authorised by the relevant NHS body may also authorise the patient's transfer to another hospital under different management. The relevant NHS body is the one which has contracted with the independent hospital to act as the responsible hospital.

Effect of a CTO on new applications for admission or guardianship under part 2 [sections 6(4) and 8(5)]

26.134 Because CTO patients can be recalled to hospital for treatment if required, it should not be necessary to make applications for their detention. In practice this may happen if the people making the application do not know that the patient is a CTO patient.

26.135 An application for admission for assessment under section 2 or 4 does not affect the patient's CTO.

26.136 But if a CTO patient is detained on the basis of an application for admission for treatment under section 3, the patient will automatically cease to be a CTO patient if, immediately before going onto the CTO, the patient had been detained on the basis of a previous application under section 3, rather than an order or direction under part 3.

26.137 The same applies if such a patient is received into guardianship as a result of an application under part 2.

26.138 That is because an application under section 3, or the reception of a patient into guardianship under part 2, automatically brings to an end any previous application for detention or guardianship under part 2.

26.139 If a patient stops being a CTO patient because of an application for admission for treatment under section 3, a new CTO would have to be made for the patient to go back onto a CTO when they no longer needed to be detained in hospital.

26.140 An application for admission for treatment under section 3 does not end a patient's CTO if, immediately before going onto CTO, the patient had been detained on the basis of a hospital order, hospital direction or transfer direction under part 3 of the Act.

Effect of new orders or directions under part 3 on CTO [section 40(5)]

26.141 If a CTO patient is admitted to hospital as the result of a hospital order, hospital and limitation direction or transfer direction, or given a guardianship order under part 3 of the Act, they automatically cease to be a CTO patient. That is because the new order or direction brings to an end the application, order or direction to which the patient was subject immediately before going onto CTO.

26.142 If a hospital order, hospital and limitation direction, or guardianship order, or the conviction on which it is based, is subsequently quashed on appeal, section 22 will apply as if the order or direction had never happened and the patient had instead been in prison since the quashed order or direction was made. This may mean that the patient automatically becomes a CTO patient again if less six months has passed since the quashed order or direction was given.

27: Discharge

Introduction

27.1 This chapter describes the provisions of the Act relating to discharge and to conditional discharge of restricted patients. See chapter 21 for more information on restricted patients generally. Only restricted patients may be conditionally discharged.

Discharge by the responsible clinician [section 23 and regulation 18]

27.2 Responsible clinicians may discharge part 2 or unrestricted part 3 patients at any time, by making a written order. They may only discharge restricted patients in this way with the consent of the Secretary of State for Justice.

27.3 The order must be sent to the hospital managers as soon as practicable after it is made, but it is effective even before it is sent to the managers.

27.4 If the patient is detained on the basis of an application for admission for treatment under section 3, the responsible clinician may, in certain circumstances, discharge the patient onto a CTO. The same applies to unrestricted part 3 patients. CTO patients remain liable to be recalled to hospital if necessary. See chapter 26.

27.5 Restricted patients and part 2 patients detained for assessment under sections 2 or 4 may not be discharged onto a CTO.

Discharge by the hospital managers [section 23]

27.6 The hospital managers may also discharge part 2 and unrestricted part 3 patients at any time by making a written order. They must always consider doing so when a responsible clinician makes a report renewing the authority for a patient's detention (see paragraph 28.21 onward). The managers may only discharge restricted patients with the consent of the Secretary of State for Justice.

27.7 Where the managers are an NHS body, or another body of persons (eg a company which owns an independent hospital), they may only delegate the discharge function as set out in figure 77. People to whom these functions are delegated, but who are not members or directors of the body in question, are sometimes termed 'associate managers' – although the Act does not use that term.

Figure 77: Delegation of discharge decisions by hospital managers

If the hospital managers are	The discharge function may be performed on their behalf by	Who are
An NHS trust	Three or more • directors of the trust board (including the Chairman), or • members of an authorised committee or sub-committee of the trust	Not employees of the trust
An NHS foundation trust	Three or more people authorised by the board of the trust	Neither executive directors of the board of the trust, nor employees of the trust
A special health authority, or local health board	Three or more • authorised members of the body (including the Chairman), or • members of an authorised committee or sub-committee of the body	Not officers of the body (within the meaning of the NHS Act 2006 or NHS (Wales) Act 2006)
Another body of persons (eg company)	Three or more • authorised members of the body, or • members of an authorised committee or sub-committee of the body	

27.8 In figure 77, 'authorised' means that the person, committee or sub-committee, as the case may be, has been authorised by the managers (ie the body in question) specifically for this purpose.

27.9 Patients can only be discharged where all three people acting on behalf of the managers agree that they should be discharged. A two to one majority decision is not sufficient.[110] If the decision is taken by more than three people, as well as a majority being in favour, the majority must consist of at least three people in favour of discharge before a decision to discharge can be made.

[110] R (on the application of Tagoe-Thompson) v The Hospital Managers of the Park Royal Centre. 2003. EWCA Civ 330. http://www.bailii.org/ew/cases/EWCA/Civ/2003/330.html

Discharge of patients by their nearest relatives [sections 23 and 25 and regulations 3 and 25]

27.10 A nearest relative may discharge a part 2 patient by making a written discharge order.

27.11 Before giving a discharge order, nearest relatives must give the hospital managers not less than 72 hours notice in writing of their intention to discharge the patient.

27.12 Neither the discharge order, nor the notice of it, has to be given in any particular form.

27.13 Although in theory the order should not be served until 72 hours after the notice has been given, in practice it is appropriate for hospital managers to accept a discharge order without prior notice as being both notice of intention to discharge the patient after 72 hours and the actual order to do so.

27.14 The notice, and the order for discharge itself must either be delivered at the hospital to an officer of the managers authorised by them to receive it, be sent by pre-paid post to those managers at that hospital, or, if the managers agree, be sent using the managers' internal mail system.

27.15 The 72 hour period starts to run from the time when the notice is:

- received by the authorised person
- if sent by pre-paid post then after the second business day following posting (first class post) or the fourth business day following posting (second class post), or
- put into the internal mail system, as the case may be.

27.16 If responsible clinicians consider that, if discharged, patients are likely to act in a manner dangerous to other persons or themselves, they may make a report to that effect under section 25 using form M2 and send it to the hospital managers before the end of the 72 hours notice period. This is sometimes known as a 'barring report'.

27.17 Unlike other statutory forms used in connection with the Act, a notice given on form M2 may be formally served on the managers, if they agree, by faxing it to them, or by emailing, or otherwise sending them, a scanned version, or other electronic reproduction, of the completed and signed form. It may not be signed electronically.

27.18 The effect of such a report is to veto the nearest relative's decision to discharge the patient. It also prevents the nearest relative from discharging the patient from detention at any time in the six months following the date of the report.

27.19 If such a report is issued in respect of a patient detained on the basis of an application for admission for treatment under section 3, the managers must arrange for the nearest relative to be informed in writing without delay. The nearest relative may then apply to the Tribunal for the patient's discharge instead – see chapter 6. There is no right to apply if the patient is detained for assessment under section 2 or 4.

27.20 If the responsible clinician does not make a report within the relevant period, the patient must be discharged in accordance with the nearest relative's order.

27.21 Nearest relatives may not discharge part 3 patients, but can make applications to the Tribunal instead in respect of unrestricted part 3 patients – see chapter 22.

Duty of managers to inform nearest relative of discharge [section 133]

27.22 Where a patient is to be discharged from detention under the Act, the hospital managers must take whatever steps are practicable to inform the person they think is the patient's nearest relative, unless the patient or the nearest relative has asked that such information should not be given, or the patient does not have a nearest relative.

27.23 If practicable, the information should be given at least seven days before the date of discharge. The obligation to inform the nearest relative does not apply where the patient is being discharged on the nearest relative's own order.

27.24 The duty on the managers applies to all patients detained in their hospitals, except CTO patients detained for up to 72 hours as a result of being recalled to hospital. By definition, restricted patients, patients remanded to hospital under section 35 or 36 and patients subject to interim hospital orders under section 38 do not have nearest relatives for the purposes of the Act.

Discharge by the Tribunal [part 5]

27.25 Part 2 and part 3 patients may also be discharged by the First-tier Tribunal (or the Upper Tribunal on appeal).

27.26 For information on this, and an explanation of the rights of patients and nearest relatives to apply to the Tribunal, see chapter 6.

27.27 In certain circumstances, hospital managers have a duty to refer patients' cases to the Tribunal. For restricted patients, these duties fall on the Secretary of State for Justice.

27.28 The Secretaries of State for Health and Justice may also refer cases to the Tribunal at any time, and in certain circumstances hospital managers should consider asking for such a reference.

27.29 See chapter 6 for further information on powers and duties to refer cases to the Tribunal.

Visiting and examination of patients in relation to use of powers of discharge [section 24]

27.30 Any doctor or approved clinician may be authorised by the nearest relative to visit and examine the patient in order to advise on the use of the nearest relative's power of discharge.

27.31 These authorised doctors and approved clinicians may visit and examine the patient in private at any reasonable time, and require any records relating to the patient's detention or treatment in any hospital, or relating to after-care services provided for the patient under section 117, to be produced for their inspection.

27.32 A person who refused, without reasonable cause, to let an authorised doctor or approved clinician see a patient in private, or inspect any relevant records, would be guilty of the offence of obstruction under section 129 (see chapter 33).

Discharge – general points

27.33 In the provisions described above, 'discharge' means discharge from liability to detention, rather than discharge from hospital. Patients may remain in hospital without being detained. Equally, patients may already have left hospital on leave of absence before they are formally discharged from detention.

27.34 Patients who have been detained on the basis of an application for admission for treatment may be entitled to mental health after-care arranged jointly by) CCGs and local authorities under section 117 of the Act when discharged. The same applies to part 3 detained patients. See chapter 29 for further information on after-care.

Conditional discharge of restricted patients [section, 42, 73, and 75]

27.35 The Secretary of State for Justice may conditionally discharge restricted patients at any time, by issuing a warrant to that effect.

27.36 The Tribunal may also conditionally discharge restricted patients (see chapter 6).

27.37 When conditionally discharging a patient, the Secretary of State will specify conditions to which the patient is to be subject. The Tribunal will typically do the same when conditionally discharging a patient, but does not have to do so. The Secretary of State may also impose, vary, or remove conditions set by the Tribunal or by the Secretary of State.

27.38 In practice, these conditions will generally include a requirement for patients to maintain contact with their mental health care team and to accept supervision from a social worker, AMHP or probation officer (a 'social supervisor'), a psychiatrist (a 'psychiatric supervisor'), or any other 'clinical supervisor'. They may also include conditions requiring patients to live at a certain place, eg accommodation that can provide a particular level of supervision or support, or to stay away from certain place, eg the place where the crime which led to their detention in hospital (their 'index offence') was committed.

27.39 The conditions of guardianship cannot amount to a deprivation of liberty, unless this is authorised under the Mental Capacity Act 2005.[111] The precise scope of the term 'deprivation of liberty' is not fixed. In its 19 March 2014 judgment[112], the Supreme Court clarified that there is a deprivation of liberty in circumstances where a person is under continuous control and supervision, is not free to leave and lacks capacity to consent to these arrangements. The Supreme Court also noted that factors which are not relevant in determining whether there is a deprivation of liberty include the person's compliance or lack of objection and the reason or purpose behind a particular placement. The relative normality of the placement, whatever the comparison made, is also not relevant. A deprivation of liberty in relation to a person who lacks capacity may be authorised by an authorisation under Schedule A1 to the Mental Capacity Act 2005 or a Court of Protection order.

27.40 While patients are conditionally discharged, the people appointed to supervise them will be required by the Secretary of State for Justice to submit a report at regular intervals. In practice, the Secretary of State normally asks for reports one month after the patient's discharge and at quarterly intervals thereafter. In some cases it may be appropriate to extend the intervals between reports but the Mental Health Casework Section (MHCS)[113] of the Ministry of Justice should be consulted in the first instance.

27.41 Conditionally discharged patients may not apply to the Tribunal for their absolute discharge until the end of the 12 months starting with the day of their conditional discharge. They may apply once in the next 12 month period and once in every subsequent two year period – see chapter 6.

27.42 Where it decides not to discharge conditionally discharged patients absolutely, the Tribunal may vary the conditions to which they are subject.

27.43 The Secretary of State may vary conditions imposed on patients, including those imposed by the Tribunal, at any time.

---

[111] Mental Capacity Act 2005. http://www.legislation.gov.uk/ukpga/2005/9/contents

[112] P v Cheshire West and Chester Council and another and P and Q v Surrey County Council. 2014. WLR 2. https://www.supremecourt.uk/decided-cases/docs/UKSC_2012_0068_Judgment.pdf

[113] Ministry of Justice Mental Health Casework Section. First Floor, Grenadier House, 99-105 Horseferry Road, London SW1P 2DD
Ministry of Justice Switchboard: 020 3334 3555
General: enquiry.mhu@noms.gsi.gov.uk

Recall to hospital [section 42(3) and (4)]

27.44 The Secretary of State may at any time recall a restricted patient to hospital.

27.45 This is done by a warrant, which will specify the hospital, or hospital unit, to which the patient is recalled. This can be any hospital or unit in England or Wales. In urgent cases, a direction recalling a patient may be given verbally outside office hours by a duty officer of the Ministry of Justice's Mental Health Casework Section on behalf of the Secretary of State. In practice, the warrant would then normally be provided on the next working day.

27.46 If the hospital, or unit, specified in the recall warrant is not the one from which patient was conditionally discharged, the original hospital order, hospital direction or transfer direction is then treated as if it had specified the new hospital or unit.

27.47 Once recalled, and until they are readmitted to hospital, patients are treated as if they were absent without leave from the hospital or unit specified in the recall warrant. The effect is that they may be taken into custody and taken to the hospital or unit in question, if necessary.

27.48 Like other restricted patients, patients who have been recalled to hospital from conditional discharge can only be discharged again by or with the Secretary of State's consent, or by the Tribunal.

Applications and references to the Tribunal by and in respect of recalled patients [sections 70 and 75(1)(b)]

27.49 The Secretary of State must refer the case of all recalled conditionally discharged patients to the Tribunal within one month of their return.

27.50 For most purposes, patients recalled to hospital are treated as if they were being detained for the first time. In particular, recall resets the periods during which patients may apply to the Tribunal.

27.51 The effect of this is that patients may not apply to the Tribunal until a further six months have passed from their return. They may then apply once during the six months following that, and once in each subsequent 12 month period. This applies to all types of restricted patients, even those who were able to make an application in the first six months of their original detention. As described above, all recalled patients will have had their cases referred to the Tribunal by the Secretary of State on their recall.

27.52 For the purpose of the rules on applications and references to the Tribunal, patients' 'return' means the day on which they arrive at, or are brought to, the hospital, or unit, to which they are recalled. If they are already in the hospital or unit at the time, it means the date of the recall warrant.

Ending of conditional discharge [sections 41, 42 and 75]

27.53 Conditionally discharged patients, unless they have been recalled to hospital, and are therefore detained again, cease to be subject to conditional discharge, and therefore to recall to hospital, if:

- they are absolutely discharged by the Tribunal or the Secretary of State
- the Secretary of State for Justice lifts their restrictions, or
- their restrictions expire.

27.54 The Tribunal may absolutely discharge a conditionally discharged patient at any time – see paragraph 6.28.

27.55 The Secretary of State for Justice has the discretion under the Act to lift a restriction order, limitation direction or restriction direction. The Secretary of State may do this if satisfied that the restrictions are no longer necessary for the protection of the public from serious harm.

27.56 In addition, there are certain circumstances in which a restriction order, limitation or restriction direction will expire automatically, as set out in figure 78.

Figure 78: Expiry of restrictions

<table>
<tr><th>Patient subject to</th><th>Restrictions end automatically at</th><th>Notes</th></tr>
<tr><td>Hospital order and restriction order</td><td>The end of period for which restriction order was imposed</td><td>This will only happen where the restriction order was given in England or Wales before 1 October 2007 and the court chose to give a restriction order for a fixed period, or where the patient is treated as subject to a restriction order of limited duration on transfer from an equivalent order imposed outside England or Wales</td></tr>
<tr><td>Hospital and limitation direction</td><td rowspan="2">On the patient's 'release date'</td><td rowspan="2">The release date is the date (if any) on which patients would have been entitled to be released from prison (or its equivalent) had they not been detained in hospital instead (see paragraph 16.16) or when the Parole Board direct the release of the individual</td></tr>
<tr><td>Restricted transfer direction (sentenced prisoner)</td></tr>
</table>

27.57 In practice, the same effect will sometimes result from a successful appeal against sentence.

27.58 When the Secretary of State lifts the restrictions on a conditionally discharged patient, or they expire automatically, the associated hospital order, hospital direction or transfer direction comes to an end as well. In other words, the patient is absolutely discharged and can no longer be recalled to hospital.

27.59 See chapter 21 for a description of the effect of the ending of restrictions on other restricted patients, including previously conditionally discharged patients who have been recalled to hospital.

28: Guardianship

Introduction

28.1 This chapter describes the provisions of the Act relating to guardianship. Guardianship enables patients to receive care outside hospital where it cannot be provided without the use of compulsory powers.

Guardianship – general

28.2 The Act allows applications to be made for people ('patients') to be placed under the guardianship of a guardian. The guardian may be a local authority, or an individual ('a private guardian'), such as a relative of the patient, who is approved by a local authority.

28.3 In most cases it should be possible for patients who need care, but do not need to be in hospital, to receive that care without being subject to the control of guardianship. In a minority of cases, the powers which may be exercised by the guardian, and the structure imposed by guardianship, may assist relatives, friends and professionals to help a mentally disordered person manage in the community.

Powers of guardians [section 8]

28.4 Guardians have three specific powers: residence, attendance and access.

28.5 The *residence power* allows guardians to require patients to live at a specified place. This may be used, for example, to discourage people from sleeping rough or living with people who may exploit or mistreat them, or to ensure that they reside in a particular hostel or other facility. This cannot be used to require a patient to reside with a specified person.

28.6 The *attendance power* lets guardians require the patient to attend specified places at specified times for medical treatment, occupation, education or training. This might include a day centre, or a hospital, surgery or clinic.

28.7 The *access power* means guardians may require access to the patient to be given at the place where the patient is living, to any doctor, approved mental health professional, or other specified person. This power could be used, for example, to ensure that patients do not neglect themselves.

28.8 The purpose of guardianship is primarily to ensure that the patient receives care and protection rather than medical treatment. Although guardians have powers to require patients to attend for medical treatment, they do not have any power to make them accept the treatment.

28.9 Only the residence power may be directly enforced by taking the patient to the place in question, if they don't go there voluntarily, although a person who refused to allow access to the patient without reasonable cause would be guilty of the offence of obstruction under section 129 (see chapter 33). So, in large part, the effectiveness of guardianship relies on the moral (rather than legal) authority of guardians and the quality of their relationship with the patient.

28.10 Guardians' powers are conferred on them to the exclusion of anyone else. In other words, no-one else may take a decision on these matters which goes against a decision of the guardian. In particular the Court of Protection lacks jurisdiction to determine the place of residence of a patient whilst that patient is subject to guardianship and there is a residence requirement in effect.[114]

28.11 Certain people do have the power to discharge patients from guardianship, which brings all the guardian's powers to an end. And the decisions of a guardian may be subject to judicial review by the courts.

No power to detain

28.12 Guardianship may be used to restrict patients' liberty (eg by determining where they are to live) but it may not be used to deprive them of their liberty (ie to detain them).

28.13 If it is in patients' best interests to be required to live at, or attend, a hospital or care home in which they will have to be deprived of their liberty, and they cannot make that decision for themselves, it may be necessary to obtain a deprivation of liberty authorisation under the Mental Capacity Act 2005 (MCA). If they are not eligible for such an authorisation, their detention could only be authorised by an application for admission, or a transfer from guardianship to hospital under the Act (see paragraphs 31.143 onwards).

28.14 Guardianship must not be used to impose restrictions that amount to a deprivation of liberty. The precise scope of the term 'deprivation of liberty' is not fixed. In its Cheshire West judgment[115] the Supreme Court clarified that there is a deprivation of liberty in circumstances where a person is under continuous control and supervision, is not free to leave and lacks capacity to consent to these arrangements. The Supreme Court also noted that factors which are not relevant in determining whether there is a deprivation of liberty include the person's compliance or lack of objection and the reason or purpose behind a particular placement. The relative normality of the placement (whatever the comparison made) is also not relevant. A deprivation of liberty in relation to a person who lacks capacity may be authorised by an authorisation under Schedule A1 to the Mental Capacity Act 2005 or a Court of Protection order.

---

[114] C v Blackburn and Darwen Borough Council. 2011. EWHC 3321 (COP). http://www.bailii.org/ew/cases/EWCOP/2011/3321.html

[115] P v Cheshire West and Chester Council and another and P and Q v Surrey County Council. 2014. WLR 2. http://www.bailii.org/uk/cases/UKSC/2014/19.html

Routes into guardianship

28.15 A person may become subject to guardianship:

- on the basis of an application for guardianship under part 2 of the Act ('a part 2 guardianship patient'), or
- by being given a guardianship order by a court under part 3 of the Act (a 'part 3 guardianship patient')

or because they are treated as if they were subject to one of the above on being:

- transferred from detention in hospital
- transferred from guardianship in Northern Ireland, the Channel Islands or the Isle of Man (but not Scotland) under part 6 of the Act.

The powers of guardians are the same in all cases. So, too, are the other arrangements, except where noted below.

Regulations about guardianship [section 9]

28.16 Section 9 allows the Secretary of State to make regulations about the way guardians exercise their powers and to impose other duties on private guardians and local authorities. The regulations include several such duties, described throughout this chapter.

Minimum age for guardianship [sections 7 and 37]

28.17 Patients may only be received into guardianship if they have reached the age of 16 years.

Responsible local authority [section 34(3)]

28.18 For the purposes of guardianship under the Act, the responsible local authority is the one which is named in the guardianship application or order as the guardian, or which has agreed to be treated as if it were, where a patient is transferred from outside England or Wales.

28.19 If there is a private guardian, the responsible local authority is the one for the area in which the guardian lives, whether or not the patient also lives in that area.

28.20 By definition, the identity of the responsible authority will change if the private guardian moves to another local authority's area. Otherwise, responsibility can be transferred between local authorities by a transfer under section 19 (see paragraph 31.134 onwards).

Delegation of functions by local authorities [section 23 and regulation 21]

28.21 With one exception, local authorities may delegate their functions in relation to guardianship, and under the Act generally, to any committee, officer or other body or person to whom they can normally delegate functions under the Local Government Act 2000, or the Local Government Act 1972, if relevant.

28.22 The one exception is local authorities' powers to discharge patients from guardianship. Decisions about discharge, including decisions not to discharge, may only be delegated in accordance with section 23 (see paragraphs 31.122 and 31.123).

Grounds for applications for guardianship under part 2 of the Act [section 7]

28.23 An application may be made for patients to be received into guardianship on the grounds that:

- they are suffering from mental disorder of a nature of degree which warrants their reception into guardianship, and
- it is necessary in the interests of their welfare, or for the protection of other persons.

28.24 Here, and in the remainder of this chapter, mental disorder does not include a learning disability unless it is associated with abnormally aggressive or seriously irresponsible conduct on the part of the patient concerned.

Making an application for guardianship [sections 7 and 11 and regulations 3 and 5]

28.25 An application may be made by the patient's nearest relative using form G1, or by an approved mental health professional (AMHP) acting on behalf of a local authority using form G2.

28.26 The most appropriate applicant is usually the AMHP rather than the nearest relative. In practice, applications by a nearest relative are rare.

28.27 The application must state who is to be the guardian, ie the name of a proposed private guardian, or the local authority. If there is to be a private guardian, the application must be accompanied by a written statement by the proposed private guardian confirming they are willing to be the guardian. In practice, this statement should be included in the part 2 of form G1 or G2, depending on which is appropriate.

28.28 The application must state the age of the patient. If applicants do not know the patient's exact age, they must state that they believe the patient to be at least 16 years old.

28.29 An application must be made to the local authority which is named as guardian. If there is to be a private guardian, it should be made to the local authority for the area in which the proposed guardian lives, whether or not the patient also lives in that area.

28.30 Applications must be delivered to the local authority itself, delivered to a person authorised by the local authority to receive it on the local authority 's behalf, sent by post to the local authority at its principal office or else, if the local authority agrees, be sent using the local authority 's internal mail system.

Local authority's duty to arrange for AMHP to consider making application [section 13]

28.31 Local authorities must arrange for an AMHP to consider a case on their behalf, if they have reason to believe that a guardianship application may need to be made in respect of a patient within their area.

28.32 AMHPs may make an application outside the area of the local authority on whose behalf they are acting. This might be appropriate if, for example, patients are temporarily being accommodated outside their home area.

AMHPs' duty to consult nearest relatives and nearest relatives' right to object [section 11]

28.33 A guardianship application cannot be made if the patient's nearest relative objects to it. The nearest relative may either lodge an objection directly with the AMHP, or with the local authority on behalf of which the AMHP is considering the patient's case. The objection does not have to be made in any particular form, provided it is clearly an objection to the proposed application being made, that patient's detention is unlawful, which can give rise to a claim for compensation.

28.34 The AMHP must consider whether, on an objective basis, there is an objection to the application. For example, should a nearest relative have objected recently, that may indicate there remains an objection to detention.

28.35 An AMHP must therefore try to consult the person (if any) who appears to be the nearest relative before making the application. Case law has established that consultation with the nearest relative can precede the obtaining of the two medical recommendations which are required for the application[116] and in suitable circumstances the approved mental health professional can carry out the duty to consult through the medium of another person.[117] The AMHP needs to provide the nearest relative with sufficient information for that person to form an opinion, and should outline to them their rights under the Act.

---

[116] Re Whitbread (Times Law Report) 14 July 1997.

[117] R v South Western Hospital Managers, ex p. M. 1994. 1 All ER 161; and B v Cygnet Healthcare. 2008. EWHC 1259 (Admin). http://www.bailii.org/ew/cases/EWHC/Admin/2008/1259.html

28.36 AMHPs do not have to consult the nearest relative if, in the circumstances, they think it is not reasonably practicable or that it would involve unreasonable delay. For practical reasons, it may not always be possible to identify, locate and contact the nearest relative within a reasonable time. But it will also not be reasonably practicable to consult with the nearest relative where – in all the circumstances – the detrimental impact of that consultation on the patient's rights under article 8 of the European Convention on Human Rights to privacy and family life would not be justified and proportionate. Consultation with the nearest relative that interferes with the patient's article 8 rights may be justified to protect the patient's article 5 rights.[118]

28.37 If the nearest relative objects, the AMHP cannot make the application. An unreasonable objection by a nearest relative is one of the grounds in section 29(3) for the county court, on application, to transfer the powers of the nearest relative to another person (see chapter 2).

Duty of AMHPs to make applications in certain cases [section 13]

28.38 As with applications for admission to hospital, AMHPs must make an application if they think that an application ought to be made and that, taking into account the views of the relatives and any other relevant circumstances, they think that it necessary and proper for them to make the application, rather than the nearest relative. This does not affect the rules about consultation with nearest relatives described above or the powers of nearest relatives to object to an application.

Medical recommendations [section 12 and mutual recognition regulations]

28.39 Like applications for admission for hospital, a guardianship application must be supported by written recommendations from two doctors who have personally examined the patient, see figure 79:

Figure 79: Medical recommendations for guardianship

One doctor	Other doctor
Approved under section 12	If the doctor approved under section 12 does not have previous acquaintance with the patient: if practical, a doctor who has previous acquaintance with the patient
	Otherwise: any doctor

[118] TW v Enfield Borough Council. 2014. EWCA Civ 362. http://www.bailii.org/ew/cases/EWCA/Civ/2014/362.html

28.40 Doctors are approved under section 12 if they have been approved as such on behalf of the Secretary of State (or the Welsh Ministers) as having special experience in the diagnosis or treatment of mental disorder. Doctors who are approved clinicians are automatically treated as being approved under section 12. See chapter 30 for more information on approvals.

28.41 At least one of the doctors should, if practicable, have had previous acquaintance with the patient. Preferably this doctor should know the patient personally, but case law has established that previous acquaintance need not involve personal acquaintance, provided the doctor in question has some knowledge of the patient and is not 'coming to them cold'.[119]

28.42 The medical recommendations must state that, in the doctors' opinion, the grounds for making the application described in paragraph 31.21 are met, and must in particular explain why guardianship is necessary for the patient's welfare or the protection of other people.

28.43 Recommendations may be made separately by each doctor using form G4, or as a joint recommendation signed by both using form G3.

28.44 If doctors making recommendations have examined the patient in Wales they must use the equivalent Welsh form on which to make their recommendations. If doctors are making a joint recommendation, and one of them examined the patient in England and one in Wales, then they may use either the English or Welsh forms.

28.45 Applications to local authorities in Wales must be made in accordance with the Welsh regulations, which will always involve using a Welsh application form.

Conflicts of interest [sections 11(1) and 12A and Conflict of Interest regulations]

28.46 AMHPs may not make an application if they have a potential conflict of interest as defined in the Act and described in figure 37. These rules are essentially the same as those for applications for admission to hospital (see chapter 11).

28.47 Similarly, doctors may not give a medical recommendation if they have a potential conflict of interest, as described in figure 38.

28.48 An application which relied on a recommendation made by a doctor who had a potential conflict of interest would again be invalid.

28.49 One of the effects of this is that three professionals involved in an application may not all be in the same clinical team, nor may any of the professionals

[119] AR (by her litigation friend JT) v Bronglais Hospital and Pembrokeshire and Derwen NHS Trust, 2001. EWHC Admin 792.

involved be in the same clinical team as the patient. This rule does not apply if the AMHP or doctor concerned thinks that it is of urgent necessity that an application be made and a delay would involve serious risk to the health or safety of the patient or others. In other words, in urgent cases it is possible for all three professionals to be from the same clinical team, or for any or all of them to be from the same clinical team as the patient.

Time limits for guardianship applications [sections 4, 6, 11 and 12]

28.50 Certain time limits apply in respect of applications, as set out in the figure 80.

Figure 80: Time limits in respect of guardianship applications

Action	Time limit	Example
Application	The applicant must personally have seen the patient within the period of 14 days ending on the day of the application.	If the applicant last saw the patient on 1 January, the application must be signed on or before 14 January.
Examination for purposes of medical recommendation for application	No more than five clear days must have elapsed between the days on which the separate examinations took place (where relevant).	If the first doctor examined the patient on 1 January, the second doctor's examination must take place on or before 7 January.
Medical recommendations in support of applications	Must be signed on or before the day of application.	If the application is signed by the nearest relative or AMHP at noon on 1 January, the medical recommendations must be signed by the doctors concerned before midnight on that day.
Application forwarded (ie sent) to the relevant local authority	Within the period of 14 days starting with the day on which the patient was last examined by a doctor for the purposes of the application.	If the patient was last examined on 1 January, the application must be sent to the local authority by the end of 14 January.

Acceptance of guardianship applications by local authorities [section 8 and regulation 5]

28.51 To be effective, the application must be accepted by the local authority to which it is sent, either on its own behalf or on behalf of the proposed private guardian. The local authority does not have to accept an application.

28.52 For an application to be accepted and confer powers on the guardian, it must be duly made in accordance with the Act and be sent to the local authority within the period of 14 days described in figure 80. An application may be acted on if it appears to be 'duly made' and founded on the necessary medical recommendations.

28.53 A document cannot be regarded as a proper application or medical recommendation if, for example:

- an application is not accompanied by the correct number of medical recommendations
- the application and the recommendations do not all relate to the same patient
- an application or recommendation is not signed at all, or is signed by someone not qualified to do so, or
- an application does not specify who is proposed to be the guardian.

28.54 Like hospital managers, local authorities do not have to seek further proof that the signatories are who they say they are, or that they have the qualification to make the application which they have signed to say they have. Nor need they seek further proof for any factual statement or opinion contained in the document.

28.55 If an application is discovered to be fundamentally flawed because of an error such as the kind set out above, there is no authority for the patient's guardianship because fundamentally defective applications cannot be retrospectively validated. In these circumstances, a new application would have to be made.

28.56 Any new application must, of course, be accompanied by medical recommendations which comply with the Act. This does not exclude the possibility of one of the two existing medical recommendations being used if the time limits and other provisions of the Act can still be complied with.

28.57 If it accepts an application, the local authority must record its acceptance using form G5, which must then be attached to the application.

28.58 If the application is accepted, the patient is received into the guardianship of the local authority or the private guardian (as applicable), and the guardian acquires the powers of residence, attendance and access described above.

Rectification of errors in guardianship applications [section 8(4)]

28.59 As with applications for admission to hospital, unless they fundamentally invalidate the application, less serious problems with applications and recommendations may be capable of being rectified and patients may continue to be subject to guardianship for a limited period while an error capable of rectification is corrected.

28.60 Faults which may be capable of rectification include the leaving blank of any spaces on the form which should have been filled in, other than the signature, or failure to delete one or more alternatives in places where the alternatives are mutually exclusive.

28.61 An application or recommendation which is found to be incorrect or defective may be amended by the person who signed it, with the consent of the local authority. In practice, if the local authority is content for the document to be amended, it should be returned to the person who signed it for amendment. Consent to the amendment should then formally be given by the local authority. The consent should be recorded in writing and can take the form of an endorsement on the document itself. If this is all done within a period of 14 days starting with the day on which the application was accepted the documents are deemed to have had effect as though originally made as amended.

28.62 If more than 14 days have elapsed from the day the application was accepted a minor mistake would not invalidate an application (a 'de minimis' mistake). If there is a fundamental error, the application should be discharged and, if appropriate, a new application made.

28.63 Unlike applications for admission to hospital, there is no procedure for obtaining a new medical recommendation if the ones that come with the application originally prove insufficient. In that case, a new application would have to be made.

Guardianship orders [section 37]

28.64 A court may make a guardianship order under part 3 in the circumstances set out in figure 81. Section 40(2) means that the effect is to make the patient subject to the guardianship of the local authority, or a person approved by a local authority, named in the order.

Figure 81: Criteria for guardianship orders

<table>
<tr><th colspan="3">Guardianship order (section 37)</th></tr>
<tr><td>May be made by</td><td colspan="2">a magistrates' court or the Crown Court</td></tr>
<tr><td rowspan="2">respect of a person who is aged 16 or over and who is</td><td>where made by a magistrates' court</td><td>where made by the Crown Court</td></tr>
<tr><td>convicted by that court of an offence punishable (in the case of an adult) on summary conviction with custody

or

charged before (but not convicted by) that court with such an offence, if the court is satisfied that the person did the act or made the omission charged</td><td>convicted before that court for an offence punishable with imprisonment (other than murder)</td></tr>
<tr><td>if the court is satisfied</td><td colspan="2">on the written or oral evidence of two doctors, at least one of whom must be approved under section 12, that the offender is 16 or over, and is suffering from mental disorder of a nature or degree which warrants the offender's reception into guardianship under the Act</td></tr>
<tr><td>and the court is of the opinion</td><td colspan="2">having regard to all the circumstances including the nature of the offence and the character and antecedents of the offender, and to the other available methods of dealing with the offender, that a guardianship order is the most suitable method of dealing with the case</td></tr>
<tr><td>and it is also satisfied</td><td colspan="2">that the local authority or proposed private guardian is willing to receive the offender into guardianship</td></tr>
</table>

28.65 The requirement that at least one of the doctors who gives evidence must be approved under section 12 is to be found in section 54(1) rather than section 37 itself.

28.66 As with hospital orders (see chapter 15), the court may not, at the same time as making a guardianship order in respect of an offender, pass a custodial sentence, impose a fine, or impose a community sentence.

28.67 Nor may it make an order for a young offender's parent or guardian to enter into a recognizance to take proper care of and exercise proper control over the offender. But otherwise the court may make any other order which it has the power to make, eg an order for compensation.

28.68 In practice, if the doctors giving evidence wish to recommend guardianship, they should consult the local authority for the offender's home area. It will be for the local authority to inform the court whether it is prepared to act as guardian.

28.69 If a private guardian is proposed, the local authority will need to inform the court that it has approved the proposed guardian and send the court a statement signed by that person confirming their willingness to act as guardian.

28.70 Courts can also make guardianship orders by virtue of certain other pieces of legislation (see chapter 22).

Duty on local authorities to provide information to the court [section 39A]

28.71 A local authority must comply with a request from a court in England or Wales to inform it whether the local authority, or another person approved by the local authority, is willing to receive an offender into guardianship and to explain, to the extent it reasonably can, how the powers conferred by the guardianship could be expected to be used.

Effect of a guardianship application or order on previous applications etc [sections 8(5), 40(5), 41(4) and 55(4)]

28.72 The acceptance of a guardianship application or the making of a guardianship order causes any previous application for admission to hospital, for assessment or treatment, any previous guardianship application to cease to have effect. In addition, the making of a guardianship order causes any previous unrestricted hospital order, unrestricted hospital direction, unrestricted transfer direction, or guardianship order to cease to have effect. It does not bring a restricted hospital order, hospital and limitation directions or a restricted transfer direction to an end.

28.73 Sometimes previous applications, orders and directions may be revived, if a guardianship order, or the convictions on which it is based, is quashed on appeal. In those cases, patients are treated as if they had been sent to prison on the day the order was made and the previous application, order or direction was still in force on that day. This means that in certain circumstances, if the patient has been subject to the guardianship order for no longer than six months, any previous application, order or direction to which they were subject will be revived – see paragraph 31.88.

28.74 Where reception into guardianship brings an application, order or direction for detention to an end, it will automatically also mean that a patient who has been discharged from that application, order or direction onto a community treatment order ceases to be a CTO patient.

Duty of private guardian to appoint nominated medical attendant [section 9(2) and regulation 22]

28.75 A private guardian must appoint a doctor to act as the patient's 'nominated medical attendant' who will care for the patient's general health and determine whether the criteria are met for renewing or confirming the patient's guardianship – see paragraph 31.92 onward.

Responsible clinician [section 34(1) and mutual recognition regulations]

28.76 Patients under the guardianship of local authorities do not have a nominated medical attendant. Local authorities need to appoint responsible clinicians to determine whether the criteria are met for renewing or confirming the patient's guardianship, as necessary.

28.77 Responsible clinicians must be approved clinicians, but otherwise it is for the responsible local authority to decide who is to act as the responsible clinician, either generally for a particular patient, or on a specific occasion or for a specific purpose.

28.78 Responsible clinicians – but not nominated medical attendants – are also amongst the people who have the authority to discharge patients from guardianship (see paragraph 31.120). Local authorities may appoint a responsible clinician for that purpose even for a patient who also has a nominated medical attendant.

28.79 If the patient happens to be living, or receiving medical treatment for mental disorder, in Wales, the local authority may appoint a person who is approved by the Welsh Ministers as an approved clinician in Wales, even if that person is not also approved as an approved clinician in England. Otherwise, the responsible clinician must be approved as an approved clinician in England.

Other duties of a private guardian [regulation 22]

28.80 Private guardians must comply with any directions given to them by the responsible local authority about the way they carry out their functions in that role under the Act or the regulations.

28.81 They must inform the responsible local authority of the name and address of the nominated medical attendant they have appointed.

28.82 When a patient is first received into their guardianship, they must inform the responsible local authority of their own address and the address of the patient. If either address is to change permanently they must inform the responsible local authority either before, or no later than seven days after, the change occurs.

28.83 If guardians themselves move to the area of another local authority, which therefore becomes the responsible local authority, they must not only inform that local authority of the change of address, but also the address of the patient and the name and address of the patient's nominated medical attendant, whether or not those details have changed. They must inform the local authority which was the responsible local authority until the move.

28.84 Guardians must also inform the responsible local authority as soon as reasonably practicable if the patient dies, or the guardianship comes to an end for any other reason.

28.85 In addition to the normal ways in which documents may be served under the regulations (see paragraph 1.49), local authorities may agree to private guardians using any other form of communication to give them information and reports required by the regulations. That can include giving the information orally (eg by telephone) or by electronic means (eg email).

Information for guardianship patients and their nearest relatives about discharge and the Tribunal [regulation 26]

28.86 When patients are received into guardianship, the responsible local authority must take whatever steps are reasonably practicable to ensure that they are informed of

- their rights, and where relevant the rights of their nearest relative, to apply to the Tribunal for their discharge – see chapter 6, and
- where relevant, the right of their nearest relative to discharge them from guardianship (see paragraph 31.118).

This should be done orally and in writing.

28.87 Whatever steps are reasonably practicable must also be taken to ensure that the person the local authority thinks is the patient's nearest relative is given the same information in writing, unless the patient has requested otherwise, or does not have a nearest relative. Information given to nearest relatives and private guardians must be in writing, but may be communicated by electronic means (eg email) if the nearest relative agrees.

Information about independent mental health advocacy for guardianship patients [section 130D]

28.88 The local authority must take steps to have patients subject to guardianship told about independent mental health advocacy. Local authorities also have a duty to take steps to give the same information to the person they think is the patient's nearest relative, unless the patient has requested otherwise, or does not have a nearest relative. This should be done as soon as practicable after the patient becomes subject to guardianship (see chapter 4 for further details).

Visits to guardianship patients [regulation 23 and mutual recognition regulations]

28.89 Responsible local authorities must arrange for patients subject to guardianship (whether of the local authority or a private guardian) to be visited on their behalf at intervals of no more than three months. At least one visit each year must be made by a doctor approved for the purposes of section 12 (in England or Wales) or by an approved clinician (approved in England). Local authorities also have a duty to arrange visits to people who are under their guardianship when they are in hospital or care home (see paragraph 31.151).

Absence without leave [section 18]

28.90 Patients who go absent without the guardian's permission from any place the guardian has required them to live are considered to be absent without leave (AWOL).

28.91 A patient who is AWOL in this way may be taken into custody under section 18(3) and returned to that place by any officer on the staff of any local authority, any police officer, or other constable, or any person authorised in writing by the patient's guardian or any local authority.

28.92 But this can only be done during the period before:

- the current period of guardianship expires, ignoring any extra time that would be allowed if the patient were to return or be taken into custody right at the end of that period – see paragraph 31.98, or
- the end of the six months starting with the first day of the absence without leave, if that is later.

28.93 For these purposes, the fact that the responsible clinician has already made a report renewing the guardianship (see paragraph 28.96) is irrelevant unless the renewed period of guardianship has already started when the patient goes absent.

28.94 Within the same time limits, these powers can also be used to take patients to the place they are required to live if they do not go there of their own accord in the first place.

28.95 If patients are taken into custody, or come voluntarily to the place they are required to live, after being AWOL for more than 28 days, ie on or after 29 January if the patient goes AWOL on 1 January, their guardianship expires at the end of the week starting with the day of their arrival at the place they are required to live unless it is confirmed by the nominated medical attendant (if there is one) or the responsible clinician (if there is not) (see paragraph 31.104).

Expiry and renewal of authority for guardianship [section 20(3) and regulations 13 and 26]

28.96 Guardianship lasts initially for six months starting with the day the patient was received into guardianship, ie when the guardianship application was accepted, or the guardianship order made, as the case may be. It can be renewed for a further six months, and then for a year at a time.

28.97 At some point during the final two months of the first and each subsequent period of guardianship, the nominated medical attendant (if there is one) or the responsible clinician (if there is not) must examine the patient in order to decide whether patient meets the criteria for renewal.

28.98 The criteria for renewal are that the patient:

- is suffering from mental disorder of a nature of degree which warrants reception into guardianship, and
- it is necessary in the interests of the patient's welfare, or for the protection of other persons, that the patient should remain under guardianship.

28.99 If nominated medical attendants or responsible clinicians think the conditions are met, they must submit a report to that effect using form G9 to both the local authority and the private guardian (if there is one).

28.100 The effect of the report is to renew the authority for guardianship detention for a further six months or a year (as applicable) from the date it would otherwise expire, not the date of the report itself.

28.101 The local authority must record its receipt of the report in part 2 of the same form G9. Unless the local authority decides to discharge the patient (see paragraph 31.122), it must arrange for the patient to be told about the renewal. It must also take reasonable steps to arrange for the person the local authority thinks is the patient's nearest relative to be informed as soon as practicable after its decision, unless the patient has requested otherwise, or does not have a nearest relative. Information given to nearest relatives must be in writing, but may be communicated by electronic means (eg email) if the nearest relative agrees.

Patients absent without leave as deadline for renewal report approaches [section 21 and 21A]

28.102 Special arrangements apply if patients are at any point during the week which ends on the day their current period of guardianship is due to expire, and a renewal report has yet to be made.

28.103 If patients have not been taken into custody under the Act, or do not come voluntarily to the place they are required to live, before the end of the period during which they can be taken into custody under section 18 (see paragraph 31.87), their period of guardianship expires, and no renewal report can be made.

28.104 If patients are taken into custody under section 18, or come to the relevant place voluntarily, within 28 days of absconding their guardianship is treated as not expiring until the end of the week starting with the day they arrive back at the place they are required to reside.

28.105 The responsible clinician or nominated medical attendant (as applicable) therefore has a week from the day of the patient's arrival at the place they are required to live to submit the report to the local authority (and, if relevant, the private guardian). So, if the patient arrives on Monday, the responsible clinician has until the end of the following Sunday to submit the report.

28.106 If patients are taken into custody, or come voluntarily to the relevant place, within the 28 days starting with the day they went AWOL (ie before the end of 28 January, if they went AWOL on 1 January), the report renewing their guardianship is to be made in the normal way under section 20 (see paragraph 31.93 onward)

28.107 If patients are taken into custody, or come voluntarily to the relevant place after more than 28 days, it is not normally necessary to make a report under section 20. That is because the patient's guardianship has anyway to be confirmed by a report under section 21B, and that report can also serve as a renewal report in place of a report under section 20 (see paragraph 31.108 onwards).

Confirmation of guardianship of patients who have been absent without leave for more than 28 days [section 21B and regulations 14 and 26]

28.108 Where patients are taken into custody, or come voluntarily to the place they are required to live, after being absent for more than 28 days, their nominated medical attendant or responsible clinician (as applicable) must examine them and, if appropriate, submit a report using form G10 to the responsible local authority confirming that the criteria for continued guardianship are met. This must be done within one week beginning with the day on which the patient is returned or returns himself to the place where he ought to be.

28.109 The criteria for continued guardianship are the same as the criteria for renewing guardianship (see paragraph 31.84).

28.110 Responsible clinicians and nominated medical attendants must submit a report, using form G10, during this period if they think that the conditions are met.

28.111 The local authority must record its receipt of the report in part 2 of the same form G10.

28.112 Unless such a report is sent to the local authority, patients' guardianship expires automatically at the end of the week starting with the day on which they arrive back at the place they are required to reside.

28.113 A report made under this procedure will renew the patient's guardianship if it would already have expired had the patient not gone absent, or if it would expire on the day the report is submitted. The local authority must take reasonable steps to inform the patient of this. It must also take such steps to inform the person it thinks is the nearest relative, unless the patient has requested otherwise (or does not have a nearest relative). The local authority must also inform the private guardian (if there is one) as soon as practicable. Information given to nearest relatives and private guardians must be in writing, but may be communicated by electronic means (eg email) if the recipient agrees.

28.114 In addition, if the patient's guardianship is due to expire during the period of two months starting with the day on which the report is given to the managers, the clinician making the report may (but need not) indicate on the form that it is to act as any renewal report which would otherwise have to be made under section 20 during that period. Unless it decides to discharge the patient (see paragraph 19.122), the local authority must take the normal steps to inform the patient and (where relevant) the nearest relative, in the same way as if it were a report under section 20 itself (see paragraph 19.97). The local authority must also inform the private guardian (if there is one) as soon as practicable.

Patients who return from absence without leave and whose guardianship would otherwise have expired [section 21A and 21B and regulation 26]

28.115 In some cases, the responsible clinician's report under section 20 or 21B renewing the guardianship of a patient who has been AWOL will be submitted on or after the day the old period of guardianship was originally due to expire. If so, that report is treated as having retrospectively renewed the guardianship from the end of the old period of guardianship in the normal way.

28.116 In the rare circumstances where the patient's guardianship would otherwise have expired twice since they went AWOL, the responsible clinician's report under section 21B is treated as having renewed the guardianship on both occasions.

28.117 If a patient's guardianship is renewed retrospectively (either once or twice) in this way, the responsible local authority must take whatever steps are reasonably practicable to arrange for the patient to be told about the renewal. They must also take such steps to arrange for the person they think is the nearest relative to be informed, unless the patient has requested otherwise (or does not have a nearest relative).

28.118 The patient must be told of the retrospective renewal both orally and in writing. Information given to nearest relatives must be in writing, but may be communicated by electronic means (eg email) if the nearest relative agrees.

Patients who are imprisoned etc [section 22]

28.119 Special rules apply to patients who are imprisoned, remanded or otherwise detained in custody by any court in the UK while subject to guardianship.

28.120 Such patients automatically cease to be liable to guardianship if they remain in prison (or the equivalent) for longer than six months in total. If they are released during that six month period, they are treated as if they had gone AWOL on the day of their release, except that they may be retaken only during the 28 days starting with that day.

28.121 Because they are treated as AWOL, if their guardianship would otherwise have expired, or is about to expire, it will not in fact expire until the end of the week starting with the day of the patient's return to the place they are required to live (provided that the patient is taken into custody or returns voluntarily during the 28 day period allowed). So if the guardianship is otherwise due to expire, nominated medical attendants and responsible clinicians (as applicable) will always have at least a week from the patient's return in which to examine the patient and submit a report renewing the patient's guardianship (if appropriate) under section 20.

Discharge of part 2 guardianship patients by their nearest relatives [section 23]

28.122 A nearest relative may discharge a part 2 guardianship patient at any time by serving a written order to that effect on the responsible local authority. The order cannot be barred and there is no need for nearest relatives to give prior notice of their intention. Nearest relatives cannot discharge part 3 guardianship patients. They do have certain rights to apply to the Tribunal instead (see chapter 6).

Visiting and examination of patients in relation to use of powers of discharge [section 24)]

28.123 Any doctor or approved clinician may be authorised by a nearest relative to visit and examine a patient in order to advise on the use of the nearest relative's power of discharge. These authorised doctors and approved clinicians may visit and examine the patient in private at any time, and (if applicable) require any records relating to the patient's detention or treatment in any hospital, or relating to after-care services provided for the patient under section 117, to be produced for their inspection. A person who refuses, without reasonable cause, to let an authorised doctor or approved clinician see a patient in private, or inspect any relevant records would be guilty of the offence of obstruction under section 129 (see chapter 33).

Discharge by the responsible clinician [section 23 and regulation 18]

28.124 Responsible clinicians may discharge patients at any time, by making a written order. The order must be sent to the guardian (whether a local authority or a private guardian) as soon as practicable after it is made (but it does not have to have been sent to the managers to be effective).

28.125 A nominated medical attendant does not have the authority to discharge a patient. Nor does a private guardian.

Discharge by the local authority [section 23]

28.126 The responsible local authority may discharge patients at any time by making a written order. It must always consider doing so when a report is made renewing the authority for detention (see paragraphs 31.101 and 31.114).

28.127 The decision may be taken on behalf of the local authority by any three or more members of the authority or of a committee or subcommittee the local authority authorises for the purpose. Those three people must be unanimous in their decision to discharge. If the decision is taken by more than three people, as well as a majority in favour, that majority must consist of at least three people in favour of discharge before a decision to discharge can be made.[120]

Discharge by the Tribunal [part 5]

28.128 Patients may also be discharged by the First-tier Tribunal (or the Upper Tribunal on appeal). For information on this, and an explanation of the rights of patients and nearest relatives to apply to the Tribunal, see chapter 6.

Guardian no longer willing or able to act as such [section 10(1) and regulation 26]

28.129 Private guardians may resign the role by notifying the responsible local authority in writing. If so, the local authority becomes the guardian, and the guardianship application or order is deemed to have named the local authority as the guardian all along. The patient is not received into guardianship anew for the purposes of calculating when guardianship needs to be renewed and such like.

28.130 The same applies if the private guardian dies.

28.131 In either case, the local authority must take whatever steps are reasonably practicable to inform the person it thinks is the patient's nearest relative, unless the patient has requested otherwise, or does not have a nearest relative. This must be done either before the transfer or as soon as practicable afterwards. Information given to nearest relatives must be in writing, but may be communicated by electronic means (eg email) if the nearest relative agrees.

---

[120] R (Tagoe-Thompson) v The Hospital Managers of the Park Royal Centre. 2003. EWCA Civ 330. http://www.bailii.org/ew/cases/EWCA/Civ/2003/330.html

Temporary guardians [section 10(2) and regulation 26]

28.132 The responsible local authority, or any person authorised by them, may act temporarily on behalf of a private guardian who is incapacitated by illness or any other reason and unable to perform the functions of guardian as a result.

28.133 If this happens, the local authority must take whatever steps are reasonably practicable to inform the person it thinks is the patient's nearest relative, unless the patient has requested otherwise, or does not have a nearest relative. This must be done either before the temporary change of guardian or as soon as practicable afterwards. Information given to nearest relatives must be in writing, but may be communicated by electronic means (eg email) if the nearest relative agrees.

28.134 The authority or person temporarily acting as guardian in these cases acts as an agent for the permanent guardian and may not go against any wishes or instructions the permanent guardian may express.

28.135 While these temporary arrangements are in place, the guardianship application or order is deemed to have named the temporary guardian all along.

Unsatisfactory private guardians [sections 10(3) and 31]

28.136 Responsible local authorities may not insist that a private guardian relinquish the position. An AMHP, acting on behalf of the responsible local authority, may make an application to the county court for the guardianship to be transferred. Proceedings in the county court are governed by the Civil Procedure Rules. The Act refers to these as the 'County Court Rules'.

28.137 If the court thinks that a private guardian has performed the role negligently or contrary to the interests of the patient, it may order the guardianship to be transferred to the local authority or any other person approved for the purpose by the local authority. The guardianship application or order is then treated as if it had always named the new guardian.

Transfers between guardians in other cases [section 19 and regulations 8 and 26]

28.138 The guardianship of a patient may be transferred to a new guardian if:

- the current guardian gives authority for the transfer using form G7
- the local authority which will be the responsible local authority after the transfer (which might be the current local authority if the transfer is to a private guardian) approves the transfer, and specifies a date for the transfer to take place, and
- if the new guardian is to a private guardian, the new guardian signs the form to record his or her agreement.

28.139 The guardianship application or order is treated as if it had always named the new guardian. Immediately after the transfer, a new private guardian must appoint a nominated medical attendant and notify the authority of the nominated medical attendant's name and address and the address at which the patient lives (as described in paragraph 31.82).

28.140 The new responsible local authority must take whatever steps are reasonably practicable to inform the person it thinks is the patient's nearest relative of the transfer as soon as practicable, unless the patient has requested otherwise, or does not have a nearest relative. This must be done before the transfer or as soon as practicable afterwards. Information given to nearest relatives must be in writing, but may be communicated by electronic means (eg email) if the nearest relative agrees.

Transfer from hospital to guardianship [section 19 and regulation 26]

28.141 Patients may also be transferred to guardianship from detention in hospital, with the agreement of the responsible local authority and, where relevant, the proposed private guardian (see paragraph 10.34 onward). On transfer, part 2 patients are treated as if subject to a guardianship application accepted on the day they were admitted to hospital on the basis of the application to which they were subject immediately before the transfer. Part 3 patients are treated as if subject to a guardianship order made on the same day as the order or direction to which they were previously subject.

28.142 If such a transfer happens, the responsible local authority must take whatever steps are reasonably practicable to inform the person it thinks is the patient's nearest relative of the transfer before or as soon as possible afterward, unless the patient has requested otherwise (or does not have a nearest relative). Information given to nearest relatives must be in writing, but may be communicated by electronic means (eg email) if the recipient agrees.

28.143 The responsible local authority has the same duties to give patients transferred to guardianship, and their nearest relatives, information about their rights and about advocacy as it has in relation to other patients newly received into guardianship (see paragraphs 31.86 and 31.87).

Admissions to hospital of patients subject to guardianship [section 6(4), 37(4) and 40(4)]

28.144 Patients subject to guardianship can be admitted to hospital in the same way as anyone else, without having to be detained under the Act. Likewise, they may also be detained under the Act on the basis of an application for admission under part 2 like anyone else, but there is also a specific procedure for transfer from guardianship to hospital (see paragraph 31.147).

28.145 Part 2 guardianship patients cease to be subject to guardianship if they are detained on the basis of an application for treatment under section 3, where there is an ineffective section 3 application, which has been found unlawful, the court has indicated it would not undermine the section 2 application that preceded it, though the court did not decide the point. Guardianship patients remain subject to guardianship if they are detained on the basis of an application for admission for assessment under section 2 or 4.

28.146 Both part 2 and part 3 guardianship patients cease to be subject to guardianship if they are given a hospital order, hospital direction or a transfer direction, subject to the rules on what happens if a hospital order or hospital direction is quashed on appeal (see paragraph 15.37).

Transfer of patients from guardianship to detention in hospital [regulation 8]

28.147 Instead of an application for admission for detention for treatment, it is also possible for the responsible local authority to authorise the transfer of a guardianship patient to detention in hospital using form G8.

28.148 Before the responsible local authority can authorise a transfer to hospital:

- an AMHP acting on behalf of a local authority must make an application that would otherwise have to be made under section 3, using the normal form A6 and following the normal rules
- that application must be supported by two medical recommendations which could be used to support an application under section 3, using the normal forms A7 or A8, or – where applicable – the equivalent Welsh forms
- the application must be accepted by the managers of the hospital to which the patient is to be admitted, and a record of admission should be made in part 2 of form G8, and
- the responsible local authority must be satisfied that arrangements have been made for the patient's admission to that hospital within the period of 14 days starting with the day the patient was last examined for the purposes of one of the medical recommendations in support of the application.

28.149 When these conditions are met, the authorisation provides the authority for an officer of the local authority or any person authorised by the local authority to convey the patient to the hospital in which the patient is to be detained. The authority lasts only until the end of the 14 days starting with the day on which the patient was last examined by a doctor for the purposes of one of the medical recommendations above.

28.150 Patients being conveyed to hospital in these circumstances are considered to be in legal custody (see chapter 23).

28.151 Transferred patients cease to be subject to guardianship when admitted to hospital. A part 2 guardianship patient is then treated as if admitted on the basis of an application for admission for treatment on the day the guardianship application was originally accepted. A part 3 guardianship patient is treated as if the guardianship order was instead a hospital order given on the same date as the guardianship order was originally given.

Transfers from England to Wales – applicable regulations [section 19 and regulation 10]

28.152 The arrangements described in paragraphs 10.5 onwards apply to transfers within England and from Wales to England.

28.153 Transfers to Wales are governed instead by the equivalent Welsh regulations, the details of which differ in some respects. A transfer is a transfer to Wales if:

- the effect of the transfer is that there will be new responsible local authority and that new responsible local authority is in Wales, or
- the patient is to be transferred to detention in a hospital in Wales.

28.154 Refer to guidance issued by the Welsh Assembly Government for details of what is required by the Welsh regulations.

Local authority visits to patients under their guardianship in hospitals or care homes [section 116]

28.155 Local authorities have a duty to arrange visits to patients who are under their guardianship when they are in hospital or a care home, whether or not they are there to receive treatment or care for mental disorder. Local authorities must also 'take such other steps in relation to the patient while in the [hospital or care home] as would be expected to be taken by [the patient's] parents'.

29: After-care

Introduction

29.1 This chapter describes the provisions in the Act requiring the NHS and local authorities to provide after-care for certain patients who have been detained. This chapter should be read in conjunction with chapters 33 and 34 of the Code of Practice on after-care and the 'care programme approach'. The ultimate aim of after-care is to maintain patients in the community, with as few restrictions as are necessary, wherever possible.

Duty to provide after-care services [section 117(2) and (6)]

29.2 Section 117 places a duty on clinical commissioning groups (CCGs) to arrange for the provision of, and local authorities to provide or arrange for the provision of, after-care for certain patients who have been detained under the Act once they leave hospital. These bodies are known collectively in this chapter as the 'responsible after-care bodies'.

29.3 After-care services are defined in the Act to mean services which have both of the following purposes: meeting a need arising from or related to the person's mental disorder; and reducing the risk of a deterioration of the person's mental condition and, accordingly, reducing the risk of the person requiring admission to a hospital again for treatment for mental disorder. After-care can encompass healthcare, social care and employment services, supported accommodation and services to meet the person's wider social, cultural and spiritual needs. Where a local authority is providing or arranging for accommodation of a type specified in the Care and Support and After-care (choice of accommodation) Regulations 2014[121] and a person expresses a preference for particular accommodation, then the local authority must provide or arrange for that accommodation under section 117A, provided that conditions prescribed in those regulations are met. If the preferred accommodation costs more than the amount the local authority would expect to be the usual cost of accommodation of that kind, then that additional cost needs to be met by the person receiving the care or another person.

29.4 The responsible after-care bodies are required to arrange or provide after-care services 'in cooperation with relevant voluntary agencies'. CCGs will, and local authorities may, commission services from other people and organisations instead of providing services themselves.

Eligible patients [section 117(1)]

29.5 The patients eligible for after-care under section 117 are set out in figure 82.

[121] Care and Support and After-care (choice of accommodation) Regulations 2014. S.I. 2014/2670.

Figure 82: Patients eligible for section 117 after-care

Patients detained on the basis of	Relevant section
An application for admission for treatment	section 3
A hospital order (with or without a restriction order)	section 37
A hospital direction (with or without a limitation direction)	section 45A
A transfer direction (with or without a restriction direction)	section 47 or 48

29.6 By definition, this includes all patients on community treatment orders (CTOs) and all conditionally discharged patients. It includes patients who are transferred back to prison or other place of custody after being detained in hospital on the basis of a transfer order under section 47 or 48.

Responsible after-care bodies [section 117(2E) and (3)]

29.7 The duty to provide or arrange for the provision of after-care services under section 117 stands by itself. It is not a duty to provide or arrange for the provision of services under other legislation (eg the Care Act 2014 or the NHS Act 2006). As a result, normal rules about NHS commissioning responsibility or ordinary residence only apply to the extent specified in section 117 and regulations made under the section.

29.8 The Act says that the responsible after-care bodies are the local authority and the CCG, or local health board, where relevant:

a) for the area in which the person was ordinarily resident immediately before being detained, or
b) if the person was not ordinarily resident in England or Wales immediately before detained, for the area in which the person is resident or to which he is sent on discharge by the hospital in which he was detained.

29.9 If there is a dispute between local authorities in England about where the person was ordinarily resident immediately before being detained, this will be determined by the process set out in section 40 of the Care Act 2014. Disputes between a local authority in England and a local authority in Wales will be determined according to arrangements between the Secretary of State for Health and Welsh ministers.[122]

29.10 The NHS body responsible for after-care will change in the circumstances set out in regulations made under section 117(2E)[123].

---

[122] These arrangements are being finalised and are expected to be published in the gov.uk website shortly.

[123] At the time of publication, see regulations 14 and 15 of the National Health Service Commissioning Board and Clinical Commissioning Groups (Responsibilities and Standing Rules) Regulations. 2008. SI 2012/2996. http://www.legislation.gov.uk/uksi/2012/2996

Preparations for after-care – particularly where conditional discharge is in view [sections 73 and 117]

29.11 The duty to provide after-care begins when patients leave hospital, which need not be at the same time as they are discharged from detention.

29.12 Case law has established that responsible after-care bodies have a power to make preparations for patients' after-care in advance of them leaving hospital, which may include paying a deposit for a place in a particular facility to be kept open for them.

29.13 As a result, responsible after-care bodies must consider making preparations in any case where they have good reason to think that there is a real possibility that the patient will be discharged if appropriate after-care can be arranged. In particular, they must use their best endeavours to put in place after-care which would allow a patient to be conditionally discharged in accordance with a provisional decision of the Tribunal (a 'deferred conditional discharge') – see paragraph 6.85 onward.

After-care and deprivation of liberty

29.14 After-care arrangements cannot amount to a deprivation of liberty, unless this is authorised under the Mental Capacity Act 2005.[124] The precise scope of the term 'deprivation of liberty' is not fixed. In its Cheshire West judgment,[125] the Supreme Court clarified that there is a deprivation of liberty in circumstances where a person is under continuous control and supervision, is not free to leave and lacks capacity to consent to these arrangements. The Supreme Court also noted that factors which are not relevant in determining whether there is a deprivation of liberty include the person's compliance or lack of objection and the reason or purpose behind a particular placement. The relative normality of the placement (whatever the comparison made) is also not relevant. A deprivation of liberty in relation to a person who lacks capacity may be authorised by an authorisation under Schedule A1 to the Mental Capacity Act 2005 or a Court of Protection order.

After-care services during leave of absence

29.15 The courts have decided that the duty to provide after-care services also applies to eligible patients when they are on leave of absence from hospital.[126] Whether they actually need any after-care services during such leave will, of course, depend on the specific circumstances of the cases.

---

[124] Mental Capacity Act 2005. http://www.legislation.gov.uk/ukpga/2005/9/contents

[125] P v Cheshire West and Chester Council and another and P and Q v Surrey County Council. 2014. WLR 2. https://www.supremecourt.uk/decided-cases/docs/UKSC_2012_0068_Judgment.pdf

[126] R v Richmond LBC ex p. W. 1999. All ER (D) 899.

Duration of after-care services [section 117(2)]

29.16 After-care services must be provided until both the responsible after-care bodies are satisfied that the patient no longer needs them. After-care services must be provided for as long as a patient is on a CTO ('CTO patient') and may still be required even after a patient is discharged from CTO.

29.17 The duty to provide after-care services does not end because patients happen to return to hospital, even if they are detained under the Act. The duty applies when patients are transferred back to prison or other place of custody after being detained on the basis of a transfer order under section 47 or 48.

29.18 If they are detained again in a way which would itself make them eligible for after-care services, eg if they are detained for treatment under section 3, that may affect the identity of the responsible after-care bodies when the patient leaves hospital again. That is because the area in which they were ordinarily resident immediately before being detained again would now determine the identity of the responsible after-care bodies. That area might not be the same as it was on the previous occasion they were detained.

29.19 In all cases, responsible after-care bodies may reassess from time to time what after-care services a person needs and change them accordingly.

No power to charge for after-care services

29.20 The Act provides no power to charge anyone for after-care services provided under section 117. They must be provided free of charge.

Professional responsibilities

This group of chapters sets out some special responsibilities and obligations of mental health professionals and hospital managers to:

- patients
- the nearest relative, and (on occasion)
- victims.

It includes the provisions in the Act relating to the approval of approved mental health professionals (AMHP), doctors approved under the Act as having special experience in the diagnosis or treatment of mental disorder, and approved clinicians.

The chapter on hospital managers and the Act covers how the Act defines hospital managers, the functions of hospital managers, how hospital managers' functions may be delegated and the scrutiny of documents and the rectification of errors.

Under the Domestic Violence, Crime and Victims Act 2004, victims of serious violent and sexual offences have the right to receive certain information about key stages in a part 3 patient's progress and treatment.

The chapter on offences describes the specific offences created by the Act, and the provisions which protect people who undertake actions under, or purporting to be under, the Act.

30: Approval of practitioners to carry out functions under the Act

Introduction

30.1 This chapter describes the provisions of the Act relating to the approval of approved mental health professionals (AMHPs), section 12 doctors and approved clinicians.

Approved mental health professionals (AMHPs) [section 114]

30.2 AMHPs are professionals who have been approved to act in that role by a local authority. AMHPs have various functions under the Act, including those set out in figure 83.

Figure 83: Main AMHP functions

AMHP function	See
Making applications for admission to hospital for assessment or treatment under part 2	chapter 8
The power to convey patients to hospital on the basis of applications for admission	chapter 8
Making applications for guardianship under part 2	chapter 28
Providing social circumstances reports on patients detained on the basis of an application for admission made by their nearest relative	Paragraph 25.24
Applying to the county court for the replacement of an unsatisfactory private guardian	Paragraph 28.136
Confirming that community treatment orders (CTOs) should be made discharging patients from detention in hospital onto CTOs and agreeing the conditions to be included in the CTO	chapter 26
Approving the extension of CTOs	chapter 26
Approving the revocation of CTOs	chapter 26
Being consulted by responsible clinicians before they make reports confirming the detention or CTOs of patients who have been absent without leave for more than 28 days	Paragraphs 25.45 and 28.105 respectively

AMHP function	See
Applying to the county court for the appointment of an acting nearest relative and the displacement of an existing nearest relative	chapter 2
Having the right to enter and inspect premises under section 115	chapter 7
Applying for warrants to enter premises under section 135	chapter 7
The power to take patients into custody and take them to the place they ought be when they have gone absent without leave (AWOL)	chapters 9, 26, and 29
The power to take and return other patients who have absconded	chapter 7

AMHPs acting on behalf of local authorities [section 145(1AC)]

30.3 When the Act refers to AMHPs it means AMHPs acting on behalf of a local authority (unless the context demands otherwise). When they carry out functions under the Act, AMHPs must be acting on behalf on a particular local authority.

30.4 In addition, local authorities have statutory duties to arrange for AMHPs to consider the cases of patients in their area with a view to making applications for admission to hospital or for guardianship under part 2 (see paragraphs 8.16 and 28.31 respectively).

30.5 Being approved by a local authority to be an AMHP is not the same as being permitted by a local authority to act on its behalf. It is for each local authority to establish its own arrangements for determining which AMHPs may act as such on its behalf and when they may do so. A local authority may arrange for AMHPs to act on its behalf even though they are approved by a different local authority.

30.6 An AMHP does not have to be employed by a local authority in order to be able to act on its behalf.

30.7 Although AMHPs act on their behalf, local authorities cannot tell AMHPs what decision they must reach in any particular case. When making decisions which the Act confers directly on AMHPs, AMHPs must reach their own independent professional judgment.

Approval by local authorities of people to act as AMHPs [section 114(3) and the AMHP regulations]

30.8 Local authorities have the power to approve people to act as AMHPs only if they are satisfied that they have appropriate competence in dealing with people who are suffering from mental disorder.

30.9 A person may only be approved as an AMHP by one local authority in England at any time, but that does not prevent them acting on behalf of any number of other local authorities.

30.10 Arrangements for approvals are set out in the Mental Health (Approved Mental Health Professionals) (Approval) (England) Regulations 2008 ('the AMHP Regulations').[127]

30.11 Only people who meet the following professional requirements (listed in schedule 1 to the AMHP Regulations) can be approved as AMHPs:

- registered social workers
- registered first level nurses, whose field of practice is mental health nursing or learning disabilities nursing
- registered occupational therapists, and
- chartered psychologists who hold a relevant practising certificate issued by the British Psychological Society.

Section 114(2) specifically prohibits doctors being approved as AMHPs.

30.12 In order to gain approval, people who have not previously been approved as AMHPs in England or Wales (or treated as such) must have completed within the previous five years an AMHP training course approved by the Health and Care Professions Council or the Care Council for Wales.

30.13 In deciding whether someone has the appropriate competence in dealing with people with mental disorders required by the Act, local authorities must take into account the factors ('key competencies') set out in schedule 2 to the AMHP Regulations. The key competencies are divided into five areas:

- application of values to the AMHP role
- application of knowledge: the legal and policy framework
- application of knowledge: mental disorder
- application of skills: working in partnership, and
- application of skills: making and communicating informed decisions.

30.14 Local authorities may approve people as AMHPs for five years at a time, after which they would need to be re-approved.

---

[127] Mental Health (Approved Mental Health Professionals) (Approval) (England) Regulations 2008.S.I. 2008/1206. http://www.legislation.gov.uk/uksi/2008/1206

30.15 Approval is conditional on each AMHP completing at least 18 hours of training in the year starting with the day of their approval and in each subsequent year. The training must be relevant to their role as an AMHP and have been agreed with the approving local authority.

30.16 Approval is also conditional on AMHPs:

- undertaking to inform the approving local authority in writing as soon as reasonably possible, if they agree to act as an AMHP on behalf of another local authority in England, and when any such agreement ends
- undertaking to stop acting as an AMHP and to notify the approving local authority immediately if their registration (or its equivalent) as any of the professionals listed in paragraph 30.11 'professional registration', is suspended and when any such suspension ends, and
- undertaking to stop acting as an AMHP and to notify the approving local authority immediately if they no longer meet at least one of the professional requirements in 30.11.

30.17 If an AMHP's professional registration is suspended, the approving local authority must suspend their approval as an AMHP for as long as the suspension of the professional registration lasts.

30.18 When the local authority is notified that the suspension of the professional registration has ended, it must end the suspension of the approval, unless it is now not satisfied that the AMHP has appropriate competence in dealing with people suffering from mental disorder.

30.19 People may not act as AMHPs while their approval as an AMHP is suspended.

30.20 Suspension of approval as an AMHP does not change the date on which that approval is due to expire.

30.21 Approving local authorities must end an AMHP's approval if:

- the AMHP notifies them in writing that they wish no longer to be approved as an AMHP, or
- they are no longer satisfied the AMHP has appropriate competence in dealing with people with mental disorder, taking into account the key competencies in the AMHP Regulations

or, they become aware that the AMHP:

- is no longer a professional who meets at least one of the professional requirements in 30.11 – but not if that is only because they are suspended from the relevant register (or equivalent)
- the AMHP is in breach of the conditions of their approval, or
- the AMHP is approved to act as an AMHP by another local authority in England.

30.22 When it ends an approval, or the approval expires, the approving local authority must notify the AMHP immediately and give the reasons. It must also notify any other local authorities in England for which it knows the AMHP has agreed to act.

30.23 A local authority which approves someone who it knows is already approved by another local authority in England must notify the old approving local authority accordingly.

30.24 Local authorities must keep records of the people they approve as AMHPs. Those records must include:

- each person's name, profession and date of approval
- details of the agreed training they undertake, any suspension of their approval, any previous approvals as an AMHP within the past five years
- the names of any other local authorities for which the approved person has an agreement to act as an AMHP, and
- where applicable, the date on which the approval ended and the reason.

30.25 Local authorities must keep those records for at least five years after the day on which the AMHP's approval ends.

30.26 There are separate regulations about approval of AMHPs in Wales.[128]

Approval of courses by Health and Care Professions Council [section 114ZA]

30.27 The Health and Care Professions Council may approve courses for people who are, or wish to become, AMHPs. The list of approved courses is published on the Council's website

30.28 As the functions of AMHPs can be performed by people from several professions, they do not count as 'relevant social work' for the purposes of the Care Standards Act 2000.[130]

AMHPs approved in England but acting in Wales (and vice versa) [section 114(10)]

30.29 AMHPs approved by an English local authority may only act on behalf of local authorities which are also in England. In order to act on behalf of local authorities in Wales, they would need also to be approved as an AMHP by a

[128] At the time of publication, Mental Health (Approval of Persons to be Approved Mental Health Professionals) (Wales) Regulations 2008, S.I. 2008/2436.
[129] The Council's list can be found at www.hcpac-uk.org/assests/documents/100414DApprovalcriteriaforapprovedmentalhealthprofessional(AMHP)programmes.pdf
[130] Care Standards Act 2000. http://www.legislation.gov.uk/ukpga/2000/14

local authority in Wales, in accordance with the corresponding regulations made by the Welsh Ministers.[131]

30.30 There is nothing to prevent an AMHP acting in Wales on behalf of an English local authority where necessary.

30.31 For example, an AMHP acting on behalf of an English local authority can make applications for admission to hospitals in Wales, or apply for a warrant under section 135 of the Act to a magistrates' court in Wales. Similarly, an AMHP acting on behalf of a Welsh local authority can make applications to hospitals in England or to English magistrates' courts.

Section 12 approved doctors [sections 12, 12ZA and 12ZB and mutual recognition regulations]

30.32 Section 12 allows the Secretary of State to approve doctors for the purposes of the Act as having special experience in the diagnosis or treatment of mental disorder.

30.33 The Secretary of State's approval function is exercised by persons with whom the Secretary of State has entered into agreements under section 12ZA or 12ZB ('approving bodies').[132]

30.34 The Secretary of State issues Instructions under section 12ZA(5) from time to time about how approving bodies should approve section 12 doctors, including the professional requirements for a section 12 doctor. These are called the Mental Health Act 1983 Instructions with respect to the Exercise of Approval Functions ('Instructions').[133] The Instructions specify the professional requirements for a section 12 doctor.

30.35 In Wales, doctors are approved under section 12 by the Welsh Ministers.

30.36 The mutual recognition regulations say that doctors approved in Wales for these purposes are treated as if approved in England as well (and vice versa).

30.37 All doctors who are approved clinicians (see below), whether in England or Wales, are automatically treated as approved under section 12 in both countries.

---

[131] This is in accordance with the Social Services and Well-being (Wales) Act 2014 which will come into effect in Wales in April 2016. http://www.legislation.gov.uk/anaw/2014/4/contents/enacted
[132] The approving bodies are listed on the Gov.uk website. https://www.gov.uk/government/publications/mental-health-act-exercise-of-approval-instructions-2013
[133] At the time of publication, the current Instructions are the Mental Health Act 1983 Instructions with respect to the Exercise of Approval Functions 2014, made on 11 February 2014. https://www.gov.uk/government/publications/mental-health-act-exercise-of-approval-instructions-2013

Approved clinicians [sections 12ZA and 145]

30.38 An approved clinician is a person approved for the purposes of the Act by the Secretary of State or another person by virtue of sections 12ZA or 12ZB. Approved clinicians have various responsibilities under the Act. This includes acting as the responsible clinician for detained and CTO patients, and so having overall responsibility for the patient's case.

30.39 The Secretary of State's approval function is exercised by persons with whom the Secretary of State has entered into agreements under section 12ZA or 12ZB ('approving bodies').[134]

30.40 The Secretary of State's Instructions specify how approving bodies should approve clinicians.

30.41 Under the Instructions, only the following professionals may be approved:

- registered medical practitioners
- registered practitioner psychologists
- registered first level nurses, whose field of practice is mental health nursing or learning disabilities nursing
- registered occupational therapists, and
- registered social workers.

30.42 The Secretary of State's Instructions specify how approving bodies should approve clinicians, including the professional requirements and relevant competencies for approved clinicians.

30.43 The Instructions set out the:

- period of approval
- conditions of approval
- circumstances in which approval is suspended or ended, and
- record keeping requirements for approving bodies.

Approved clinicians approved in England but acting in Wales (and vice versa) [section 142A and mutual recognition regulations]

30.44 An approved clinician approved by the Secretary of State or an approving body is only an approved clinician in England. To be an approved clinician in Wales, a practitioner must be approved by, or on behalf of, the Welsh ministers.

30.45 Approved clinicians in one country may act as such in the other country if they are doing so:

---

[134] The approving bodies are listed on the Gov.uk website. https://www.gov.uk/government/publications/mental-health-act-exercise-of-approval-instructions-2013

- in relation to a patient who is liable to be detained in a hospital under the Act in the country in which they are approved, or
- in relation to a CTO patient whose responsible hospital is in the country in which they are approved, or
- as the responsible clinician for a guardianship patient whose responsible local authority is in the country in which they are approved.

and the patient happens to be in the other country.

30.46 Similarly, in certain cases, a clinician approved as an approved clinician in Wales, but not England, may be authorised by the responsible English local authority to be a guardianship patient's responsible clinician.

30.47 The responsible local authority may only do this if the patient is either in or receiving medical treatment for mental disorder in Wales. An English local authority can be responsible for a patient who lives in Wales if the patient has a private guardian who lives in England.

30.48 A Welsh approved clinician authorised in this way may carry out the duties of the responsible clinician (eg examining the patient with a view to making a renewal report under section 20) whether the patient happens to be in England or Wales at the time.

30.49 A clinician approved as an approved clinician in England (but not Wales) may be authorised by a responsible Welsh local authority to be a guardianship patient's responsible clinician if the patient is either in or receiving medical treatment for mental disorder in England.

30.50 All doctors who are approved clinicians, whether in England or Wales are automatically treated as approved under section 12 in both countries. This does not apply to approved clinicians who are not doctors.

31: Hospital managers

Introduction

31.1 This chapter is concerned with various aspects of administering the Act. It deals with the definition of hospital managers, a group who are frequently referred to in the Act, usually in the context of their responsibilities to carry out various actions. This chapter brings together in one place a list of the functions of hospital managers although other chapters also include information for hospital mangers and the whole Reference Guide is relevant to them. The Act mentions the delegation of the powers of managers and this has to be done in a prescribed manner in order to be valid. In the course of administering the Act there is always the possibility that forms may be completed incorrectly and the possibility of rectifying a mistake varies with the nature of the error. It should be read in conjunction with chapters 37 and 38 of the Code of Practice.

Definition of hospital managers [section 145]

31.2 Hospital managers have various powers and duties under the Act. In this context, 'managers' does not mean the management team of the hospital, but the people or body whose hospital it is, as set out in figure 84.

Figure 84: Identification of hospital managers

For a hospital which is	The managers are
Vested in an NHS trust	The NHS trust as a body
Vested in an NHS foundation trust	The NHS foundation trust as a body
Vested in a local health board (LHB) in Wales	The LHB as a body
An independent hospital/provider	The person or persons registered as a service provider under chapter 2 of part 1 of the Health and Social Care Act 2008[135] in respect of the regulated activity (within the meaning of that part) relating to the assessment or medical treatment of mental disorder carried out by the hospital

[135] Health and Social Care Act 2008. http://www.legislation.gov.uk/ukpga/2008/14

31.3 For the most part, hospital managers do not have to perform their functions personally, eg by decision of the board of an NHS trust, but may delegate them to officers, ie members of their staff, and, in some cases, to other people. Delegation is discussed in more detail below.

Functions of hospital managers

31.4 The formal duty to ensure that patients subject to the Act, and their nearest relatives, have been informed about their legal situation and rights falls to the hospital managers. In practice, it would usually be more appropriate for professionals working with the patient to provide them with the information.

31.5 In order to fulfil their statutory duties hospital managers should have policies in place to ensure that:

- the correct information is given to patients and their nearest relatives
- information is given in accordance with the requirements of the legislation, at a suitable time and in an accessible format, where appropriate with the aid of assistive technologies and interpretative and advocacy services
- information must be provided in a format and or language that the individual understands, eg Braille, easy-read or Moon
- people who give the information have received adequate and appropriate training and guidance and, if relevant, have specialist skills in relation to people with learning disability, autism and or children and young people
- a record is kept of the information given, including how, when, where and by whom it was given, and an assessment made of how well the information was understood by the recipient
- regular checks are made that information has been properly given to each patient and understood by them
- although the Act does not impose any duties to give information to informal patients, these patients should have their legal position and rights explained to them
- informal patients should be provided with relevant information, eg about how to make a complaint and consent requirements for treatment
- certain patients are referred to the Tribunal if six months have passed since they were first detained, or transferred to detention from outside England and Wales, the details are set out in figure 56
- the cases of detained patients, unless they are restricted patients, and community treatment order (CTO) patients in the circumstances set out in figure 19 are referred to the Tribunal
- the cases of patients whose CTOs have been revoked, as soon as possible after the CTO is revoked are referred to the tribunal
- patients are informed of their right to make an application to the Tribunal
- patients must be informed about the role of the Care Quality Commission (CQC) and their right to meet visitors appointed by the CQC in private
- patients must be informed about the process of making a complaint to the CQC

- such steps are taken as are practicable to give the patient's nearest relative a copy of the information given to the patient in writing, unless the patient requests otherwise, and
- the patient's nearest relative are told of the patient's discharge from detention or CTO, unless the patient or the nearest relative has requested otherwise.

31.6 This list is not definitive.

Delegation of hospital managers' functions [section 32(3), section 142B and regulation 3 and 19]

31.7 Hospital managers' functions under parts 2, 3 and 6 of the Act can be delegated in accordance with the regulations, or, in the cases of discharge decisions under section 23, in accordance with section 23 itself (see paragraphs 31.9 to 31.17 in particular). Hospital managers' functions in respect of patients' correspondence under section 134 of the Act may be delegated in accordance with regulation 29 (see paragraph 5.9).

31.8 Hospital managers may delegate their other functions under the Act in any way they can normally delegate their functions – which will depend on the constitution of the body concerned and (in the case of NHS trusts and NHS foundation trusts) the relevant NHS legislation.

31.9 The provisions described in this chapter include various duties on the hospital managers. The meaning of hospital managers is described in paragraph 31.2.

31.10 As hospital managers are, in most cases, people or a body, they do not have to perform their functions personally.

31.11 In some cases, the relevant section of the Act (or the regulations) says how and to whom the hospital managers may delegate their functions.

31.12 In particular, wherever the hospital managers are required by the regulations to make a record or report of anything, that record can be made on their behalf by any officer they have authorised for the purpose.

31.13 When they are required by the regulations to give information to patients (or their nearest relatives) or to take steps to arrange for them to be given information, the managers may authorise officers to do that on their behalf.

31.14 Similarly, wherever the regulations say that people are allowed to use a particular method of communication – eg the managers' internal mail system, fax or email – to serve a report or information on the managers only with the managers' permission, the managers may authorise any officer to take that decision on their behalf.

31.15 Officers can be clinical as well as administrative staff, and can include patients' responsible clinicians (see paragraph 25.26 onward below).

31.16 Unless otherwise stated, hospital managers may delegate the other functions described in this chapter to anyone their constitution, or, in the case of NHS bodies, the relevant NHS legislation, allows.

31.17 Section 142B of the Act means that where rules in the Act (and regulations) permit managers to delegate to other people, those freedoms apply to foundation trusts as well, provided the particular trust's constitution allows it.

Fundamental errors in applications

31.18 Whilst some less serious problems with application are capable of rectification under the Act, fundamental errors are incapable of remedy and therefore invalidate the application.

31.19 Examples of fundamental errors are:

- a review of detention or CTO not taking place before it expires leading to an illegal deprivation of liberty (see also Code of Practice paragraphs 32.10 and 38.50)
- an application or medical recommendation which is unsigned, or
- an application signed by a person not qualified to complete it, ie an application not signed by an AMHP, a nearest relative, or a person authorised to exercise the nearest relative's functions, or
- a medical recommendation by a person without power to make such a recommendation, ie a medical recommendation from someone disqualified from making one by reason of section 12, section 12A or the Mental Health (Conflicts of Interest) (England) regulations 2008[136] (see further 28.83).

31.20 Where an application suffers from a fundamental error, the application is of no effect at all.

31.21 If this occurs, the hospital managers or the responsible clinician should discharge the patient pursuant to section 23. It would then be open for the patient to be made subject of a report pursuant to section 5(2) (report by registered medical practitioner or approved clinician) or 5(4) (report by nurse), which would allow detention for a limited time: see further 28.83. During this time, authorisation for further detention can be sought through a fresh application.

Rectification of minor errors in applications [section 15 and regulation 4]

31.22 Less serious problems with applications and recommendations may be capable of being rectified and patients may continue to be detained for a limited period while that is done.

---

[136] Mental Health (Conflicts of Interest) (England) regulations. 2008. SI 2008/1205. http://www.legislation.gov.uk/uksi/2008/1205

31.23 Examples of errors capable of rectification include:

- leaving blank spaces on the form, which should have been completed, other than the space for signing it or for recording the doctor's reasons for believing the statutory criteria are satisfied
- failure to delete one or more alternative clauses in places where only one can be correct
- errors in the spelling of names, addresses or places, and
- discrepancies in the spelling of a patient's name, in circumstances where there is no doubt the documents refer to the same person.

31.24 An application or recommendation which is found to be incorrect or defective can be amended by the person who signed it, with the consent of the managers of the hospital, within the period of 14 days starting with the day of the patient's admission.

31.25 A faulty emergency application (made under section 4) may not be corrected after the patient has been detained for 72 hours on the basis of that application, unless a second medical recommendation has been received and the application has become in effect a section 2 application. In other words, errors in emergency applications cannot be put right retrospectively once the application will inevitably have ceased to be effective.

31.26 In practice, any document found to contain faults of this sort should be returned to the person who signed it for amendment. When the amended document is returned to the hospital it should again be scrutinised to check that it is now in the proper form, following which consent can be given by the hospital managers (managers may authorise officers to consent to amendments on their behalf). The consent should be recorded in writing and can take the form of an endorsement on the document itself.

31.27 Provided this is all done within a period of 14 days starting with the day on which the patient was admitted, or – in the case of a patient who was already in hospital – the day on which they were treated as admitted as a result of the application, the documents are deemed to have had effect as though originally made as amended.

31.28 Where an error is not corrected in 14 days, an application will not necessarily be invalid. The hospital managers are required to decide whether the error is trivial and therefore falls within the 'de minimis' principle. Particular emphasis will be placed on the consequence of any error.

Replacement of insufficient medical recommendations [section 15(2) and (3) and regulation 4]

31.29 If one of the medical recommendations on which an application is based is found to be insufficient, or the two medical recommendations taken together are insufficient, it may be possible to correct the error by having a new recommendation submitted.

31.30 A medical recommendation may be insufficient because:

- it has been signed after the date on which the application was made, or
- the doctor's reasons in the form do not appear to be sufficient to support the conclusions stated in it (but do not suggest that the conclusions are wrong or have no proper basis)

and recommendations taken together may be insufficient because

- longer than 5 clear days has elapsed between the patient being examined by the first and second doctor, or
- neither doctor is approved under section 12.

31.31 If any of these problems turn out simply to be errors in the way the forms were completed (eg a date was entered incorrectly), they can be corrected with the consent of the managers as described above.

31.32 Otherwise, the application is invalid, unless the position can be rectified by a fresh recommendation.

31.33 In that case, the managers may notify in writing the approved mental health professional (AMHP) or nearest relative who made the application that the recommendation will have to be disregarded unless it can be replaced, managers may authorise officers to do this on their behalf. In practice, it would be helpful also to notify the doctor concerned. If the problem is with two recommendations taken together, the notice can be given in respect of either, but not both.

31.34 The applicant has 14 days starting with the day of the patient's admission to arrange for a replacement recommendation to be provided to the hospital managers. The replacement recommendation does not necessarily have to be from the same person as who provided the first recommendation.

31.35 The new recommendation must comply with all the requirements with which the original recommendation should have complied, except the deadlines by which the original recommendation had to be signed or by which the examination it was based on had to take place.

31.36 If a correct replacement medical recommendation is received by, or on behalf of, the managers before the end of the 14 day period starting with the day the patient was admitted, then the application is to be treated as if it were, and always had been, properly supported by the necessary medical recommendations. If not, the application ceases to provide any authority to detain the patient as of the end of the 14 day period.

31.37 As with rectification of minor mistakes, an emergency application (made under section 4) may only be corrected in the first 72 hours, unless a second medical recommendation has been received and the application has, in effect, been converted into a section 2 application. This is for the same reason as below at paragraph 32.25.

Rectification of errors in guardianship applications [section 8(4)]

31.38 Minor errors in an application for guardianship can be rectified using the same procedure as for applications for admission to hospital pursuant to section 15(1), and as outlined above at paragraphs 32.23 to 32.29. During the 14 day period during which an error capable of rectification is corrected, patients may continue to be subject to guardianship.

31.39 Unlike applications for admission to hospital, there is no procedure for obtaining a new medical recommendation if the ones that come with the application originally prove insufficient. In that case, a new application would have to be made.

32: Information for victims

Introduction

32.1 Since the end of the 1990s successive governments have introduced a number of ways of protecting victims and the wider public from people who have been convicted of sexual and violent offences. For example, mental health trusts are under wider legal obligations to inform the local multi-agency public protection board when certain patients are released regardless of their status under the Act. The Code of Practice for Victims of Crime[137] sets out the rights of victims of restricted and unrestricted hospital order patients. The Code of Practice: Mental Health Act 1983[138] also contains detailed information about the National Probation Service Victim Contact Scheme[139] as it operates in respect of restricted and unrestricted patients (see Code of Practice chapter 40).

Victim Contact Scheme and the Victim's Code

32.2 The Victim Contact Scheme (VCS) arises from section 69 Criminal Justice and Courts Services Act 2000,[140] updated by sections 35–45 Domestic Violence Crime and Victims Act 2004 (DVCVA).[141]

32.3 The VCS requires that probation contacts and offers the VCS to victims of offenders who have committed a specified serious violent or sexual offence, for which the offender has been sentenced to 12 months or more in custody or detained under the Act, with or without restrictions.

32.4 Victims who choose to participate in the VCS may make representations about the offender's licence or discharge conditions, to whoever is responsible for making that decision, and receive certain information about key stages of the offender's sentence from their probation Victim Liaison Officer (VLO). If the patient is unrestricted and a victim wishes to receive information, the VLO will pass on the victim's details to the hospital and all future contact will be between the provider and the patient.

32.5 Since April 2014, victims of restricted patients are being told if a patient has been granted leave from hospital by the Mental Health Casework Section (MHCS), unless there are exceptional reasons not to disclose this information (see Code of Practice paragraph 40.13).

---

[137] The Code of Practice for Victims of Crime. Ministry of Justice. 2013. https://www.gov.uk/government/publications/the-code-of-practice-for-victims-of-crime

[138] Mental Health Act 1983: Code of Practice of Practice 2015. https://www.gov.uk/government/uploads/system/uploads/attachment_data/file/396918/Code_of_Practice.pdf

[139] Victim Contact Scheme Guidance Manual - www.justice.gov.uk/.../probation.../pi-11-2013-vicitim-contact-scheme-guidance(1).doc

[140] Criminal Justice and Courts Services Act 2000. http://www.legislation.gov.uk/ukpga/2000/43

[141] Domestic Violence Crime and Victims Act 2004. http://www.legislation.gov.uk/ukpga/2004/28

33: Offences and protection for acts done

Introduction

33.1 This chapter describes the specific offences created by the Act, and the provisions which provide protection for certain people against civil and criminal proceedings for their actions under the Act. The offences are in part 9 of the Act.

Forgery, false statements etc [section 126]

33.2 Section 126 creates offences in connection with documents purporting to be applications for admission or guardianship, any medical or other recommendations or reports under the Act, and any other documents required or authorised to be made for any of the purposes of the Act.

33.3 It is an offence for any person or any body of persons (such as a corporation), without lawful authority or good excuse, to have such documents in their custody or under their control, which are – and which they know or believe to be – false. A statement or entry may be false because of what it omits, conceals or implies, even though the statement or entry itself is literally true.[142] It is also an offence to make or have in their custody or under their control a document so closely resembling such a document as to be calculated to deceive.[143] Deception also includes inducing someone to believe something is false which is in fact true.[144]

33.4 It is an offence wilfully to make any false entry or statement in any application, recommendation, report or other document required or authorised to be made for any purposes of the Act, or to make use of such an entry or statement with intent to deceive, knowing it to be false.

Ill-treatment of patients [section 127]

33.5 It is an offence for any of the managers of a hospital, independent hospital or care home, or any officer on its staff or otherwise employed in it, to ill-treat or wilfully neglect a patient, whether or not detained, who is for the time being receiving treatment for mental disorder as an in-patient in that hospital or home. The ill-treatment or wilful neglect of an in-patient need not have taken place on the premises of that hospital or home.

---

[142] R v Lord Kylsant. 1932. 1 KB 442.

[143] In: Re London and Globe Finance Corporation. 1903. 1 Ch 728, 732, Mr Justice Buckley said: '*To deceive is…to induce a man to believe that a thing is true which is false, and which the person practising the deceit knows or believes to be false*'.

[144] Welham v DPP. 1961. AC 103.

33.6 The same applies to a patient receiving outpatient treatment for a mental disorder when they are on the premises of the hospital or care home, or premises of which the hospital or care home forms a part.

33.7 It is also an offence for individuals to ill-treat or wilfully neglect a mentally disordered patient who is for the time being subject to their guardianship under the Act, or otherwise in their custody or care, whether by virtue of a legal or moral obligation, or otherwise. A mentally disordered patient is someone who either is or appears to be suffering from a mental disorder; he or she need not have had a history of in-patient treatment or to have been a detained patient or a detained patient on leave of absence from a hospital.

33.8 'Ill-treatment' encompasses a wide range of conduct: there is no need to show that the treatment caused actual injury to the victim.[145]

33.9 'Wilful' is used to describe the mental element, which must be proved in addition to the fact of neglect. The primary meaning of 'wilful' is 'deliberate' but it may also include recklessness.[146]

33.10 Taken as a whole, the meaning of the expression 'wilful neglect' may vary according to context; however, generally, the expression should be taken to mean that there has been an intentional or purposive omission to do something that the person in question knows he or she has a duty to do.

Assisting patients to absent themselves without leave etc [section 128]

33.11 It is an offence for any person or any body of persons (such as a corporation) to induce or knowingly assist another person who is liable to be detained or is subject to guardianship under the Act, or is a community treatment order (CTO) patient, to absent himself without leave, or to induce or knowingly assist a person in legal custody by virtue of section 137 to escape.

33.12 It is also an offence knowingly to harbour a patient who is absent without leave or is otherwise at large and liable to be retaken under the Act, or to give such patients any assistance with intent to prevent, hinder or interfere with their being taken into custody, or returned to the hospital or other place where they ought to be.

Obstruction [section 129]

33.13 It an offence for a person or any body of persons (such as a corporation) without reasonable cause to:

- refuse to allow the inspection of any premises
- refuse to allow people authorised to do so by or under the Act to visit, interview or examine any person, or to refuse them access to that person

[145] R v Newington 1990. 91 Cr App R 247.
[146] R v Sheppard. 1981. AC 394 HL.

- refuse to produce any records or documents required for inspection by a person who is authorised to require them to be produced
- fail to provide the Care Quality Commission (CQC) or authorised person with such information as it or he may reasonably request for, or in connection with, the exercise of their duties and powers for the general protection of relevant patients (but this only applies to managers of a hospital within the meaning of part 2 of the Act (including a registered establishment), a local authority, or persons of any other description prescribed in regulations), or
- otherwise obstruct authorised people in the exercise of their functions under the Act.

33.14 It is an offence to insist on being present when required to withdraw by a person authorised under the Act to interview or examine someone in private.

Maximum penalties for offences

33.15 The maximum penalties for these offences are set out in figure 86.

Figure 86: Maximum penalties for offences under the Act

Offence	On summary conviction (ie in a magistrates' court)	On conviction on indictment (ie in the Crown Court)
Forgery, false statements etc (section 126)	Imprisonment for a term not exceeding six months,[147] or a fine[148] or both.	Imprisonment for a term not exceeding two years, or a fine of any amount, or both.
Ill-treatment etc (section 127)	Imprisonment for a term not exceeding six months,[21] or a fine[22] or both.	Imprisonment for a term not exceeding five years, or a fine of any amount, or both.
Assisting patients to go AWOL etc (section 128)	Imprisonment for a term not exceeding six months,[21] or a fine[22] or both.	Imprisonment for a term not exceeding two years, or a fine of any amount, or both.
Obstruction (section 129)	Imprisonment for a term not exceeding three months or to a fine not exceeding level 4 on the standard scale, or both.[149]	

[147] When section 282 of the Criminal Justice Act 2003 comes into force (on a date to be appointed at the time of publication), these maximum sentences will be increased from six to 12 months.

[148] Since section 85 of the Legal Aid Sentencing and Punishment of Offenders Act 2012 came into force on 12 March 2015, magistrates' courts are able to impose a fine of any amount for offences punishable on summary conviction. Section 85 removes the maximum fine limit of £5,000 or more for an offence which is punishable on summary conviction.

[149] When schedule 25 to the Criminal Justice Act 2003 comes into force (on a date to be appointed at the time of publication), the maximum penalty for this offence will be a fine not exceeding level 4 on the standard scale. The scope to imprison in respect of this offence will be removed.

Prosecution of offences under the Act [section 130]

33.16 A prosecution under section 127 may only be instituted by, or with the consent of, the Director of Public Prosecutions.

33.17 Subject to that, a local authority may prosecute any of these offences, but see further commentary on section 139 below.

Other proceedings relating to the Act – protection for acts done [section 139]

33.18 People or any body of persons (such as a corporation) are not liable for civil or criminal proceedings in respect of any act done (or purporting to be done) under the Act, or any regulations or rules made under it, so long as the act in question was not done in bad faith or without reasonable care.

33.19 This section offers protection even if the person either acted without jurisdiction or misconstrued the Act, so long as the misconstruction was one which the Act was reasonably capable of bearing.[150]

33.20 Criminal proceedings in respect of such an act may only be brought by or within the consent of the Director of Public Prosecutions. Civil proceedings against any person, in any court, in respect if any such act, require the leave of the High Court. Failure to obtain that leave renders any proceedings a nullity.[151]

33.21 This section does not prevent a patient bringing, without leave, a claim for judicial review, nor a claim for damages for unlawful detention where that detention has purportedly been made under the Act.[152] Nor does it prevent a patient from applying to the Court to be released if he claims to have been unlawfully detained.

33.22 The protections in this section do not apply to proceedings against a Secretary of State, NHS trust, NHS foundation trust, NHS Commissioning Board (NHS England), clinical commissioning group, special health authority, or a local health board. Nor do they apply to prosecution for an offence of ill-treatment.

[150] Richardson v London County Council [1957] 1 WLR 751.
[151] Seal v Chief Constable of South Wales Police. 2007. 1 WLR 1910. http://www.bailii.org/uk/cases/UKHL/2007/31.html
[152] TTM v London Borough of Hackney. 2011. 1 WLR 2873. http://www.bailii.org/ew/cases/EWCA/Civ/2011/4.html

Transfer of patients between jurisdictions

On occasions it is necessary to transfer patients to different parts of the United Kingdom, the Channel Islands or the Isle of Man or abroad. These chapters look at the provisions within the Act which govern whether, and if so how, this may be done. For transfers between England and Wales, see chapter 10.

34: Transfer of patients from outside England and Wales

Introduction

34.1 This chapter describes the provisions of the Act which deal with the transfer of patients from Scotland, Northern Ireland, the Isle of Man or any of the Channel Islands. These are mainly to be found in part 6 of the Act. Details to do with transfers between England and Wales are included in chapter 10.

Relevant sections of the Act

34.2 The sections of the Act which deal with the transfer of patients (or responsibility for patients) to England (and Wales) from corresponding or similar provision elsewhere are set out in figure 89.

Figure 89: Sections of the Act dealing with cross border transfers to England

From	Scotland	Northern Ireland	Isle of Man/ Channel Islands
Detention in hospital	section 80B	section 82	section 85
Community treatment	section 80C	n/a	section 85ZA
Conditional discharge	section 80D	section 82A	section 85A
Guardianship	n/a	section 82	section 85

General rules applicable to transfers from all jurisdictions

34.3 Although some of the precise details differ, the following basic rules apply in all cases.

Transfer to detention in hospital

34.4 When the equivalent of part 2 patients are transferred to detention under the Act, they are treated on their admission to hospital in England or Wales as if they had been admitted on that date as a result of a corresponding application for admission under part 2 of the Act. In other words, they are treated as if they were a newly detained patient.

34.5 If patients were subject to the equivalent of a hospital order, hospital direction or a transfer direction before being transferred, then instead of being treated as detained on the basis of an application, they are treated as if subject to the corresponding order or direction under part 3 of the Act given on the date of their admission.

34.6 This means that these patients are also, for the most part, treated as if they had been newly detained under part 3 of the Act. There are some differences, described below. In particular, patients treated as becoming subject to an unrestricted hospital order on their transfer may apply to the Tribunal in the six months following their transfer, even though such patients would normally not be able to apply unless or until their detention had been renewed after six months (see section 69(2)) (see chapter 6).

34.7 If they were restricted patients, or the equivalent, before they were transferred, they are treated on admission to hospital as if they are also subject to a restriction order, limitation direction, or restriction direction as applicable.

34.8 If they were subject to the equivalent of hospital and limitation directions or a transfer direction under section 47, the associated sentence of imprisonment, or equivalent, is treated as if it had been imposed by a court in England or Wales. If there is more than one associated sentence, they are all treated in that way. Similarly, the restriction order or direction will cease on the date that the first restriction order or direction would have ceased.

Transfer to a CTO

34.9 When patients are transferred from the equivalent of a community treatment order (CTO), they are treated as if they had been detained and then immediately discharged onto a CTO on the day they arrive at the place they are to live in England or Wales. Specifically, they are treated as if, on that day:

- an application for their admission under part 2, or an order or direction for their detention under part 3, as applicable, had been made equivalent to the authority to which they were subject before being transferred
- they had been admitted to the hospital whose managers have agreed to be the responsible hospital, and
- their responsible clinician then immediately made a CTO.

34.10 The hospital from which they are treated as having been discharged onto a CTO becomes their responsible hospital.

Transfer to guardianship

34.11 When patients from Jersey or the Isle of Man are transferred from guardianship, they are treated as if a guardianship application under part 2 was accepted, or a guardianship order under part 3 was made, as applicable, on the day they arrive at the place they are to live in England or Wales.

Transfer of responsibility for conditionally discharged patients

34.12 Responsibility for conditionally discharged patients can only be transferred if the Secretary of State for Justice agrees to take over that responsibility.

34.13 Where the Secretary of State agrees to the transfer of responsibility, patients are treated as if they:

- are subject to a hospital order and restriction order, or hospital and limitation directions, or a transfer direction and restriction direction, depending on which corresponds to their position before transfer, and
- had been conditionally discharged on the day responsibility is transferred.

Restricted patients (detained or conditionally discharged)

34.14 None of the above affects the date on which a restriction order, limitation direction or restriction direction is due to expire, if the equivalent to which a patient was previously subject outside England or Wales was due to expire on a fixed date.

Arrangements for transfers

34.15 It is up to the authorities in the jurisdiction from which the patient is being transferred to decide whether to authorise the transfer in accordance with the local legislation.

34.16 The authorities will almost certainly require evidence that arrangements have been made for the patient to be received in England before they will agree to the transfer. In practice, they will generally ask the Department of Health (or the Ministry of Justice for restricted patients) to confirm this with the relevant English hospital or local authority.

34.17 The Secretary of State for Justice will not, in practice, agree to the transfer of a restricted patient to England unless satisfied that the proposed arrangements will enable the patient's safe management in England.

Record of transfer – managers' and guardians' duties [regulation 15]

34.18 Hospital managers in England are required to record the admission of patients transferred to detention in their hospitals from outside England or Wales using form M1. The managers must then take whatever steps are reasonably practicable to inform the person they think is the patient's nearest relative of the patient's admission, unless the patient has asked that such information not be given or does not have a nearest relative. Restricted patients, by definition, will not have a nearest relative.

34.19 The managers of the responsible hospital must similarly record the arrival of patients transferred to a CTO using form M1. In this case, arrival means the day on which the patient arrives at the place they are to live in England or Wales. The managers must then take whatever steps are reasonably practicable to inform the person they think is the patient's nearest relative that the patient is now a CTO patient, unless the patient has asked that such information not be given or does not have a nearest relative.

34.20 In both cases, the record on form M1 may be made by an officer authorised by the managers to do so.

34.21 Guardians (whether local authorities or private guardians) must record the arrival of patients transferred to their guardianship using form M1. Again, arrival means the day on which the patient arrives at the place they are to live in England or Wales. The guardian must then take whatever steps are reasonably practicable to inform the person they think is the patient's nearest relative that the patient is now subject to guardianship in England, unless the patient has asked that such information not be given or does not have a nearest relative.

34.22 A private guardian must also inform the responsible local authority of their own address, the patient's address and the name and address of the patient's nominated medical attendant (see paragraph 28.75).

34.23 These duties are in addition to the normal duties that hospital managers and local authorities have to give information to patients who are newly detained, or who become CTO patients or guardianship patients, and their nearest relatives.

Patients transferred to a CTO – responsible clinician's duty to set conditions [sections 80C and 85ZA and regulation 16]

34.24 As soon as practicable after patients are treated as having become CTO patients, the responsible clinician must specify the conditions which are to be included in their CTO under section 17B of the Act (see paragraphs 15.16 onward). Those conditions must first be agreed by an approved mental health professional (AMHP). The conditions which are specified are deemed to be included in the patient's CTO.

34.25 The responsible clinician must specify those conditions using form CT09 and the AMHP must confirm agreement using the same form.

Transfers from Scotland – further detail [sections 80B, 80C and 80D]

34.26 Transfers to England and Wales can only take place with the approval of Scottish Ministers in accordance with regulations made under the following provisions of the Mental Health (Care and Treatment) (Scotland) Act 2003:[153]

Section 289	Patients who are not subject to a measure authorising detention in hospital, ie the equivalent of CTO patients.
Section 290	Patients who are liable to be detained (including those who are on the equivalent of leave of absence) and conditionally discharged patients.

[153] Mental Health (Care and Treatment) (Scotland) Act 2003. http://www.legislation.gov.uk/asp/2003/13

34.27 An application for a transfer should be made to the Scottish Government.

34.28 In practice, the Scottish Government will generally ask the Department of Health (or the Ministry of Justice for restricted patients) to confirm that arrangements have been made. The Secretary of State for Justice will not, in practice, agree to the transfer of a restricted patient to England unless satisfied that the proposed arrangements will enable the patient's safe management in England.

34.29 Although the Act does not specify which of its provisions are to be considered equivalent to those in Scotland, they are likely to be as set out in figure 88.

Figure 88: Transfers from Scotland: likely corresponding provisions

Scotland	England and Wales
Emergency detention certificate under section 36 of the Mental Health (Care and Treatment) (Scotland) Act 2003	Emergency application (section 4)
Short term detention certificate under section 44 of the Mental Health (Care and Treatment) (Scotland) Act 2003	Application for admission for assessment (section 2)
Compulsory treatment order under section 64 of the Mental Health (Care and Treatment) (Scotland) Act 2003 authorising detention in hospital	Application for admission for treatment (section 3)
Compulsory treatment order under section 64 of the Mental Health (Care and Treatment) (Scotland) Act 2003 not authorising detention in hospital	CTO following detention under an application for admission for treatment (sections 3 and 17A)
Compulsion order under section 57A of the Criminal Procedure (Scotland) Act 1995 authorising detention in hospital, without a restriction order	Hospital order (section 37)
Compulsion order under section 57A of the Criminal Procedure (Scotland) Act 1995 authorising detention in hospital, with a restriction order under section 59 of that Act	Hospital order (section 37) with restriction order (section 41)
Compulsion order under section 57A of the Criminal Procedure (Scotland) Act 1995 not authorising detention in hospital	CTO following detention under an unrestricted hospital order (sections 37 and 17A as applied by part1 of schedule 1)

Scotland	England and Wales
Hospital direction under section 59A of the Criminal Procedure (Scotland) Act 1995	Hospital and limitation directions (section 45A)
Transfer for treatment direction under section 136 of the Mental Health (Care and Treatment) (Scotland) Act 2003	Restricted transfer direction for sentenced prisoner (sections 47 and 49)

34.30 At the time of publication, Scottish regulations do not permit the transfer of patients subject to treatment orders, assessment orders, interim compulsion orders, temporary compulsion orders or remands for inquiries into their mental condition. Between them, these are roughly equivalent to remands under section 35 or 36 of the Act, interim hospital orders under section 38 and transfer directions for unsentenced prisoners under section 48.

Transfer from Northern Ireland – further details [sections 82 and 82A]

34.31 Transfers from Northern Ireland must be approved by the Department of Health, Social Services and Public Safety (DHSSPS) for Northern Ireland under section 82 of the Act, unless the patient is restricted. At the time of publication, transfers of restricted detained patients, and transfers of conditionally discharged patients under section 82A, must be approved by the Department of Justice in Northern Ireland.

34.32 Before authorising a transfer, the DHSSPS or the Department of Justice in Northern Ireland, as applicable, must deem or judge it to be in the patient's interests after all appropriate investigations and assessments have been completed. The level of investigation and assessment required would depend on the gravity of the decision involved. More serious decisions, including decisions to transfer a patient against his ascertainable wishes and those of his family, would require the highest level of informed scrutiny.

34.33 In practice, the Northern Ireland authorities will generally ask the Department of Health (or the Ministry of Justice for restricted patients) to confirm that arrangements have been made for the patient to be admitted to hospital or received into guardianship in England or Wales. The Secretary of State for Justice will not, in practice, agree to the transfer of a restricted patient to England unless satisfied that the proposed arrangements will enable the patient's safe management in England.

34.34 Section 82 specifies the provision to which certain patients are to be treated as subject if transferred to England or Wales, as set out in figure 89.

Figure 89: Transfers from Northern Ireland: corresponding provisions as set out in section 82

Liable to be detained in Northern Ireland immediately before the transfer on the basis of	To be treated as liable to be detained in England and Wales on the basis of
A report under article 12(1) or 13 of the Mental Health (Northern Ireland) Order 1986[154]	An application for admission for treatment (section 3)
An application for assessment under article 4 of that Order	An application for admission for assessment (section 2)

34.35 Although the Act does not specify which of its provisions are to be considered equivalent to those in Northern Ireland in other cases, they are likely to be as set out in figure 90.

Figure 90: Transfers from Northern Ireland: likely corresponding provisions in other cases

Northern Ireland (Mental Health (Northern Ireland) Order 1986)	England and Wales
Liable to be detained under article 44 without restrictions on discharge	Hospital order (section 37)
Liable to be detained under 44, with restrictions under article 47	Hospital order (section 37) and restriction order (section 41)
Liable to be detained under article 53 without restrictions on discharge	Transfer direction for sentenced prisoner (section 47)
Liable to be detained under article 53, with restrictions under article 57	Transfer direction for sentenced prisoner (section 47) with restriction direction (section 49)
Liable to be detained under article 54 without restrictions on discharge	Transfer direction for unsentenced prisoner (section 48)
Liable to be detained under 54, with restrictions under article 57	Transfer direction for unsentenced prisoner (section 48) with restriction direction (section 49)
Subject to guardianship on the basis of an application under article 18	Guardianship application (section 7)
Subject to guardianship order under article 44	Guardianship order (section 37)

[154] Mental Health (Northern Ireland) Order. 1986. NISI 1986/595. http://www.legislation.gov.uk/nisi/1986/595

Transfer from Isle of Man or the Channel Islands – further details [sections 85, 85ZA and 85A]

34.36 Transfers from the Isle of Man or any of the Channel Islands require the approval of the relevant island authorities, in accordance with local legislation.

34.37 In practice, the island authorities will generally ask the Department of Health (or the Ministry of Justice for restricted patients) to confirm that arrangements have been made. The Secretary of State for Justice will not, in practice, agree to the transfer of a restricted patient to England unless satisfied that the proposed arrangements will enable the patient's safe management in England.

34.38 Patients transferred from the Isle of Man or the Channel Islands are treated on their arrival in England or Wales as if subject to the application, order or direction which corresponds to the provisions to which they were subject in the island in question. Advice should be sought from the island authorities or from the Department of Health or the Ministry of Justice, as applicable, if there is doubt about what the relevant corresponding provision is. Patients subject to the equivalent of remand to hospital under sections 35 or 36, or an interim hospital order under section 38, cannot be transferred.

34.39 For patients transferred from the Isle of Man who become subject to the equivalent of hospital directions or restriction directions in England, detention under sections 53 and 54 of the Mental Health Act 1998[155], is treated, where relevant, as if it were a sentence of imprisonment which has been given by a court in England or Wales.

Offenders found insane in Isle of Man or the Channel Islands [section 84]

34.40 Under section 84, the Secretary of State for Justice may direct that an offender be removed to a hospital in England or Wales if the offender:

- has been found insane by a court in the Isle of Man or any of the Channel Islands, or to have been insane at the time of the alleged offence, and
- has been ordered to be detained during Her Majesty's pleasure.

34.41 When admitted to the hospital in England or Wales, the patient is treated as if subject to a hospital order and restriction order. The Secretary of State may subsequently direct that the patient be returned to the island, to be dealt with as if never transferred in the first place.

[155] Mental Health Act 1998. https://www.gov.im/media/13725/mentalhealthact1998.pdf

Related material

Scotland
Directorate for Population Health Improvement Mental Health, St Andrews House, Regents Road, Edinburgh, EH1 3DG
Telephone: 0131 244 5668
Email: andy.lawson2@scotland.gsi.gov.uk

For cases concerned with criminal proceedings email:
restrictedpatients@scotland.gsi.gov.uk

Northern Ireland
Mental Health Unit, Department of Health, Social Services and Public Safety, D1.4 Castle Buildings, Stormont Estate, Belfast BT4 3SQ
Telephone: 028 9052 2562
Fax: 028 9052 2500
Email: mentalhealthunit@dhsspsni.gov.uk

States of Jersey
Community Mental Health Service, 20 La Chasse, St Helier, Jersey, Channel Islands, JE24UE
Tel: 01534 445841
Fax: 01534 445140
Email: health@gov.je

Bailiwick of Guernsey
Corporate Headquarters, Rue Mignot, St Andrews, Guernsey, Channel Islands, GY6 8TW
Tel: 10481 725241
Fax: 01481 235341
Email: healthandwellbeing@gov.gg

Isle of Man
Department of Health and Social Care, Mental Health Service, Cronk Coar, Noble's Hospital, Braddan, Isle of Man, IM4 4RF
Telephone: 01624 656015
Fax: 01624 642805
Email: mentalhealthcustomerservices.dh@gov.im

35: Transfer of patients to Scotland

Introduction

35.1 This chapter describes the provisions of the Act under which patients may be transferred from detention, a community transfer order (CTO) or conditional discharge in England to the equivalent in Scotland. The provisions in question are mainly to be found in part 6 of the Act.

Purpose of transfers under the Act

35.2 A transfer under the Act is only necessary where the patient concerned needs to remain subject to detention, conditional discharge or the equivalent of a CTO on arrival in Scotland.

Transfer of detained patients to Scotland [sections 80 and 92]

35.3 The Secretary of State may issue a warrant ('a transfer warrant') authorising the transfer of the detained patients from England to Scotland if they are detained on one of the provisions set out in figure 91.

Figure 91: Detained patients who may be transferred to Scotland

Patients liable to be detained on the basis of	Relevant section
An application for admission for assessment	section 2 or 4
An application for admission for treatment	section 3
A hospital order (with or without a restriction order under section 41)	section 37 (or 51)
A hospital direction (with or without a limitation direction)	section 45A
a transfer direction (with or without a restriction direction under section 49)	section 47 or 48
and Patients treated as detained on the basis of one of the above (eg as a result of transfer from guardianship or from outside England or Wales)	

35.4 A warrant cannot be issued for the transfer of patients remanded to hospital under section 35 or 36, subject to an interim hospital order under section 38, or detained in a hospital as a place of safety under section 135 or 136. In practice, it is unlikely that a warrant would be issued for the transfer of patients detained in hospital under the 'holding powers' in section 5.

35.5 A warrant may only be issued if the Secretary of State thinks it is in the patient's interests to be removed to Scotland and that arrangements have been made for the patient to be admitted to hospital in Scotland or (if the patient is not, in fact, to be admitted immediately to hospital) for the possibility of the patient's detention in hospital to be authorised under the relevant Scottish legislation.

Requesting a transfer warrant for Scotland for a detained patient

35.6 In practice, a request for a transfer warrant should be made by, or on behalf of, the managers of the hospital in which the patient is detained in England.

35.7 The request should explain why the hospital thinks the transfer would be in the patient's interests, not the interests of the hospital, and the arrangements that have been agreed for the patient to be received in Scotland.

35.8 For patients other than restricted patients, a pro-forma to be used for such requests is available from the Department of Health.

35.9 Requests for the transfer of restricted patients should be made to the Ministry of Justice. The Act only provides for the transfer of patients between hospitals in different jurisdictions but not the transfer between a prison in one jurisdiction and a hospital in another. If such a transfer is being contemplated, it will need to be undertaken in two stages. Either the patient will be transferred from prison to hospital and from there to a hospital in the other jurisdiction or from prison to another prison and then prison to hospital. Although this might appear complicated, it can be agreed in principle with the patient only having to move once.

35.10 For patients detained under section 2 of the Act, the Scottish authorities require there to be at least 10 days and preferably 14 days remaining on the section 2 when the transfer takes place. This means that the pro-forma for such a transfer should be completed as soon as it is known that the patient is to be transferred to Scotland and the hospital in England has been advised that there is a bed available for the patient at the receiving hospital in Scotland. The completed pro-forma should be faxed or emailed to the Department of Health by day 11 (day 14 at the very latest) and the hospital in England would need to transfer the patient by day 18 (preferably by day 14). A warrant issued for a patient detained under section 2 would not be valid beyond day 18 of the patient's detention.

35.11 Transfer to Scotland requires the approval of Scottish Ministers in accordance with Scottish legislation. The Department of Health (or the Ministry of Justice) will seek this directly from the Scottish Government. If necessary, they may need to ask the hospital in England for any further information which the Scottish Ministers require.

Conveyance of detained patients to Scotland [section 80 and 137]

35.12 If the Secretary of State issues a warrant, it will include any necessary directions allowing the patient to be conveyed to the relevant hospital (or other place) in Scotland by specified people (normally anyone authorised by the hospital managers) within a fixed period. This is normally 14 days, unless the patient's current period of detention is due to expire sooner or, in a section 2 case, day 18 will be reached in less than 14 days.

35.13 The Scottish Ministers may also give directions about the patient's conveyance once in Scotland under Scottish regulations (or authorise the patient's intended responsible medical officer in Scotland to do so).

35.14 While being conveyed to Scotland in accordance with the transfer warrant, the patient is considered to be in legal custody under the Act (see chapter 11).

Effect of transfer of a detained patient [section 91]

35.15 When the transfer is completed, the application, order or direction on the basis of which the patient was detained in England ceases to have effect and cannot be revived.

35.16 The transfer is completed when the patient is admitted to the relevant hospital in Scotland. If the patient is not in fact to be detained, eg because the patient is to be given the equivalent of leave of absence under Scottish legislation without first being admitted to the new hospital, the transfer is completed when the possibility of detention is authorised under the relevant Scottish legislation.

35.17 The patient will then be subject to the relevant legislation in Scotland – which differs in many respects from that in England.

35.18 For the patient to return to England a further transfer would be necessary, in accordance with Scottish legislation, which will require the agreement of the Scottish Ministers (see chapter 34).

Transfer of responsibility for conditionally discharged patients to Scotland [section 80A and 92]

35.19 If the Secretary of State for Justice thinks it would be in the patient's interests, the Secretary of State may agree with the relevant Scottish Minister that the latter will take over responsibility for a conditionally discharged patient. If responsibility is transferred to the Scottish Minister in this way, the patient will become subject to the arrangements for conditional discharge under the relevant legislation in Scotland.

Transfer of responsibility for patients on a CTO to Scotland [section 80ZA and 91]

35.20 The Secretary of State for Health may authorise the transfer of responsibility for a patient on a CTO to Scotland.

35.21 Such a transfer of responsibility may only be authorised if the Secretary of State thinks that it is in the patient's interests and that arrangements have been made for the patient to be made subject to provisions under Scottish legislation which correspond or are similar to CTOs. At the time of publication, the relevant legislation is the Mental Health (England and Wales Cross-border transfer: patients subject to requirements other than detention) (Scotland) Regulations 2008 (SSI 2008/356).[156]

35.22 In practice, this means a CTO under the Mental Health (Care and Treatment) (Scotland) Act 2003[157] (or a compulsion order under the Criminal Procedure (Scotland) Act 1995)[158] which does not authorise the patient's detention in hospital.

35.23 The Secretary of State may not authorise a transfer of responsibility for patients on a CTO while they are recalled to hospital (which includes any period during which they are absent without leave from the hospital while recalled).

35.24 If the Secretary of State authorises a transfer of responsibility, responsibility for the patient passes to the appropriate body in Scotland from whatever time is specified in the authority. When responsibility passes to Scotland, the patient's CTO ceases to have effect and the patient ceases to be a patient on a CTO. In other words, the patient is no longer liable to recall to or detention in hospital in England or Wales. The patient will then be subject to the relevant legislation in Scotland.

35.25 In practice, a request for the transfer of a patient on a CTO should be made to the Department of Health by, or on behalf of, the managers of the patient's responsible hospital using the same pro-forma as for detained patients.

35.26 A transfer of responsibility for a patient on a CTO does not give anyone any power to convey the patient to Scotland against the patient's will.

---

[156] Mental Health (England and Wales Cross-border transfer: patients subject to requirements other than detention) (Scotland) Regulations. 2008 SSI 2008/356. http://www.legislation.gov.uk/all?title=Mental%20Health%20%28England%20and%20Wales%20Cross-border%20transfer%3A%20patients%20subject%20to%20requirements%20other%20than%20detention%29%20%28Scotland%29%20Regulations%202008%20%28SSI%202008%2F356%29%20.

[157] Mental Health (Care and Treatment) (Scotland) Act 2003. http://www.legislation.gov.uk/asp/2003/13

[158] Criminal Procedure (Scotland) Act 1995). http://www.legislation.gov.uk/ukpga/1995/46

Transfer of guardianship patients to Scotland

35.27 It is not possible to transfer guardianship patients to guardianship (or any other form of compulsory measure) in Scotland.

> Related material
>
> **England**
> For advice on proposals to transfer a patient from England to another jurisdiction please contact:
> Department of Health, Richmond House, 79 Whitehall, London SW1A 2NS
> Telephone: 020 7210 5359 or 020 7210 5775

36: Transfer of patients to Northern Ireland

Introduction

36.1 This chapter describes the provisions of the Act under which patients may be transferred from detention, a CTO, guardianship or conditional discharge in England to the equivalent in Northern Ireland. The provisions in question are mainly to be found in part 6 of the Act.

Purpose of transfers under the Act

36.2 A transfer under the Act is only necessary where the patient concerned needs to remain subject to detention, guardianship, conditional discharge or the equivalent of a CTO on arrival in Northern Ireland.

Transfer of detained patients to Northern Ireland [section 81 and 92]

36.3 The Secretary of State may issue a warrant ('a transfer warrant') authorising the transfer of detained patients from England to Northern Ireland if they are detained on one of the provisions set out in figure 91.

Figure 91: Detained patients who may be transferred to Northern Ireland

Patients liable to be detained on the basis of	Relevant section
An application for admission for assessment	section 2 or 4
An application for admission for treatment	section 3
A hospital order (with or without a restriction order under section 41)	section 37 (or 51)
A hospital direction (with or without a limitation direction)	section 45A
A transfer direction (with or without a restriction direction under section 49)	section 47 or 48
and Patients treated as detained on the basis of one of the above (eg as a result of transfer to or from guardianship, or from outside England or Wales)	

36.4 A warrant cannot be issued for the transfer of patients remanded to hospital under section 35 or 36, or subject to an interim hospital order under section 38 or detained in a hospital as a place of safety under section 135 or 136. And, in practice, it is very unlikely that a warrant would be issued for the transfer of patients detained in hospital under the 'holding powers' in section 5.

36.5 A transfer warrant may only be issued if the Secretary of State thinks that it is in the patient's interests to be removed to Northern Ireland and that arrangements have been made for the patient to be admitted to hospital in Northern Ireland.

Requesting a transfer warrant for Northern Ireland for a detained patient

36.6 In practice, a request for a transfer warrant should be made by, or on behalf of, the managers of the hospital in which the patient is detained in England.

36.7 The request should explain why the hospital thinks the transfer would be in the patient's interests, not the interests of the hospital, and the arrangements that have been agreed for the patient to be received in Northern Ireland.

36.8 For patients other than restricted patients, a pro-forma to be used for such requests is available from the Department of Health.

36.9 Requests for the transfer of restricted patients should be made to the Ministry of Justice. The Act only provides for the transfer of patients between hospitals in different jurisdictions but not the transfer between a prison in one jurisdiction and a hospital in another. If such a transfer is being contemplated, it will need to be undertaken in two stages. Either the patient will be transferred from prison to hospital and from there to a hospital in the other jurisdiction or from prison to another prison and then prison to hospital. Although this might appear complicated, it can be agreed in principle with the patient only having to move once.

Conveyance of detained patients to Northern Ireland [section 81 and 137]

36.10 If the Secretary of State issues a warrant, it will include any necessary directions allowing the patient to be conveyed to the relevant hospital in Northern Ireland by specified people (normally anyone authorised by the hospital managers) within a fixed period (normally 14 days, unless the patent's current period of detention is due to expire sooner).

36.11 While being conveyed in accordance with the warrant, the patient is considered to be in legal custody, whether in England or Northern Ireland – see chapter 11.

Effect of transfer of a detained patient [section 91]

36.12 When the transfer is completed, the application, order or direction on the basis of which the patient was detained in England ceases to have effect and cannot be revived. For the patient to return to England a further transfer would be necessary, in accordance with section 82 of the Act (see chapter 34).

36.13 The transfer is completed when the patient is admitted to the relevant hospital in Northern Ireland. From that point the patient is treated as if subject to the corresponding provision of legislation in force in Northern Ireland. In particular:

Figure 92: Transfer of a detained patient to Northern Ireland

If the patient, immediately before being transferred to Northern Ireland was liable to be detained on the basis of	The patient is treated, on admission to hospital in Northern Ireland, as if
An application for admission for assessment (section 2)	Admitted to the hospital on the basis of an application for assessment under article 4 of the Mental Health (Northern Ireland) Order 1986[159] made on the date of his admission to that hospital
An application for admission for treatment (section 3)	Detained for treatment under part2 of the Mental Health (Northern Ireland) Order 1986 by virtue of a report under article 12(1) of that Order made on the date of his admission

36.14 Patients subject to a hospital direction or to a transfer direction under section 47 given while they were serving a prison sentence (as defined in section 47(5)) imposed by a court in England or Wales are treated on their transfer as if the associated prison sentence(s) had been imposed by a court in Northern Ireland.

36.15 If they were subject to a restriction direction or a limitation direction due to end on a fixed date (eg because they are serving a prison sentence of fixed duration, rather than a life sentence), the equivalent restriction direction will still expire on that date. The same applies to patients who were subject to a restriction order of limited duration before their transfer.

Transfer of responsibility for conditionally discharged patients to Northern Ireland [section 81A and 92]

36.16 If the Secretary of State for Justice thinks it would be in the patient's interests, the Secretary of State may agree with the Secretary of State for Northern Ireland that the latter will take over responsibility for a conditionally discharged patient.

36.17 If a transfer of responsibility is agreed, patients are treated as if they were subject to a hospital order and restriction order, or transfer direction and restriction direction (as applicable) under the corresponding legislation in

[159] Mental Health (Northern Ireland) Order. 1986. NISI 1986/595. http://www.legislation.gov.uk/nisi/1986/595

Northern Ireland, and as if they had been conditionally discharged on the day of the transfer.

36.18 The transfer does not affect the day on which the patient's restriction order or direction expires, if it was due to expire on a fixed date.

Transfer of patients on a CTO to Northern Ireland [section 81ZA]

36.19 At the time of publication, there is no equivalent of a CTO under Northern Ireland legislation, so responsibility for patients on a CTO may not be transferred to a hospital in Northern Ireland.

36.20 If it is in their interests, patients on a CTO may instead be transferred to detention in Northern Ireland under a transfer warrant as described earlier in this chapter, as if (in effect) they had never become a patient on a CTO.

36.21 In practice, a request for the transfer of a patient on a CTO should be made to the Department of Health by, or on behalf of, the managers of the patient's responsible hospital.

Transfer of guardianship patients to Northern Ireland [section 81]

36.22 The Secretary of State may also issue a transfer warrant authorising the transfer of a guardianship patient to guardianship in Northern Ireland. This may only be done if the Secretary of State thinks that it is in the patient's interests to be removed to Northern Ireland and that arrangements have been made for the patient to be received into guardianship in Northern Ireland.

36.23 In practice, a request for a transfer warrant should be made by, or on behalf of, the patient's responsible local authority in England to the Department of Health using the same pro-forma as for detained patients. The request should explain why the transfer would be in the patient's interests, the arrangements that have been agreed for the patient to be received into guardianship in Northern Ireland, and whether, and if so why, the patient needs to be kept in custody while being taken there.

36.24 If the Secretary of State for Health issues a warrant, it will include directions allowing the patient to be conveyed to the place where they are to live in Northern Ireland, so that the patient is treated as being in legal custody on the journey – see chapter 11.

36.25 The transfer is complete once the patient has arrived at that place. From then on, a patient who was previously subject to guardianship on the basis of a guardianship application under the Act is treated as if subject to guardianship on the basis of a corresponding application made under the legislation in Northern Ireland on the day the transfer was completed. Similarly, a patient previously subject to a guardianship order under the Act is treated as if given an equivalent order or direction under Northern Ireland legislation on that day.

Related material

England
For advice on proposals to transfer a patient from England to another jurisdiction please contact:
Department of Health, Richmond House, 79 Whitehall, London SW1A 2NS
Telephone: 020 7210 5359 or 020 7210 5775

37: Transfer to the Isle of Man or the Channel Islands

Introduction

37.1 This chapter describes the provisions of the Act under which patients may be transferred from detention, a CTO, guardianship or conditional discharge in England to the equivalent in the Isle of Man or any of the Channel Islands. The provisions in question are mainly to be found in part 6 of the Act.

Purpose of transfers under the Act

37.2 A transfer under the Act is only necessary where the patient concerned needs to remain subject to detention, or the equivalent of a CTO, guardianship or conditional discharge on arrival in the island in question if equivalent arrangements are available there.

Transfer of detained patients to the Isle of Man or the Channel Islands [section 83 and 92]

37.3 The Secretary of State may issue a warrant ('a transfer warrant') authorising the transfer detained patients from England to the Isle of Man or any of the Channel Islands if they are detained on one of the provisions set out in figure 93.

Figure 93: Detained patients who may be transferred to the Isle of Man or Channel Islands

Patients liable to be detained on the basis of	Relevant section
An application for admission for assessment	section 2 or 4[160]
An application for admission for treatment	section 3
A hospital order (with or without a restriction order (section 41))	section 37 (or 51)
A hospital direction (with or without a limitation direction)	section 45A
A transfer direction (with or without a restriction direction (section 49))	section 47 or 48
and Patients treated as detained on the basis of one of the above (eg as a result of transfer to or from guardianship or from outside England or Wales)	

[160] In practice transfers are unlikely to be made before a patient is detained under section 2 of the Act.

37.4 A warrant cannot be issued for the transfer of patients remanded to hospital under section 35 or 36, subject to an interim hospital order under section 38, or detained in hospital as a place of safety under section 135 or 136. And in practice it is very unlikely that a warrant would be issued for the transfer of patients detained in hospital under the 'holding powers' in section 5.

37.5 A transfer warrant may only be issued if the Secretary of State thinks that it is in the patient's interests to be removed to the island in question and that arrangements have been made for the patient to be admitted to hospital there.

Requesting a transfer warrant for the Isle of Man or the Channel Islands for a detained patient

37.6 In practice, a request for a transfer warrant should be made by, or on behalf of, the managers of the hospital in which the patient is detained in England.

37.7 The request should explain why the hospital thinks the transfer would be in the patient's interests, not the interests of the hospital and the arrangements that have been agreed for the patient to be received in the island in question.

37.8 For patients other than restricted patients, a pro-forma to be used for such requests is available from the Department of Health.[161]

37.9 Requests for the transfer of restricted patients should be made to the Ministry of Justice. The Act only provides for the transfer of patients between hospitals in different jurisdictions but not the transfer between a prison in one jurisdiction and a hospital in another. If such a transfer is being contemplated, it will need to be undertaken in two stages. Either the patient will be transferred from prison to hospital and from there to a hospital in the other jurisdiction or from prison to another prison and then prison to hospital. Although this might appear complicated, it can be agreed in principle with the patient only having to move once.

37.10 Transfers may require the approval of the relevant island authorities in accordance with the local legislation.[162] The Department of Health (or the Ministry of Justice) will seek this as necessary. They may need to ask the hospital in England for any further information which island authorities require.

---

[161] The form is currently available from https://www.gov.uk/government/uploads/system/uploads/attachment_data/file/191482/Transfer_of_non-restricted_patients_to_a_hospital_outside_England_and_Wales.rtf

[162] At the time of publication, the relevant local legislation in respect of the Isle of Man is the Isle of Man Mental Health Act 1998 (https://www.gov.im/media/13725/mentalhealthact1998.pdf), and in respect of the Channel Islands is the Jersey Mental Health Act 1969 (https://www.jerseylaw.je/law/Display.aspx?url=%2Flaw%2Flawsinforce%2Fconsolidated%2F20%2F20.650) and the Guernsey Mental Health (Bailiwick of Guernsey) Law 2010 (http://www.guernseylegalresources.gg/article/95741/Mental-Health-Bailiwick-of-Guernsey-Law-2010).

Conveyance to the Isle of Man or the Channel Islands of detained patients [section 83 and 137]

37.11 If the Secretary of State issues a warrant, it will include any necessary directions allowing the patient to be conveyed to the relevant hospital (or other place) in the island by specified people (normally anyone authorised by the hospital managers) within a fixed period (normally 14 days, unless the patent's current period of detention is due to expire sooner).

37.12 While being conveyed in accordance with the warrant, the patient is considered to be in legal custody while in England or Wales – see chapter 11. Once the patient reaches the territory of the relevant island, local legislation governs whether they may be kept in custody and whether, by whom and during what period, they may be retaken if they abscond. The receiving hospital or the island authorities may be asked to advise on this as necessary.

Effect of transfer of a detained patient [section 91]

37.13 When the transfer is completed, the application, order or direction on the basis of which the patient was detained in England ceases to have effect and cannot be revived. For the patient to return to England a further transfer would be necessary, in accordance with section 85 of the Act (see chapter 34).

37.14 The transfer is completed when the patient is admitted to the relevant hospital in the island in question. The patient will then be subject to the relevant local legislation – which may be significantly different from that in England.

Transfer of responsibility for conditionally discharged patients to Isle of Man or the Channel Islands [section 83A and 92]

37.15 If the Secretary of State for Justice thinks it would be in the patient's interests, the Secretary of State may agree with the relevant authorities in the Isle of Man or any of the Channel Islands that those authorities will take over responsibility for a conditionally discharged patient. If responsibility is transferred in this way, the patient will become subject to arrangements corresponding to conditional discharge under the relevant local legislation.

Transfer of responsibility for patients on a CTO to Isle of Man or the Channel Islands [section 83ZA]

37.16 If the local legislation in force in the Isle of Man or any of the Channel Islands includes provisions corresponding or similar to a CTO, the Secretary of State for Health may authorise the transfer of responsibility for a patient on a CTO to that island.

37.17 Such a transfer of authority may only be authorised if the Secretary of State thinks that it is in the patient's interests and that arrangements have been made for the patient to be made subject to the relevant local provisions.

37.18 The Secretary of State may not authorise a transfer of responsibility for patients on a CTO while they are recalled to hospital, which includes any period during which they are absent without leave while recalled.

37.19 If the Secretary of State authorises a transfer of responsibility, responsibility for the patient passes to the appropriate authority or person in the island from whatever date is specified in the authority, and at that point the patient's CTO ceases to have effect and the patient ceases to be a patient on a CTO. In other words, the patient is no longer liable to recall to or detention in hospital in England or Wales. Instead they become subject to the local legislation, which may be different in significant respects.

37.20 A transfer of responsibility for a patient on a CTO does not give anyone any power to convey the patient to the island against the patient's will. The island authorities should be able to advise on what, if any, powers would be available if the patient did not arrive as expected.

37.21 If there is no equivalent of a CTO in the island in question, patients on a CTO may instead be transferred to detention in the island under a transfer warrant as described earlier in this chapter, as if (in effect) they had never become a patient on a CTO.

37.22 In practice, a request for the transfer of a patient on a CTO should be made to the Department of Health by, or on behalf of, the managers of the patient's responsible hospital. At the time of publication the Isle of Man legislation contains provision for 'After-care under supervision' (section 28 *et seq*). The Jersey Mental Health Act 1969 contains no provision equivalent to the CTO.

The Mental Health Law 2010 of the Bailiwick of Guernsey does contain provision for CTOs (section 26 *et seq*).

Transfer of guardianship patients to Isle of Man or the Channel Islands [section 83]

37.23 The Secretary of State may also issue a transfer warrant authorising the transfer of a guardianship patient to guardianship in the Isle of Man or Jersey. This may only be done if the Secretary of State thinks that it is in the patient's interests to be removed to the island and that arrangements have been made for the patient to be received into guardianship there.

37.24 In practice, a request for a transfer warrant should be made by, or on behalf of, the patient's responsible local authority in England to the Department of Health. The request should explain why the transfer would be in the patient's interests, the arrangements that have been agreed for the patient to be received into guardianship in the island in question, and whether, and if so why, the patient needs to be kept in custody while being taken there. The transfer may also have to be agreed with the relevant island authorities in accordance with local legislation.

37.25 If the Secretary of State for Health issues a warrant, it will include directions allowing the patient to be conveyed to the relevant island. Those directions have the same effect as directions in a transfer warrant for a detained patient (see paragraph 37.12).

37.26 The transfer is complete once the patient has been placed under guardianship in the island. From that point, the patient is no longer subject to guardianship or a guardianship order in England or Wales, but is subject to the relevant local legislation instead, which may be different.[163]

> ### Related material
>
> **England**
> For advice on proposals to transfer a patient from England to another jurisdiction please contact:
> Department of Health, Richmond House, 79 Whitehall, London SW1A 2NS
> Telephone: 020 7210 5359 or 020 7210 5775

[dr u] Isle of Man Mental Health Act 1998. https://www.gov.im/media/13725/mentalhalthact1998.pdf
Jersey Mental Health Act 1969.
https://www.jersey.je/law/Display.aspx?url=%2%Flawsinforce%2Fconsoloidated%2F20%2F20.650_MentalHealthLaw1969_RevisedEdition_1January2013.pdf
Guernsey Mental Health (Bailiwick of Guernsey) Law 2010.
http://guernseylegalresources.gg/CHttpHandler.ashx?id=79818&p=0

38: Removal of foreign patients

Introduction

38.1 This chapter describes the provisions in part 6 of the Act under which certain detained in-patients may be repatriated (or otherwise moved) to a jurisdiction outside the UK, the Isle of Man and the Channel Islands.

Purpose of these provisions

38.2 A removal warrant under the Act is only necessary where patients are not willing to travel or need to be kept in custody on the journey. A warrant is not necessary if patients are willing to travel and it is safe for them to do so without being in legal custody.

Secretary of State's power to authorise removal of patient [section 86]

38.3 The Secretary of State may authorise a person's removal to a place in a jurisdiction outside the UK, the Isle of Man or the Channel Islands if that person is:

- neither a British citizen nor a Commonwealth citizen with the right of abode in the United Kingdom
- receiving in-patient treatment in hospital for mental disorder in England or Wales, and
- detained pursuant to an application for admission for treatment, a hospital order, a hospital direction or a transfer direction.

38.4 This may only be done if the Secretary of State thinks that removal is in the interests of the patient and that proper arrangements have been made for:

- the patient's removal to the country or territory outside the United Kingdom, the Isle of Man and the Channel Islands, and
- care or treatment for the patient there

and the proposed removal has been agreed by the First-tier Tribunal (or the Upper Tribunal on appeal), or the Mental Health Tribunal for Wales, or the Mental Health Review Tribunal for Northern Ireland ('the Tribunal').

38.5 In practice, this provision is not likely to be used often, not least because of the difficulty of being sure that patients who need to remain detained can and will be detained under the legislation of the country to which it is proposed they be removed.

Proposals for removal

38.6 Proposals for the removal of a patient detained on the basis of an application for admission under part 2 should be made to the Department of Health. If the patient is detained under part 3, the Ministry for Justice should be contacted instead.

38.7 The Ministry of Justice guidance document 'Foreign national restricted patients: Guidance on repatriation' (25 March 2009)[164] states that 'use of s. 86 is not appropriate where the patient is likely to be discharged within 6 months' (p.4).

38.8 Before deciding whether to seek the agreement of the Tribunal, the Department of Health or the Ministry of Justice will need to have details of the reasons for the proposed transfer and the arrangements that have or could be made for the patient's transport (in the UK and abroad) and for the patient's subsequent care and treatment. In practice, the Departments will expect the managers of the hospital in which the patient is detained to provide this information and (if the case is referred to the Tribunal) to provide any further information which the Tribunal requires.

Effect of Secretary of State's warrant

38.9 If the Secretary of State obtains the Tribunal's approval and decides to authorise the patient's transfer, the Secretary of State will issue a warrant which directs that the patient is taken directly to the point of embarkation and which may also include any appropriate directions to allow the patient to be conveyed, while remaining in legal custody, out of the UK. This includes being kept in custody while en route to another country, eg on a plane or ship. But the Secretary of State cannot authorise the patient being kept in custody or detained once the patient has arrived in another country – so any escort arrangements for the rest of the journey would have to be made under the law of that country, if that is allowed.

Effect of removal from England [section 91]

38.10 In most cases, when patients are removed from England and Wales under these arrangements, the authority for their detention ceases to have effect when they are received into hospital (or another institution) in the country to which they have been removed. But where the patient is subject to a restricted hospital order, it will remain in force so that it will apply again should the patient return to England or Wales, unless the restriction order is for a fixed period, in which case both it and the hospital order will expire at the end of that period.

Alternative means of repatriation

38.11 In many cases, it may be more appropriate and more practicable for patients who have no legal right to remain in the UK to be repatriated under other powers (eg immigration legislation). Case law has established that it is

[164] 'Foreign national restricted patients: Guidance on repatriation' (25 March 2009). https://www.justice.gov.uk/downloads/offenders/mentally-disordered-offenders/guidance-repatriation.pdf

possible to remove people who are detained under the Act but who are not entitled to remain in the UK without using section 86.[165]

38.12 It may also be possible to arrange repatriation of certain patients detained in hospital under part 3 of the Act under the Repatriation of Prisoners Act 1984.[166] Advice should be sought from the Ministry of Justice.

[165] R (on the application of X) v Secretary of State for the Home Office. 2001. 1 WLR 740 ; and MJ (Angola) v Secretary of State for the Home Office. 2011. 1 WLR 2699. http://www.bailii.org/ew/cases/EWCA/Civ/2010/557.html

[166] Repatriation of Prisoners Act 1984. http://www.legislation.gov.uk/ukpga/1984/47

ANNEXES

Annex A – Key words and phrases used in this Guide

Absent without leave (AWOL)	A patient being absent, without permission, from the place they ought to be under the Act.
The Act	The Mental Health Act 1983, as amended over time.
Acting nearest relative	A person appointed by a court to act as a patient's nearest relative, either in place of the person who would otherwise be the nearest relative, or because no nearest relative can be identified. See chapter 2 in particular.
Admission (to hospital)	In the Act, admission to hospital generally implies admission as an in-patient.
Advance decision	A decision, under the Mental Capacity Act 2005, to refuse specified treatment made in advance by a person who has capacity to do so. This decision will then apply at a future time when that person lacks capacity to consent to, or refuse the specified treatment. The meaning and general effect of advance decisions are set out in sections 24 to 26 of the Mental Capacity Act 2005. In the Mental Health Act, advance decisions are particularly relevant to section 58A treatments and to the treatment of CTO patients under Part 4A. See chapters 23 and 24 in particular.
Advocacy	In this Reference Guide, advocacy generally refers to independent mental health advocacy (IMHA) services established under sections 130A to 130D of the Act. See chapter 4 in particular.
After-care	In this Reference Guide, after-care refers to the after-care services which section 117 of the Act requires clinical commissioning groups (CCGs) (and, in some circumstances, the NHS Commissioning Board) and local authorities to provide for certain patients who have been detained under the Act, after they leave hospital. It is also known as 'section 117 after-care'. See chapter 29. The duty applies to community patients and conditionally discharged restricted patients, as well as those who have been fully discharged.
AMHP Regulations	The Mental Health (Approved Mental Health Professionals) (Approval) (England) Regulations 2008 (No. 1206) which deal with the approval by local authorities of approved mental health professionals.

Application	Application is used in the Act (and this Reference Guide) in several different contexts. Depending on the context, it generally means: • an application to have a patient detained in hospital or received into guardianship under Part 2 of the Act – see chapters 8 and 28 respectively; • an application to the Tribunal by a patient (or their nearest relative) seeking their discharge from detention etc - see chapter 2; or • an application to a court under the Act, eg to have an acting nearest relative appointed or a private guardian replaced – see chapters 2 and 28 respectively.
Application for admission to hospital	An application to the managers of a hospital for a patient to be detained there under Part 2 of the Act. See chapter 8 in respect of making applications and chapter 9 (in particular) for their effect. As well as being the means of requesting a patients detention, the application itself (when properly completed and submitted) becomes the legal authority on the basis of which the patient is detained.
Application for admission for assessment	An application for admission under section 2 of the Act for the patient to be detained in hospital for up to 28 days to be assessed (or assessed and treated). See chapter 8 in respect of making applications, and chapter 9 (in particular) for their effect. An emergency application under section 4 is also a form of application for admission for assessment.
Application for admission for treatment	An application for admission under section 3 of the Act for a patient to be detained in hospital for medical treatment. See chapter 8 in respect of making applications, and chapter 9 (in particular) for their effect.
Application for guardianship	See guardianship application.
Appropriate medical treatment	The Act defines appropriate medical treatment as medical treatment is which is appropriate in the patient's case, taking into account the nature and degree of the patient's mental disorder and all the other circumstances of the case. See paragraph 8.8 in particular. A requirement that such treatment must be available forms part of the criteria in the Act for detention in many cases (though not the criteria for an application for admission for assessment). See chapters 2, 6, 9, 15 to 19, and 20. It also forms part of the criteria for CTOs – see chapters 6 and 23.
Approved clinician	A mental health professional approved by the Secretary of State or a person or body exercising the approval function of the Secretary of State[167], or by the Welsh Ministers to act as an approved clinician for the purposes of the Act. See chapter 30. Certain decisions under the Act can only be made by approved clinicians. In particular, medical treatment cannot (in general) be given without a patient's consent unless an approved clinician is in charge of it – see chapters 23 and 24. Only approved clinicians can be responsible clinicians.

[167] A person with whom the Secretary of State for Health has made an agreement under section 12ZA of the Act, or a body on whom the Secretary of State has imposed a requirement under section 12ZB of the Act

Approved mental health professional (AMHP)	A social worker or other professional approved by a local authority to perform a variety of functions under the Act. See chapter 30. Those functions including making applications for admission to hospital and guardianship applications, and agreeing that patients should become patients supervised on a community treatment order. References in the Act to AMHPs are to AMHPs acting on behalf of a local authority (unless that does not make sense in context).
Attorney	Someone appointed, in accordance with the Mental Capacity Act 2005, under a lasting power of attorney (LPA), who has the legal right to make decisions within the scope of the authority conferred by that LPA on behalf of the person (the donor) who made the LPA. Also called a 'donee' of lasting power of attorney. In the context of the Mental Health Act, this means people whose authority extends to make personal welfare decisions on behalf of donors who now lack capacity to make those decisions themselves. They are particularly relevant to section 58A treatment and to the treatment of patients on CTO under Part 4A - see chapters 23 and 24 in particular.
Capacity	The ability to take a decision about a particular matter at the time the decision needs to be made. Some people may lack capacity to take a particular decision (eg to consent to treatment) because they cannot understand, retain, use or weigh the information relevant to the decision. A legal definition of lack of capacity for people aged 16 or over is set out in section 2 of the Mental Capacity Act 2005. See also competence to consent.
Care programme approach (CPA)	A system of care and support for individuals with complex needs which includes an assessment, a care plan and a care coordinator. It is used mainly for adults in England who receive specialist mental health care and in some Children and Adolescent Mental Health services (CAMHS). There are similar systems for supporting other groups of individuals including, children and young people (children's assessment framework), older adults (single assessment process) and people with learning disabilities (person centred planning).
Care Quality Commission (CQC)	The regulator established by the Health and Social Care Act 2008 of all providers of regulated health and social care. This includes care provided under the Mental Health Act 1983.
Certificate required	Whether or not part 4A patients consent to treatment, there are certain treatments they can only be given if they have been approved by a SOAD on a 'part 4A certificate' (see paragraph 24.22). The Act refers to this as the 'certificate requirement', which is above and beyond the requirements described above, which the Act calls the 'authority' to give treatment. Broadly speaking, the certificate requirement applies to any treatment for which a certificate would be necessary under section 58 or 58A of the Act were the patient detained instead (see chapter 23).
Child (and children)	A person under the age of 16.

Clinical commissioning group (CCG)	The NHS body responsible for commissioning (arranging) NHS services for a particular part of England from NHS trusts, NHS foundation trusts and independent sector providers. CCGs replaced primary care trusts from 1 April 2013. CCGs' commissioning plans are reviewed by the NHS Commissioning Board (NHS England). CCGs are generally responsible for commissioning mental healthcare, except for specialist care commissioned by the NHS Commissioning Board.
Code of Practice	Under section 118 of the Act, the Secretary of State must publish a Code of Practice for the guidance of certain people who make decisions under the Act. The Welsh Ministers must do the same in relation to Wales. See chapter 3.
Community patient	A patient who is supervised on a community treatment order. See chapter 26 in particular.
Community treatment order (CTO)	An order made by a patient's responsible clinician under section 17A of the Act discharging a patient from detention in hospital, subject to the possibility of recall to hospital. A CTO is the legal authority for the patient's discharge from detention, subject to the possibility of recall. Community patients are expected to comply with the conditions specified in the CTO. See chapter 26 in particular for CTOs generally and chapter 24 for medical treatment of community patients.
Competence to consent	Similar to capacity to consent, but specifically about a child's ability to make particular decisions. A child may be unable to make the particular decision in question due to their mental condition or because they do not have the maturity to do so. See also 'Gillick competent'.
Compulsory measures	Things which can be done to people under the Act without their agreement. This includes detention in hospital, a community treatment order and guardianship. The term is not used in the Act.
Compulsory treatment	Medical treatment for mental disorder given under the Act, which may be against the wishes of the patient.
Conditional discharge	The discharge from hospital by the Secretary of State for Justice or the Tribunal of a restricted patient subject to conditions. The patient remains subject to recall to hospital by the Secretary of State.
Conditionally discharged patient	A restricted patient who has been given a conditional discharge by the Secretary of State for Justice or the Tribunal. See chapter 27 in particular.
Confirmation (of detention, CTO or guardianship)	In this Reference Guide, 'confirmation' refers to the decision that responsible clinicians and others make under section 21B that patients continue to meet the criteria for continued detention, CTOs or guardianship when they return from being AWOL after more than 28 days. See chapters 9, 26 and 28 respectively. The term is not used in the Act itself.
Conflict of Interest Regulations	The Mental Health (Conflicts of Interest) (England) Regulations 2008 (No. 1205) which set out when AMHPs may not make applications for detention or guardianship under Part 2 of the Act and when doctors may not make medical recommendations in support of those applications. See paragraphs 8.55 to 8.59 (detention) and 28.46 to 28.49 (guardianship).

Convey and conveyance	The Act uses the term 'convey' to mean transporting a patient under the Act to hospital (or anywhere else), while keeping them in custody.
Court of Protection	The specialist court established under section 45 of the Mental Capacity Act 2005 to deal with issues relating to people who lack capacity to make specific decisions for themselves. The Court is most relevant to the Mental Health Act in relation to section 58A treatment and to the treatment of community patients under Part 4A - see chapters 4, 23 and 24 in particular.
Custody	See Legal custody.
Deprivation of liberty	References to 'deprivation of liberty' in the Mental Capacity Act have the same meaning as Article 5 of the European Convention on Human Rights (ECHR). 'Deprivation of liberty' means the circumstances in which a person's freedom is taken away. Its meaning has been developed through case law.
Deputy	Someone appointed under the Mental Capacity Act 2005 by the Court of Protection with ongoing legal responsibility, within the bounds set by the Court, to make specified decisions on behalf of a person who lacks capacity to make those decisions for themselves. They are most relevant to the Mental Health Act in relation to section 58A treatment and to the treatment of community patients under Part 4A - see chapters 4, 23 and 24 in particular.
Detained patient	Broadly speaking, a patient who is detained (or is liable to be detained) in hospital. The term is not used in the Act. In this Reference Guide it is used as a short-hand way of referring collectively to patients who are (or could be) detained in hospital – but the precise groups of patients covered varies from chapter to chapter (as explained in those chapters).
Detention	Being detained in a hospital (or other place) under the Act. A person who is detained may be kept in the hospital or other place against their wishes.
Detention for assessment	The detention of a person in order to carry out an assessment. Can normally only last for a maximum of 28 days. Also known as 'section 2 detention'.
Detention for medical treatment	The detention of a person in order to give them the medical treatment for mental disorder they need. There are various types of detention for medical treatment in the Act. It most often means detention as a result of an application for detention under section 3 of the Act. But it also includes several types of detention under part 3 of the Act, including hospital directions, hospital orders and interim hospital orders.

Discharge	Discharge means different things in different contexts in the Act (and this Reference Guide). But more often than not, it refers to the discharge of a patient from being subject to detention or another compulsory measure under the Act. In the context of detention, it means discharge from being liable to be detained under the Act – which may or may not be accompanied by discharge from hospital in the normal sense. In the context of CTOs, it means discharge from the community treatment order and therefore the possibility of recall to hospital. The Act (and this Reference Guide) distinguishes this from cases where community patients are allowed to leave hospital before the end of the maximum 72 hour period for which they can be detained on recall. That is referred to as release. For nearest relatives and hospital managers' powers of discharge from detention, CTOs and guardianship respectively, see chapters 25, 26 and 28. For the Tribunal's power of discharge see chapter 6. See also conditional discharge.
Displacement (of nearest relative)	The provision under section 29 of the Act, under which the County Court can order that the functions of the nearest relative be carried out by another person or by a local authority (as defined by the Care Act 2014).
Doctor	A fully registered medical practitioner. For simplicity, this Reference Guide uses doctor where the Act itself uses the term 'medical practitioner', which is defined in the Interpretation Act 1982.
Doctor approved under section 12	A doctor who has been approved under the Act by the Secretary of State for Health as having special experience in the diagnosis or treatment of mental disorder, or by a body which the Secretary of State has authorised to exercise the approval function under the Act, or by Welsh Ministers. Some medical recommendations and medical evidence to courts under the Act can only be made by a doctor who is approved under section 12. (Doctors who are approved clinicians are automatically treated as though they have been approved under section 12.)
Donee (of lasting power of attorney)	See Attorney.
Electro-convulsive therapy (ECT)	A form of medical treatment for mental disorder in which a small, carefully controlled electric current is introduced into the brain. It is administered in conjunction with a general anaesthetic and muscle relaxant medications and is occasionally used to treat very severe depression.
Emergency application	An application for detention for assessment made under section 4 with only one supporting medical recommendation in cases of urgent necessity. The patient can only be detained for a maximum of 72 hours unless second medical recommendation is received. Also known as a section 4 application.
Escorted leave	Leave to be absent from hospital granted on condition that the patient concerned remains in the custody of someone else while away from the hospital. See paragraphs 25.2 to 25.7 and 11.14 to 11.16 in particular.
Equality Act 2010	A law making it unlawful (either directly or indirectly) to discriminate against a person on the basis of a protected characteristic (as defined in that Act). Imposes a public sector equality duty on public bodies.

European Convention on Human Rights (ECHR)	The European Convention for the Protection of Human Rights and Fundamental Freedoms. The substantive rights it guarantees are largely incorporated into UK law by the Human Rights Act 1998.
Extension (of CTO)	Authorising the extension of a community treatment order when it would otherwise expire. See paragraphs 26.72 to 26.102 in particular. Extension is the equivalent of renewal of detention or guardianship.
First-tier Tribunal	An independent judicial body with the power to discharge detained patients, community patients, guardianship patients and conditionally discharged patients. See chapter 6.
Guardian	Unless otherwise stated, the person on whom certain powers are conferred in respect of a patient who has been received into their guardianship. See chapter 28 in particular. In the vast majority of cases, the guardian is the local authority, but there can be a private guardian instead.
Guardianship	Unless otherwise stated, the regime established by the Act under which patients may become and remain subject to the guardianship of an individual or body (the guardian) who has certain powers, including the power to decide where the patient should live. See chapter 28. Guardianship is generally authorised by means of a guardianship application under Part 2 of the Act. But it can also be imposed by a court under Part 3 of the Act as an alternative to punishment for a criminal offence. Only the latter is correctly referred to as a guardianship 'order'.
Guardianship application	An application to a local authority for a patient to be received into the guardianship of the local authority or of a private guardian. See chapter 28. As well as being the means of requesting a patient's reception into guardianship, the application itself (when properly completed and accepted by the local authority) becomes the legal authority for the powers of the guardian.
Guardianship order	An order made by a court under Part 3 of the Act that a mentally disordered offender should be received into the guardianship of the local authority or private guardian named in the order. The order is the legal authority for the guardian to exercise powers of guardianship over the patient. See chapter 28.
Guardianship patient	A person subject to guardianship under the Act.
High Security Psychiatric Hospital	Hospitals approved by the Secretary of State for the treatment of patients detained under the Act who require special security because of their dangerous, violent or criminal propensities. At the time of publication there are three such hospitals – Ashworth, Broadmoor and Rampton. Most of the provisions in section 134 relating to the withholding of patients correspondence (see chapter 5) apply exclusively to patients in these hospitals.

Holding powers	The powers in section 5 of the Act to detain hospital in-patients temporarily to allow time to make the applications necessary to detain them under the Act in the normal way. There are two powers. Under section 5(2) the doctor or approved clinician in charge of a patient's treatment (whether or not for mental disorder) may detain them for up to 72 hours. Under section 5(4) certain nurses may detain patients already being treated for mental disorder for up to six hours, pending the arrival of the doctor or approved clinician who could exercise the power in section 5(2). See chapter 8. These are often referred to as 'holding powers', but the Act itself does not use that term.
Hospital and limitation directions	An order of a court under section 45A of the Act that a mentally disordered offender should be detained in hospital for medical treatment (the hospital direction), subject to special restrictions (the limitation direction) that apply to restricted patients under the Act. See chapter 16 in particular. These directions can only be given where the court also passes a sentence of imprisonment. (For that reason, they have sometimes been known in the past as 'hybrid orders'.) Initially, a hospital direction cannot be given without a limitation direction. But it is possible for the limitation direction to end, or be lifted, while the hospital direction remains in place – see chapter 21.
Hospital direction	See Hospital and limitation directions.
Hospital managers	The individual or body responsible for a particular hospital. In the context of detention, it generally refers to the managers of the hospital in which a patient is (or is liable to be) detained. In the context of CTOs, it generally (but not always) refers to the managers of the responsible hospital. In the context of hospital managers' power to discharge patients, it generally means the three or more individuals to whom the body concerned delegates the task of holding 'managers' hearings' and deciding whether to exercise the power of discharge from detention or the CTO. See chapters 26 and 27 respectively.
Hospital order	An order of a court under section 37 (or 51) of the Act that a mentally disordered offender should be detained in hospital for medical treatment, instead of being punished for the offence. See chapter 15. A hospital order may be given on its own, or with a restriction order under section 41. Where a restriction order is in force alongside a hospital order, this Reference Guide refers to it as a restricted hospital order for convenience. A hospital order without a restriction order is referred to as an unrestricted hospital order.

Immediately necessary	In certain circumstances, some of the rules in Part 4 and Part 4A of the Act regarding medical treatment do not apply to treatment which is immediately necessary. Although, for convenience, it is often equated with an 'emergency', immediately necessary has a specific definition in the Act – which varies according to the type of treatment. See paragraphs 23.56 to 23.61, 24.12 to 24.13 and 24.30 in particular.
Independent hospital	In practice, this means a hospital which is not managed by an NHS body.
Independent mental capacity advocate (IMCA)	An advocate able to offer help to patients who lack capacity under arrangements which are specifically required to be made under the Mental Capacity Act 2005.
Independent mental health advocate (IMHA) and independent mental health advocate services	Independent mental health advocacy means the advocacy services for detained (and various other patients) to be provided under sections 130A to 130D of the Act. An independent mental health advocate is an individual assisting patients as part of such a service. See chapter 4.
Informal patient	A patient who is not subject to any compulsory measure under the Act. In other words, a patient who is not a detained patient, a community patient, a guardianship patient or a conditionally discharged patient. The term is not used in the Act. A few of the provisions of the Act apply to informal patients generally, or to certain groups of them. These are summarised in chapter 13.
Interim hospital order	An order made by a court under section 38 of the Act that a mentally disordered offender be detained in hospital. A court can only make such an order as an interim measure prior to deciding whether to make a hospital order or give hospital and limitations directions, or to deal with the offender in another way. See chapters 15, 16 and 18.
Learning disability qualification	The rule which says that, for certain (but not all) purposes of the Act, a learning disability is not to count as a mental disorder unless it is associated with abnormally aggressive or seriously irresponsible conduct on the part of the person concerned. See paragraphs 1.12 to 1.15.
Leave of absence	Permission to be absent from hospital, granted under section 17 of the Act by a patient's responsible clinician. Patients remain under the powers of the Act when they are on leave and can be recalled to hospital if necessary in the interest of the patient's health or safety or for the protection of other people. See paragraphs 25.2 to 25.12.
Legal custody	Section 137 of the Act states that, in certain circumstances, patients being detained, conveyed etc under the Act are deemed to be in legal custody. This confers certain powers on the person in whose custody they are (or ought to be). It also means that if they abscond they may be taken back into custody. See chapter 11.

Liable to be detained	Broadly speaking, a person is liable to be detained under the Act if they either are, or could be, detained in hospital, because a specific authority for that is in force in respect of them, eg a relevant application for admission to hospital under Part 2, or an order or direction under Part 3. As such, it includes patients who are on leave of absence from hospital – or who are absent without leave – as well as those who are actually detained. For drafting reasons, the Act uses it to include conditionally discharged patients, but not community patients, even though both are subject – in different ways – to recall to hospital. As explained in paragraphs 1.37 and 1.38, this Reference Guide tends to use 'detained' to cover both 'detained' and 'liable to be detained' in the terms of the Act. But references to detained patients in the Guide never include conditionally discharged patients.
Limitation direction	See Hospital and limitation directions.
Local authority	The local authority responsible for care and support services in a particular area of England, which is a local authority for the purpose of the Care Act 2013 (except where otherwise indicated).
Magistrates' remand patient	A defendant remanded in custody by a magistrates' court who has subsequently been transferred to detention in hospital by a transfer direction made by the Secretary of State under section 48. See chapter 20. This term is not used in the Act.
Managers	See Hospital managers.
Medical recommendation	A recommendation made by a doctor, in the form set out in regulations, in support of an application for admission to hospital or a guardianship application. See chapters 8 and 28 respectively. An application is not valid unless it is supported by the proper medical recommendation(s).
Medical treatment	Medical treatment as defined for the purposes of the Act covers more than what might normally be meant by the term. In the Act, it includes nursing, psychological intervention and specialist mental health habilitation, rehabilitation and care. See paragraphs 1.17 to 1.21 for the definition, and chapters 23 and 24 for the rules in the Act relating to specific treatments and to treatment without consent.
The MCA	The Mental Capacity Act 2005, which provides a legal framework for decision-making in relation to people who lack capacity to take particular decisions for themselves. For all purposes relevant to the Mental Health Act, the MCA does not apply to people aged under 16.
Mental disorder	The Act defines mental disorder as any disability or disorder of the mind (apart from dependence on alcohol or drugs). As well as mental illnesses, it includes conditions like personality disorders, autistic spectrum disorders and learning disabilities. See chapter 1.
Mental Health Review Tribunal (MHRT) for Wales	The tribunal which exercises in Wales the functions under the Act exercised in England by the First-tier Tribunal.

Mutual Recognition Regulations	The Mental Health (Mutual Recognition) Regulations 2008 (No. 1204) which set out when approved clinicians and section 12 approved doctors approved in England may act as such in Wales, and vice versa. See chapter 30 in particular (and chapter 28 in relation to guardianship specifically).
NHS body	A NHS trust, NHS foundation trust, clinical commissioning group, the NHS Commissioning Board or (in Wales) a local health board.
NHS Commissioning Board (NHS England)	The NHS Commissioning Board (also known as NHS England) reviews the commissioning plans of CCGs and assures the Secretary of State that the plans will deliver a comprehensive health service. The NHS Commissioning Board took over most of the functions of Strategic Health Authorities from 1 April 2013.
NHS patient	A patient whose care in or by an independent hospital is being funded by an NHS body. Where an NHS patient is a detained patient in an independent hospital, or a community patient whose responsible hospital is an independent hospital, the NHS body which has contracted for the patients care has the same power as the managers of the independent hospital itself to discharge the patient or transfer them to another hospital under different managers – see paragraphs 10.13 to 10.15, 26.51 to 26.118 in particular. The term is not used in the Act.
Nearest relative	Nearest relative is defined in section 26 of the Act. It often does not mean the same thing as next-of-kin and need not mean a relative at all (in the normal sense). The nearest relatives of many (but not all) detained patients, community patients and guardianship patients have various rights under the Act. See chapter 2 for nearest relatives generally, and chapters 8 and 9, 26 and 28 for their main functions in relation to detained patients, community patients and guardianship patients respectively.
Nominated medical attendant	A doctor appointed by a private guardian for a guardianship patient. The nominated medical attendant has certain powers and duties, eg in respect of renewal of the patient's guardianship. See chapter 28.
Nurses Order	The Mental Health (Nurses) (England) Order 2008 (No. 1207) which sets out which nurses are of the 'prescribed class' to exercise the holding power under section 5(4) of the Act. See paragraphs 8.80 to 8.85.
Part 2	The part of the Act which deals mainly with detention, CTOs and guardianship for 'civil patients' (rather than mentally disordered offenders or suspected offenders). Some aspects of Part 2 also applies to some patients who have been detained or made subject to guardianship by the courts but who have been transferred from prison to detention in hospital by the Secretary of State for Justice under part 3 of the Act.
Part 2 guardianship patient	A patient subject to guardianship on the basis of a guardianship application under Part 2 of the Act (rather than a guardianship order under Part 3). See chapter 28 in particular. The term is not used in the Act.

Part 2 patient	Broadly speaking, a 'civil patient' – ie someone who is a detained patient, a community patient or a guardianship patient under Part 2 of the Act, rather than as a result of the criminal justice related provisions in Part 3. The term is not used in the Act. Its precise meaning in this Reference Guide varies from chapter to chapter (as explained in each case). The term is not used in the Act.
Part 2 community patient	A community patient who was discharged from detention onto a CTO which was based on an application for admission for treatment under part 2 of the Act. See chapter 26 in particular. The term is not used in the Act.
Part 3	The part of the Act which deals with mentally disordered offenders and defendants in criminal proceedings. Among other things, it allows courts to detain people in hospital for treatment instead of punishing them, where particular criteria are met. It also allows the Secretary of State for Justice to transfer people from prison to detention in hospital for treatment. See chapters 14 to 22 and 27 in particular.
Part 3 patient	Broadly speaking, someone who is a detained patient, a community patient or a guardianship patient as result of the criminal justice related provisions in part 3 of the Act, rather than the provisions for 'civil patients' in part 2. part 3 patients are also sometimes known as 'forensic patients'. The term is not used in the Act. Its precise meaning in this Reference Guide varies from chapter to chapter (as explained in each case).
Part 3 guardianship patient	A patient subject to guardianship on the basis of a guardianship order under part 3 (rather than a guardianship application under part 2 of the Act). See chapter 28 in particular. The term is not used in the Act.
Part 3 community patient	A community patient who was discharged from detention onto a CTO which was based on an unrestricted hospital order, unrestricted hospital direction or unrestricted transfer direction under part 3 of the Act.
Part 4	The part of the Act which deals mainly with medical treatment for mental disorder – especially medical treatment without consent of patients detained under the Act and of community patients on recall to hospital. See chapter 23 and 24.
Part 4A	The part of the Act which deals mainly with the medical treatment for mental disorder of community patients who have not been recalled to hospital. See chapter 23.
Part 4A certificate	A certificate issued by a SOAD approving the administration of section 58 type treatments and section 58A type treatments to community patients who have not been recalled to hospital. A part 4A certificate may also approve section 58 treatments and section 58A treatments to be given should the patient be recalled to hospital. See paragraphs 24.23 to 24.27 in particular.
Patient	The Act defines a patient as a person who is, or who appears to be, suffering from mental disorder – see paragraph 1.22. For consistency, the Reference Guide uses the term in the same way. This use of the term is not a recommendation that the term patient should be used in practice in preference to other terms such as 'service user', 'client' or similar terms. It is just a reflection of the terminology used in the Act itself.

Place of safety	Broadly speaking, the Act uses place of safety to mean somewhere where a patient may be detained temporarily. In particular it is used in relation to patients who are removed from public places by the police under section 136, or from a private place on the basis of a magistrates' warrant under section 135, and who need to be detained temporarily so that they can be assessed to see if an application should be made under part 2. See paragraph 7.10.
Private guardian	A guardian who is not a local authority. Such a guardian can (but need not be) a relative of the patient concerned. Private guardians are (in effect) under the supervision of the responsible local authority and have certain specific duties as well as powers – see chapter 28.
Recall and recalled (to hospital)	An enforceable order requiring a patient who has previously been released from detention to come back to hospital (though not necessarily the same hospital in which they were previously detained). Recall happens in three separate contexts in the Act: recall of detained patients from leave of absence (section 17); recall of conditionally discharged patients (section 42); and recall of community patients (section 17E). The criteria, procedures and effects are different in each case. See paragraphs 25.16 to 25.20 (leave of absence), 26.31 to 26.39 (CTOs) and 27.44 to 27.52 (conditional discharge).
Recommendation	See Medical recommendation.
Reference (to Tribunal)	A request from hospital managers or the Secretary of State for the First-tier Tribunal to consider a patient's case. Hospital managers are under a duty to make references in certain cases, as is the Secretary of State. The Secretary of State also has the discretion to do so in other cases. See chapter 6. For most purposes, a reference has the same effect as an application to the Tribunal by a patient (or a nearest relative).
Regulations (or regulation X or Y)	Unless it says otherwise, in this Reference Guide references to the regulations (and references to regulation X or Y) are to the Mental Health (Hospital, Guardianship and Treatment) (England) Regulations 2008 (No. 1184). Those regulations include (amongst other things) the statutory forms which must be used for applications for admission for treatment, medical recommendations, CTOs and various other purposes.
Release date	The day on which patients subject to hospital and limitation directions and sentenced prisoners subject to restricted transfer directions would have been entitled to be released from prison (or its equivalent) had they not be detained in hospital instead. If the patient is serving a life sentence, or an indeterminate sentence, the release date is the date (if any) on which the person's release is ordered by the Parole Board. When the release date is reached, limitation directions and restriction directions cease to have effect – which means (amongst other things) that these patients are not longer liable to be removed to prison to complete their sentences. See paragraphs 16.15 to 16.18 (limitation directions) and 19.14 to 19.17 (restriction directions).

Release from hospital	Community patients who have been recalled to hospital may be detained for a maximum of 72 hours (unless their CTO is then subject to revocation). When their responsible clinician agrees that they may leave the hospital again, patients are described in the Act as having been 'released' (to distinguish between that and discharge from the CTO itself). See paragraphs 26.64 to 26.66 in particular.
Remand for report	An order by a court under section 35 of the Act that a defendant be remanded to detention in hospital pending trial or sentencing, so that a report may be compiled on the defendant's mental condition. Such patients may not be treated without their consent. See chapter 14.
Remand for treatment	An order by a court under section 36 of the Act that a mentally disordered defendant be remanded to detention in hospital for medical treatment while awaiting trial or sentencing. See chapter 14.
Remand patient	A patient who is detained in hospital as a result of a remand for report or remand for treatment under sections 35 or 36 of part 3 of the Act. See chapter 14.
Renewal (of detention, guardianship etc)	Authorising the continuation of the authority to detain a detained patient, or to keep someone subject to guardianship, for a further period after the existing authority is due to expire. See paragraphs 26.29 to 26.58 (detention) and 28.96 to 28.118 (guardianship). The authority that is to be renewed may be either an application under part 2 or an order or direction under part 3. Renewal is the equivalent of extension of a CTO.
Responsible after-care bodies	The clinical commissioning group (or in some circumstances, the NHS Commissioning Board) and local authority responsible for providing a patient with after-care under section 117 of the Act. See chapter 29.
Responsible clinician	For (most) detained patients and community patients, the responsible clinician is the approved clinician in overall charge of the patient's case. Responsible clinicians have various specific powers and duties under the Act in respect of their patients. See chapters 8 and 26 in particular. Responsible clinician has a different meaning for guardianship patients – for which see chapter 28.
Responsible hospital	The hospital whose managers have various powers and duties under the Act in respect of community patients. See chapter 26 in particular. Initially, the responsible hospital is the one in which the patient was liable to be detained immediately before being discharged onto the CTO. But responsibility may subsequently be assigned to a different hospital.
Responsible local authority	The local authority responsible for a guardianship patient. If the local authority is itself the guardian, it will be the responsible local authority. If there is a private guardian, the responsible local authority will be the one for the area in which the guardian lives (regardless of where the patient lives). Responsible local authorities have various powers and duties, including the power to discharge guardianship patients. See chapter 28.

Restricted hospital order	See Hospital order.
Restricted patient	A patient who is subject to a restriction order, limitation direction or restriction direction, imposing special restrictions, in addition to those imposed normally by detention in hospital under the Act. Those special restrictions are primarily designed to protect the public from harm. The effect of the restrictions is summarised in chapter 21. Restricted patients are subject to ongoing case management by the Mental Health Casework Section of the Ministry of Justice on behalf of the Secretary of State. They are also the only patients who may be conditionally discharged from detention.
Restricted transfer direction	See Transfer direction.
Restrictions	The special restrictions to which restricted patients are subject. See chapter 21.
Restriction direction	A direction under section 49 imposing special restrictions on a patient made by the Secretary of State when directing the patient's transfer from prison (or another form of custody) to detention in hospital for medical treatment by means of a transfer direction under part 3. See chapters 15 to 21 in particular.
Restriction order	An order under section 41 imposing special restrictions on a patient which is made by a court together with a hospital order detaining an mentally disordered offender in hospital for medical treatment. See chapters 15 to 21 in particular.
Revocation (of a community treatment order)	A decision by a responsible clinician to revoke a community patient's community treatment order (CTO). Its effect is that the patient ceases to be a community patient and becomes a detained patient again. See paragraphs 26.56 to 26.63. Revocation can only happen when a community CTO patient has been recalled to hospital.
Second opinion appointed doctor (SOAD)	A doctor appointed by the Care Quality Commission to provide an independent second medical opinion on whether it is appropriate for certain types of medical treatment for mental disorder to be given to patients under part 4 and part 4A of the Act. Certain treatments cannot be given unless the SOAD has issued a SOAD certificate approving their administration. See chapters 23 and 24.
SOAD certificate	A certificate given by a SOAD approving the administration of specified treatments. See chapters 23 and 24. A SOAD certificate will always be needed for section 57 treatments and (if the patient is under 18) section 58A treatments. It is also needed for section 58A treatments for detained patients aged 18 or over if they cannot consent and for section 58 treatments for detained patients of all ages who either cannot, or do not consent. A part 4A certificate is a form of SOAD certificate specifically for community patients.
Secretary of State	The Secretary of State for Health or the Secretary of State for Justice (but see paragraph 1.47). In practice, the Secretaries of State act through the Department of Health and the Ministry of Justice respectively.

Section 2	See Application for admission for assessment.
Section 3	See Application for admission for treatment.
Section 4	See Emergency application.
Section 5	See Holding powers.
Section 12 approved doctor	A doctor approved by the Secretary of State for Health or persons with whom the Secretary of State has entered into agreements under section 12ZA or 12ZB of the Act[168] (or the Welsh Ministers) to carry out certain functions under the Act. See paragraphs 30.32 to 30.37 respectively. At least one of the medical recommendations required to support an application for admission or a guardianship application under part 2 must be made by a section 12 doctor - see chapters 11 and 31 respectively. Similarly, medical evidence required by courts or the Secretary of State under part 3 must often come, at least in part, from a section 12 approved doctor - see chapters 14 to 20. All approved clinicians who are doctors are automatically treated as approved under section 12.
Section 37	See Hospital order.
Section 41	See Restricted hospital order.
Section 45A	See Hospital and limitation directions.
Section 47	See Transfer direction (for sentenced prisoners).
Section 48	See Transfer direction (for unsentenced prisoners).
Section 49	See Restriction direction.
Section 57 treatment	A treatment for mental disorder which may not be given to any patient (whether or not detained) except in accordance with section 57. The main such treatment is neurosurgery for mental disorder ('psychosurgery'). See chapter 23.
Section 58 treatment	A treatment for mental disorder which may not be given to a detained patient except in accordance with section 58. This applies, in particular, to medication for mental disorder (after an initial three month period). See chapter 23.
Section 58 type treatment	Broadly speaking, a treatment to be given to a community patient which would be a section 58 treatment if the patient were detained. See chapter 24.
Section 58A treatment	A treatment for mental disorder which may not be given to a detained patient (or any patient under 18) except in accordance with section 58A. See chapter 23. The main such treatment is electro-convulsive therapy (ECT).

[168] The approving bodies are listed on the Gov.uk website. https://www.gov.uk/government/publications/mental-health-act-exercise-of-approval-instructions-2013

Section 58A type treatment	A treatment to be given to a community patient which would be a section 58A treatment if the patient were detained. See chapter 24.
Section 117	See after-care.
Sentenced prisoner	A prisoner who is serving a sentence of imprisonment following conviction for an offence. The rules for giving, and ending, transfer directions for sentenced prisoners differ from those for unsentenced prisoners in certain respects. See chapter 19.
Special restrictions	See Restrictions.
Statutory forms	Forms which the Regulations say must be used to make applications, medical recommendations and to record various other decisions and events. If the regulations say that a particular statutory form must be used, a form whose wording corresponds to the wording in Schedule 1 to the Regulations must be used.
Transfer direction	A warrant issued by the Secretary of State for Justice directing that a prisoner be removed to a hospital and detained there. Transfer directions for sentenced prisoners are given under section 47, those for unsentenced prisoners under section 48. See chapters 19 and 20 respectively, in particular. A transfer direction may (and often must) be accompanied by a restriction direction under section 49 imposing special restrictions on the patient. For convenience, this Reference Guide refers to the result as a restricted transfer direction and to a transfer direction without a restriction direction as an unrestricted transfer direction.
Transfer warrant	A warrant issued by the Secretary of State authorising the transfer of a patient to Scotland, Northern Ireland, the Isle of Man or any of the Channel Islands. See chapters 35 to 37.
Tribunal	Depending on the context, the First-tier Tribunal or the Upper Tribunal on appeal (and sometimes both). See chapter 6 in particular. The Tribunal is a judicial body which has the power to discharge patients from detention, community treatment orders, guardianship and conditional discharge. Sometimes it also includes the Mental Health Review Tribunal (MHRT) for Wales.
Tribunal Rules	The procedural rules by which the First-tier Tribunal and the Upper Tribunal operate.[169] See chapter 6.
Upper Tribunal	An independent judicial body with the power to determine appeals on a point of law against decisions of the First-tier Tribunal (and the Mental Health Review Tribunal (MHRT) for Wales). See chapter 6.

[169] The Rules are available at http://www.justice.gov.uk/tribunals/rules.

Unrestricted part 3 patient	Broadly speaking, a part 3 patient who is not subject to special restrictions. More specifically, a patient who is liable to be detained in hospital on the basis of a hospital order or transfer direction who either never was, or is no longer, subject to a restriction order or restriction direction, or a patient subject to a hospital direction where the associated limitation direction is no longer in effect. See chapters 15 and 18, 19, 20 and 21 in particular.
Unrestricted hospital direction	A hospital direction where the associated limitation direction is no longer in effect. See chapter 18 in particular.
Unrestricted hospital order	A hospital order which either never was, or is no longer, accompanied by a restriction order. See chapter 20.
Unrestricted patient	See Unrestricted part 3 patient.
Unsentenced prisoner	A prisoner (or other detainee) who is not serving a sentence of imprisonment following conviction for an offence. The rules for giving, and ending, transfer directions for unsentenced prisoners differ from those for sentenced prisoners in certain respects. See chapter 20 in particular.
Unrestricted transfer direction	A transfer direction which either never was, or is no longer, accompanied by a restriction direction. See chapters 19 and 20 in particular.
Welsh Ministers	Ministers in the Welsh Assembly Government.

Annex B: List of Statutory Forms

Form		Regulation
A1	Section 2 - application by nearest relative for admission for assessment	4(1)(a)(i)
A2	Section 2- application by an approved mental health professional for admission for assessment	4(1)(a)(ii)
A3	Section 2 - joint medical recommendation for admission for assessment	4(1)(b)(i)
A4	Section 2 - medical recommendation for admission for assessment	4(1)(b)(ii)
A5	Section 3 - application by nearest relative for admission for treatment	4(1)(c)(i)
A6	Section 3- application by an approved mental health professional for admission for treatment	4(1)(c)(ii)
A7	Section 3 - joint medical recommendation for admission for treatment	4(1)(d)(i)
A8	Section 3 - medical recommendation for admission for treatment	4(1)(d)(ii)
A9	Section 4 – emergency application by nearest relative for admission for assessment	4(1)(e)(i)
A10	Section 4 – emergency application by an approved mental health professional for admission for assessment	4(1)(e)(ii)
A11	Section 4 – medical recommendation for emergency admission for assessment	4(1)(f)
H1	Section 5(2) – report on hospital in-patient by registered medical practitioner or approved clinician or person nominated to act for them	4(1)(g)

Form		Regulation
H2	Section 5(4) – record of hospital in-patient by nurse prescribed for the purposes of section 5(4)	4(1)(h)
H3	Sections 2, 3, and 4 – record of admission to hospital	4(4) and (5)
H4	Section 19 – authority for transfer from one hospital to another under different managers	7(2)(a) and 7(3)
H5	Section 20 – renewal of authority for detention	13(1), (2) and (3)
H6	Section 21B – authority for detention after absence without leave for more than 28 days	14(1)(a) and (b)
G1	Section 7 – guardianship application by nearest relative	5(1)(a)(i) and (1)(b)
G2	Section 7 – guardianship application by an approved mental health professional	5(1)(a)(ii) and (1)(b)
G3	Section 7 – joint medical recommendation for reception into guardianship	5(1)(c)(i)
G4	Section 7 – medical recommendation for reception into guardianship	5(1)(c)(ii)
G5	Section 7 - record of acceptance of guardianship application	5(2)
G6	Section 19 – authority for transfer from hospital to guardianship	7(4)(a), (d) and (e)
G7	Section 19 – authority for transfer of a patient from the guardianship of one guardian to another	8(1) (a), (d) and (e)
G8	Section 19 – authority to transfer from guardianship to hospital	8(2) and (4)
G9	Section 20 – renewal of authority for guardianship	13(4) and (5)
G10	Section 21B - authority for guardianship after absence without leave for more than 28 days	14(2)(a) and (b)

Form		Regulation
M1	Part 6 - date of reception of a patient in England	15(2), (4)(a) and 16(2)
M2	Section 25 – report barring discharge by nearest relative	25(1)(a) and (b)
T1	Section 57 - certificate of consent to treatment and second opinion	27(1)(b)
T2	Section 58(3)(a) – certificate of consent to treatment	27(2)
T3	Section 58(3)(b) – certificate of second opinion	27(2)
T4	Section 58A(3) – certificate of consent to treatment (patients at least 18 years old)	27(3)(b)
T5	Section 58A(4) – certificate of consent to treatment and second opinion (patients under 18)	27(3)(b)
T6	Section 58A(5) – certificate of second opinion (patients who are not capable of understanding the nature, purpose and likely effects of the treatment)	27(3)(b)
CTO1	Section 17A - community treatment order	6(1)(a), (b) and 6(2)(a)
CTO2	Section 17B - variation of conditions of a community treatment order	6(2)(b)
CTO3	Section 17E – community treatment order: notice of recall to hospital	6(3)(a)
CTO4	Section 17E – community treatment order: record of patient's detention in hospital after recall	6(3)(d)
CTO5	Section 17F(4) - revocation of community treatment order	6(8)(a) and (b)
CTO6	Section 17F(2) –authority for transfer of recalled community patient to a hospital under different managers	9(3)(a) and (5)
CTO7	Section 20A – community treatment order: report extending community treatment period	13(6)(a) and (b) and 13(7)

Form		Regulation
CTO8	Section 21B – authority for extension of community treatment period after absence without leave for more than 28 days	14(3)(a) and (b)
CTO9	Part 6 – community patients transferred to England	16(4) and (5)
CTO10	Section 19A - authority for assignment of responsibility for community patient to a hospital under different managers	17(3)(a) and (d)(i) and (ii)
CTO11	Section 64C(4) - certificate of appropriateness of treatment to be given to community patient not recalled to hospital ('part 4A certificate')	28(1)
CTO12	Section 64B(2)(b) or 64E(2)(b) – certificate of capacity (or competence if under 16) to consent to treatment for community patient not recalled to hospital	28(1A)

Annex C: Related material

Publications

Related material	Chapter
Procedure for the Transfer from Custody of Children and Young People to and from Hospital under the Mental Health Act 1983 in England. Department of Health and Youth Justice Board, 2011. https://www.gov.uk/government/uploads/system/uploads/attachment_data/file/215496/dh_128855.pdf	12
Standards on the use of section 136 of the Mental Health Act 1983 (England and Wales). Royal College of Psychiatrists CR159. 2011. http://www.rcpsych.ac.uk/usefulresources/publications/collegereports/cr/cr159.aspx	7
The Legal Aspects of the Care and Treatment of Children and Young People with Mental Disorders: a guide for professionals. National Institute for Mental Health in England. 2009. http://www.chimat.org.uk/resource/item.aspx?RID=94476	12
Working Together to Safeguard Children: a guide to inter-agency working to safeguard and promote the welfare of children. Department for Children, Schools and Families. 2010. http://www.workingtogetheronline.co.uk/resources.html	12

Useful addresses and contact information

Scotland
Directorate for Population Health Improvement Mental Health, St Andrews House, Regents Road, Edinburgh, EH1 3DG
Telephone: 0131 244 5668
Email: andy.lawson2@scotland.gsi.gov.uk

For cases concerned with criminal proceedings email: restrictedpatients@scotland.gsi.gov.uk

Northern Ireland
Mental Health Unit, Department of Health, Social Services and Public Safety, D1.4 Castle Buildings, Stormont Estate, Belfast BT4 3SQ
Telephone: 028 9052 2562
Fax: 028 9052 2500
Email: mentalhealthunit@dhsspsni.gov.uk

States of Jersey
Community Mental Health Service, 20 La Chasse, St Helier, Jersey, Channel Islands, JE24UE
Tel: 01534 445841
Fax: 01534 445140
Email: health@gov.je

Bailiwick of Guernsey
Corporate Headquarters, Rue Mignot, St Andrews, Guernsey, Channel Islands, GY6 8TW
Tel: 10481 725241
Fax: 01481 235341
Email: healthandwellbeing@gov.gg

Isle of Man
Department of Health and Social Care, Mental Health Service, Cronk Coar, Noble's Hospital, Braddan, Isle of Man, IM4 4RF
Telephone: 01624 656015
Fax: 01624 642805
Email: mentalhealthcustomerservices.dh@gov.im

England
For advice on proposals to transfer a patient from England to another jurisdiction please contact:
Department of Health, Richmond House, 79 Whitehall, London SW1A 2NS
Telephone: 020 7210 5359 or 020 7210 5775

Ministry of Justice Mental Health Casework Section. First Floor, Grenadier House, 99-105 Horseferry Road, London SW1P 2DD
Ministry of Justice Switchboard: 020 3334 3555
General: enquiry.mhu@noms.gsi.gov.uk

Annex D: Figures: written description

This annex provides a written description of figures 94 to 96 which refer to decisions described in chapters 23 and 24. The written explanations are to assist those with visual impairments to access this material.

Figure 94 Treatment with medication for mental disorder[170] of detained patients[171] under the Act

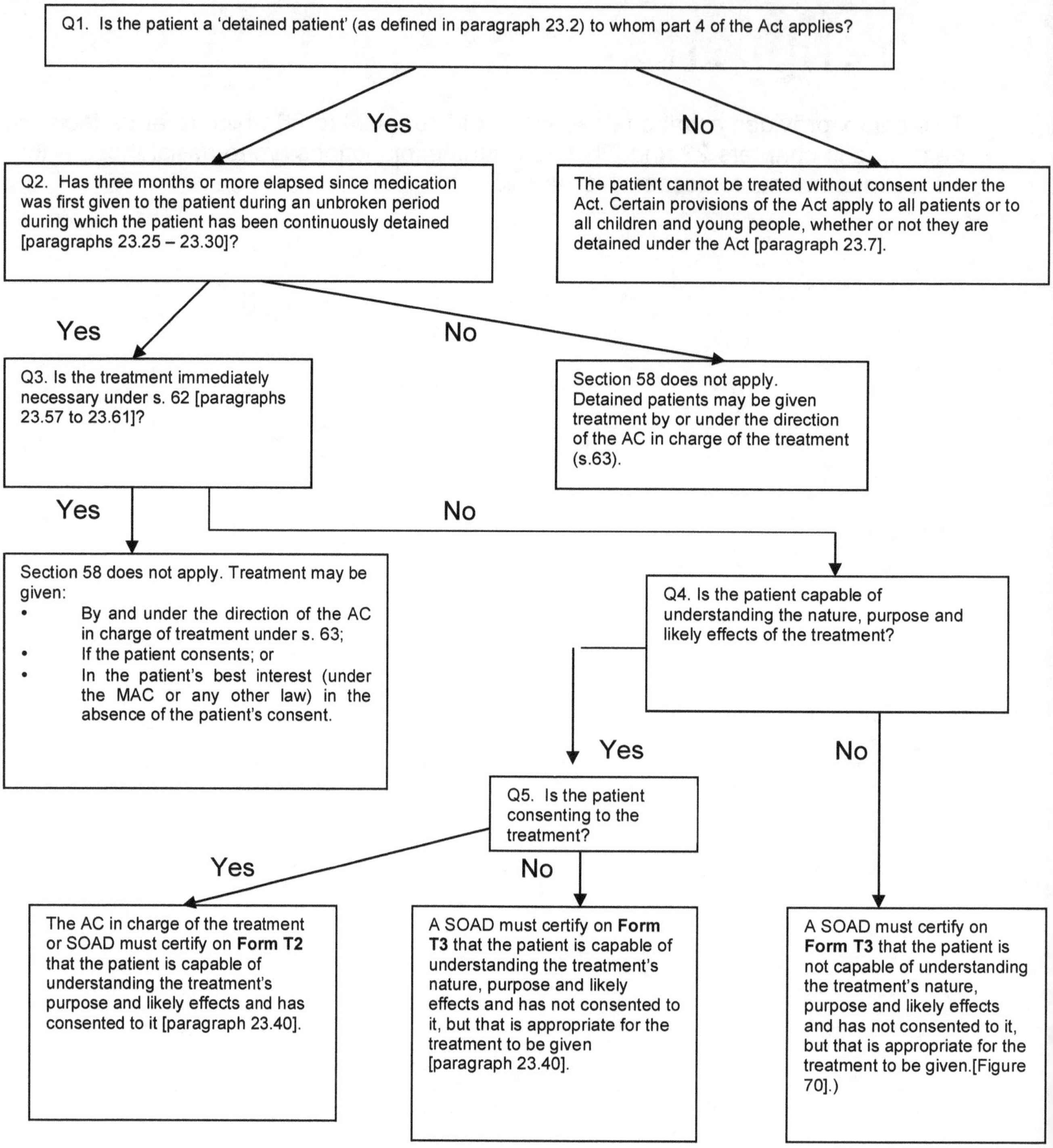

---

dMA Excluding medication administered as part of ECT ('section 58A treatment'): refer to paragraphs 23.41 to 23.56 and section 57 treatment.

[171] A 'detained patient' as defined in paragraph 23.2

Written explanation of Figure 94: Treatment with medication for mental disorder[172] of detained patients[173] under the Act

The first question to be answered is whether or not the patient is a 'detained patient' as defined in paragraph 23.2 to whom part 4 of the Act applies?

If the answer to the first question is 'No', then the patient cannot be treated without consent under the Act. Although certain provisions of the Act apply to all patients or to all children and young people whether or they are detained under the Act as defined in paragraph 23.2.

If the answer to the first question is 'Yes', then the second question is whether three or more months have elapsed since medication was first given to the patient during an unbroken period during which the patient has been continuously detained as explained in paragraphs 23.25 – 23.30.

If the answer to the second question is 'No', then section 58 does not apply and detained patients may be given treatment, by or under, the direction of the approved clinician in charge of the treatment (see section 63 of the Act).

If the answer to the second question is 'Yes', then the third question is whether or not the treatment is immediately necessary under section 62, which is explained in paragraphs 23.57 – 23.61.

If the answer to the third is 'Yes', then section 58 does not apply and treatment may be given (i) by and under the direction of the approved clinician in charge of the treatment under section 63 (ii) if the patient consents or (iii) in the patient's best interest (under the Mental Capacity Act 2005) in the absence of the patient's consent.

If the answer to the third question is 'No', the fourth question is whether the patient is capable of understanding the nature, purpose and likely effects of the treatment?

If the answer to the fourth question is 'No', then a SOAD must certify on Form T3 that the patient is not capable of the understanding the nature, purpose and likely effects of the treatment, but that it is appropriate for the treatment to be given.

If the answer to the fourth question is 'Yes', then the fifth question is whether the patient is consenting to the treatment.

If the answer to the fifth question is 'Yes', then the approved clinician in charge of the treatment or the SOAD must certify on Form T2 that the patient is capable of understanding the nature, purpose and likely effects of the treatment and has consented to it (paragraph 23.40).

If the answer to the fifth question is 'No', then the SOAD must certify on Form T3 that the patient is capable of understanding the treatment's nature, purpose and likely effects and has not consented to it, but that is appropriate for the treatment to be given.

---

[172] Excluding medication administered as part of ECT ('section 58A treatment'): refer to Reference Guide 23.41 – 23.56.
[173] A 'detained patient' as defined in Reference Guide 23.2

Figure 95: Treatment with medication for mental disorder[174] under the Act of CTO patients[175] not recalled to hospital[176] ('section 58 type treatment' under part 4A)

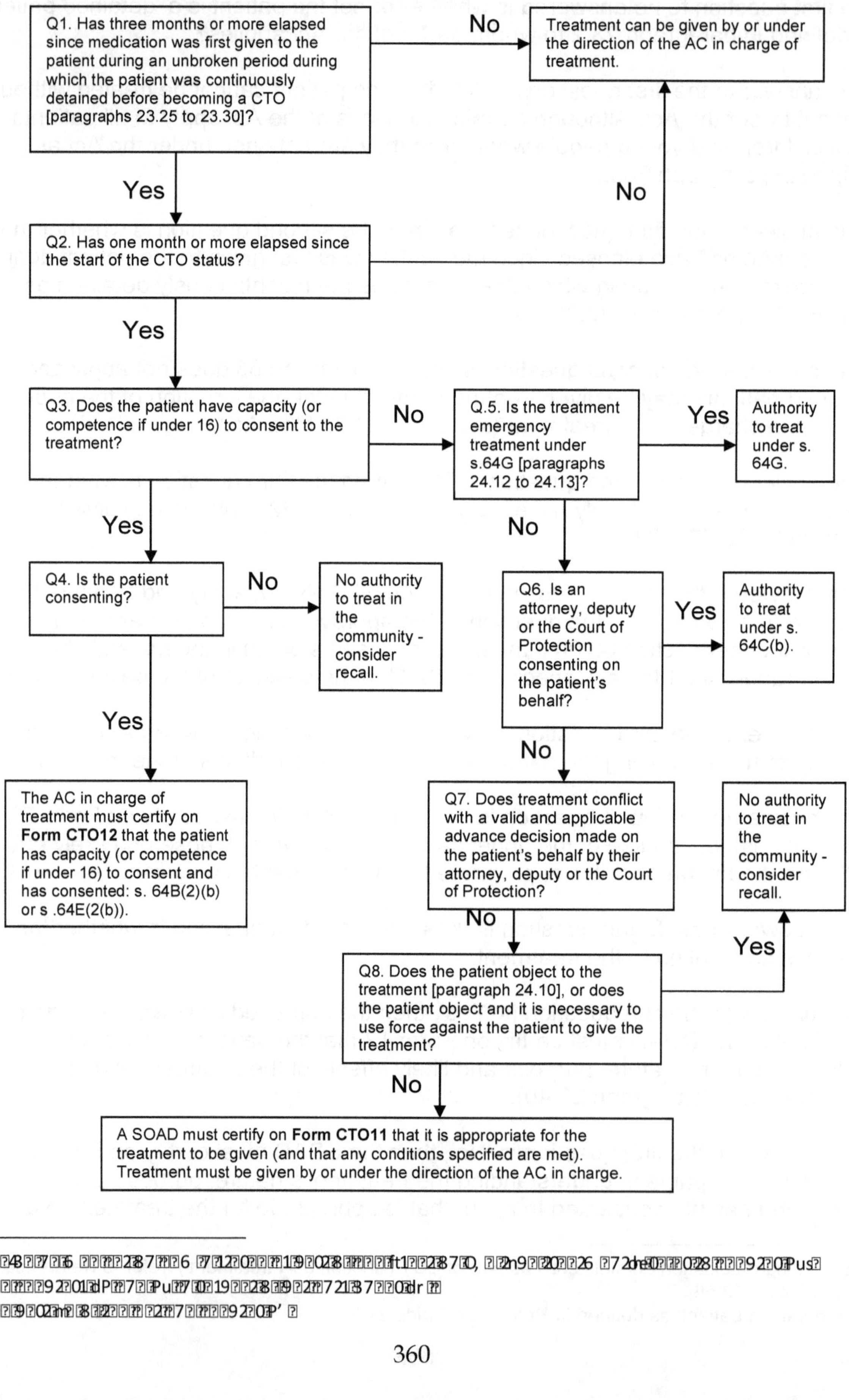

---

174 [illegible]

175 [illegible]

176 [illegible]

Written explanation of Figure 95: Treatment with medication for mental disorder under the Act of CTO patients not recalled to hospital ('section 58 type treatment' under part 4A)

The first question to be asked is whether three months or more have elapsed since medication was given to the patient during an unbroken period in which the patient was continuously detained before becoming a CTO patient.

If the answer to the first question is 'No', then treatment can be given by the approved clinician in charge of treatment even without the patient's consent.

If the answer to the first question is 'Yes', then the second question is whether one month or more has elapsed since the CTO was made.

If the answer to the second question is 'No', then treatment can be given by or under the direction of the approved clinician in charge of treatment.

If the answer to the second question is 'Yes', then the third question is whether the patient has the capacity (or if the patient is under 16, the competence) to consent to the treatment?

If the answer to the third question is 'Yes', then the fourth question is whether the patient consents to the treatment? If the answer is 'No' and the patient does not consent then there is no authority to treat the patient in the community but recall can be considered. If the answer is 'Yes' and the patient does consent then the approved clinician in charge of the treatment must certify on Form CTO12 that the patient has the capacity (or competence, if under 16) to consent to the treatment and has consented.

If the answer to this third question is 'No', then the fifth question is whether or not the treatment is 'emergency treatment' under section 64G (as in paragraphs 24.12 to 24.13)?

If the answer to the fifth question is 'Yes', then treatment can be given in accordance with that section.

If the answer to the fifth question is 'No', then the sixth question is whether an attorney, deputy or the Court of Protection is consenting on the patient's behalf?

If the answer to the sixth question is 'Yes', then there is authority to treat based on that consent (under section 64C(2)(b).

If the answer to the sixth question is 'No', then the seventh question is whether the treatment conflicts with a valid and applicable advance decision made by the patient or a decision made on the patient's behalf by their attorney or deputy or the Court of Protection?

If the answer to the seventh question is 'Yes', there is no authority to treat the patient in the community and recall from the CTO should be considered.

If the answer to the seventh question is 'No', then the eighth question is whether the patient objects to the treatment or whether the person objects and it is necessary to use force against the patient to give the treatment.

If he answer to the eighth question is 'Yes', then there is no authority to treat the patient in the community and recall from the CTO should be considered.

If the answer to the eighth question is 'No', then a SOAD must certify on Form CTO11 that it is appropriate for the treatment to be given and that any conditions specified in the certificate are met). Treatment must be given by or under the direction of the approved clinician in charge of the treatment.

Figure 96: Treatment with medication for mental disorder[177] under the Act of CTO patients upon recall to hospital or the revocation of the CTO[178]

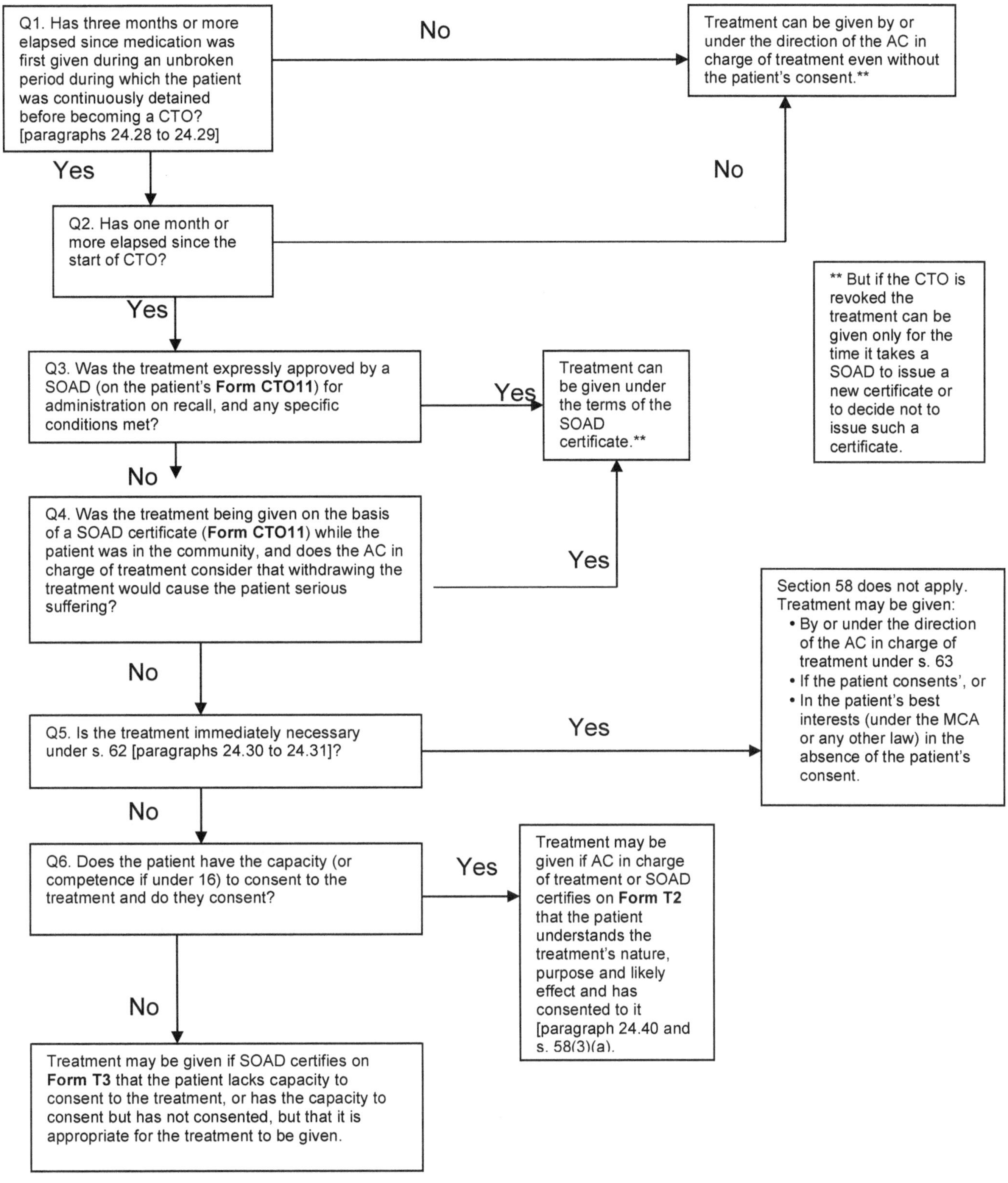

[177] Excluding medication administered as part of ECT ('section 58A treatment') see paragraphs 24.28 to 24.31.

[178] Refer to section 62A and paragraphs 24.32 to 24.42.

Written explanation of Figure 96: Treatment with medication for mental disorder under the Act of CTO patients upon recall to hospital or the revocation of the CTO

The first question is whether three or more months have elapsed since medication was first given to the patient during an unbroken period during which the patient was detained before they became a CTO patient?

If the answer to the first question is 'No', then treatment can be given by the approved clinician in charge of treatment even without the patient's consent.

If the answer to the first question is 'Yes', then the second question is whether one month or more has elapsed since the CT Order was made?

If the answer to the second question is 'No', then treatment can be given by or under the direction of the approved clinician in charge of the treatment even without the patient's consent.

If the answer to the second question is 'Yes', the third question is whether the treatment is expressly approved by a SOAD (on the patient's Form CTO11) for administration on recall, and whether any specific conditions have been met?

If the answer to the third question is 'Yes' then treatment can be given under the terms of the SOAD certificate.

If the answer to the third question is 'No', then the fourth question is whether the treatment was being given on the basis of a SOAD certificate (Form CTO11) while the patient was in the community, and does the AC in charge of treatment consider that withdrawing the treatment would cause the patient serious suffering?

If the answer to the fourth question is 'Yes', then treatment can be given under the terms of the SOAD certificate.

If the answer to the fourth question is 'No', then the fifth question is whether the treatment is immediately necessary under section 62? [paragraphs 24.30 to 24.31]. If the answer to this question is 'Yes' then Section 58 does not apply. Treatment may be given:

- by or under the direction of the AC in charge of treatment under s.63;
- if the patient consent; or
- in the patient's best interests (under the Mental Capacity Act 2005 or any other law) in the absence of the patient' consent.

If the answer to the fifth question is 'No', the sixth question is whether the patient has the capacity or (competence if they are under 16) to consent to the treatment and do they consent? If the answer is 'Yes' then treatment may be given if the approved clinician in charge of treatment or SOAD certifies on Form T2 that the patient understands the treatment's nature, purpose and likely effect and has consented to it [Paragraph 26.40 and section 58(3)(a)]. If the answer is 'No' then treatment may be given if a SOAD certifies on Form T3 that the patient lacks capacity to consent to the treatment, or has the capacity to consent but has not consented, but that it is appropriate for the treatment to be given.

Where the answers to the second question is 'No' and fourth question is 'Yes' treatment may be given, if a CTO has been revoked then treatment can be given only until a new certificate can be arranged, or it is decided not to issue such a certificate.

Annex E
Index by sections and schedules of the Act

Section No.	Heading	See in particular	See in Code of Practice
1	Application of Act: 'mental disorder'	Paragraphs 1.2, 1.7 to 1.15	Paragraphs 2.4 to 2.8
2	Admission for assessment	Paragraphs 8.2 to 8.5, 8.12 to 8.14, 9.5	Chapter 14
3	Admission for treatment	Paragraphs 8.6 to 8.14	Chapter 14
4	Admission for assessment in cases of emergency	Paragraphs 8.46 to 8.54, 8.61 to 8.64, 28.51	Chapter 15
5	Application in respect of patient already in hospital	Paragraphs 8.70 to 8.85, 9.5	Paragraphs 18.3 to 18.11, 18.19 to 18.40
6	Effect of application for admission	Paragraph 8.60, 8.66 to 8.69, 8.86 to 8.101, 26.134 to 26.140, 28.51, 28.145 to 28.147	Paragraphs 17.7 to 17.21, 37.12 to 37.13
7	Application for guardianship	Paragraphs 28.17, 28.23 to 28.30	Paragraphs 30.8 to 30.15, 35.14 to 35.15 35.18 to 35.20
8	Effect of guardianship application, etc	Paragraphs 26.134 to 26.140, 28.4 to 28.11, 28.52 to 28.64, 28.73 to 28.75, 32.38 to 32.39	
9	Regulations as to guardianship	Paragraphs 28.16, 28.76	
10	Transfer of guardianship in case of death, incapacity, etc of guardian	Paragraphs 28.130 to 28.138	
11	General provisions as to applications	Paragraphs 8.12 to 8.14, 8.21 to 8.30, 8.55 to 8.60, 28.25 to 28.30, 28.33 to 28.37, 28.46 to 28.51	
12	General provisions as to medical recommendations	Paragraphs 8.38 to 8.45, 8.55 to 8.60, 28.39 to 28.44, 28.51, 30.32 to 30.43	
12A	Conflicts of interest	Paragraphs 28.46 to 28.50	Chapter 39

Section No.	Heading	See in particular	See in Code of Practice
13	Duty of mental health professionals to make applications for admission or guardianship	Paragraphs 8.16 to 8.19, 8.31 to 8.37, 28.31 to 28.32, 28.38	Paragraphs 14.49 to 14.70, 29.22 to 29.26, 30.10 to 30.11
14	Social reports	Paragraphs 9.25 to 9.26	
15	Rectification of applications and recommendations	Paragraphs 32.22 to 32.37	Chapter 35
17	Leave of absence from hospital	Paragraphs 11.21 to 11.22, 25.2 to 25.7, 25.13 to 25.20	Chapter 27, Paragraphs 22.57 to 22.60, 31.4 to 31.5, 33.2
17A	Community treatment orders	Chapter 26	Chapters 29 and 31
17B	Conditions		
17C	Duration of community treatment order		
17D	Effect of community treatment order		
17E	Power to recall to hospital		
17F	Powers in respect of recalled patients		
17G	Effect of revoking community treatment order		
18	Return and readmission of patients absent without leave	Paragraphs 11.12 to 11.13, 25.21 to 25.28, 26.67 to 26.71, 28.91 to 28.96	Paragraphs 28.3 to 28.10
19	Regulations as to transfer of patients	Paragraphs 10.5 to 10.12, 10.20 to 10.23, 10.29 to 10.38, 28.139 to 28.144, 28.153 to 28.155	Paragraphs 22.61 to 22.63
19A	Regulations as to assignment of responsibility for community patients	Paragraphs 26.126 to 26.133	Paragraph 37.31
20	Duration of authority	Paragraphs 9.5, 25.29 to 25.35, 28.97 to 28.102	Paragraphs 32.1 to 32.16, 32.19 38.50
20A	Community treatment period	Paragraphs 26.72 to 26.79	Paragraphs 32.11 to 32.16
20B	Effect of expiry of community treatment order	Paragraphs 26.72 to 26.79	

Section No.	Heading	See in particular	See in Code of Practice
21	Special provisions as to patients absent without leave	Paragraphs 25.36 to 25.41, 26.67 to 26.71, 26.80 to 26.85, 26.94 to 26.104, 28.103 to 28.108	
21A	Patients who are taken into custody or return within 28 days	Paragraphs 25.36 to 25.41, 25.50 to 25.53, 26.80 to 26.85, 26.94 to 26.104, 28.103 to 28.108, 28.116 to 28.119	
21B	Patients who are taken into custody or return after more than 28 days	Paragraphs 25.21 to 25.28, 25.42 to 25.53, 26.86 to 26.97, 28.109 to 28.119	
22	Special provisions as to patients sentenced to imprisonment, etc	Paragraphs 25.54 to 25.58, 28.120 to 28.122	
23	Discharge of patients	Paragraphs 25.64 to 25.83, 26.105 to 26.118, 28.21 to 28.22, 28.123, 28.125 to 28.128	Chapter 38, paragraphs 29.75 to 29.77, 32.17 to 32.21, 32.26
24	Visiting and examination of patients	Paragraphs 25.92 to 25.94, 26.123, 28.124	Paragraphs 11.7 to 11.10
25	Restrictions on discharge by nearest relative	Paragraphs 25.64 to 25.75, 26.105 to 26.114	Paragraphs 32.22 to 32.25
26	Definition of 'relative' and 'nearest relative'	Paragraphs 1.23 to 1.28, 2.6 to 2.17	Paragraphs 5.2 to 5.4
27	Children and young persons in care	Paragraphs 2.20 to 2.21, 12.6 to 12.19	Paragraph 5.3
28	Nearest relative of minor under guardianship, etc	Paragraphs 2.22 to 2.24, 12.20 to 12.22	
29	Appointment by court of acting nearest relative	Paragraphs 2.37 to 2.57	Paragraphs 5.7 to 5.24
30	Discharge and variation of orders under section 29	Paragraphs 2.58 to 2.60	
31	Procedure on applications to county court	Paragraph 2.61	
32	Regulations for purposes of Part II	Paragraphs 2.25 to 2.36, 26.7 to 26.8, 31.7 to 31.17	
33	Special provisions as to wards of court	Paragraphs 8.15, 12.12 to 12.15	

Section No.	Heading	See in particular	See in Code of Practice
34	Interpretation of Part II	Paragraphs 1.29 to 1.31, 9.27 to 9.29, 28.18 to 28.20, 28.77 to 28.80	
35	Remand to hospital for report on accused's mental condition	Paragraphs 14.2 to 14.7, 14.17 to 14.24, 25.61 to 25.63	Paragraphs 22.13, 22.16 to 22.24
36	Remand of accused person to hospital for treatment	Paragraphs 14.8 to 14.13, 14.17 to 14.24, 25.61 to 25.63	Paragraph 22.40
37	Powers of courts to order hospital admission or guardianship	Paragraphs 15.2 to 15.10, 15.22 to 15.26, 28.17, 28.65 to 28.71, 28.145 to 28.147	Paragraphs 22.53 to 22.56, 30.38 to 30.39,
38	Interim hospital orders	Paragraphs 15.21, 18.2 to 18.9, 18.12 to 18.16, 25.61 to 25.63	Paragraphs 22.15, 22.36, 38.2
39	Information as to hospitals	Paragraphs 14.14 to 14.15, 15.11 to 15.12	
39A	Information to facilitate guardianship orders	Paragraph 28.72	
40	Effect of hospital orders, guardianship orders and interim hospital orders	Paragraphs 11.20, 15.30, 15.34 to 15.39, 15.42 to 15.44, 18.10 to 18.11, 18.13 to 18.16, 19.26 to 19.27, 26.141 to 26.142, 28.73 to 28.75, 28.145 to 28.147	Chapters 30 and 31, paragraphs 22.13, 22.24, 22.27, 22.28.
41	Power of higher courts to restrict discharge from hospital	Paragraphs 15.13 to 15.20, 15.40 to 15.44, 21.3 to 21.6, 21.11 to 21.16, 21.19 to 21.24, 25.59 to 25.60, 27.20 to 27.26, 28.73 to 28.75	
42	Powers of Secretary of State in respect of patients subject to restriction orders	Paragraphs 21.3 to 21.6, 21.7 to 21.14, 21.17 to 21.18, 21.25 to 21.26, 27.2 to 27.15, 27.20 to 27.26	Paragraphs 22.78 to 22.84
43	Power of magistrates' courts to commit for restriction order	Paragraphs 17.2 to 17.3, 17.10 to 17.12	
44	Committal to hospital under section 43	Paragraphs 17.4 to 17.9	
45	Appeals from magistrates' courts	Paragraphs 15.27 to 15.29, 16.2 to 16.7, 16.9, 16.12 to 16.14, 18.6 to 18.9	Paragraphs 22.22 to 22.74

Section No.	Heading	See in particular	See in Code of Practice
45A	Power of higher courts to direct hospital admission	Chapter 16, Paragraphs 25.59 to 25.60	Paragraphs 22.70 to 22.74
45B	Effect of hospital and limitation directions	Chapter 16	
47	Removal to hospital of persons serving sentences of imprisonment, etc	Paragraphs 19.2 to 19.5, 19.8 to 19.13, 19.26 to 19.27	Paragraphs 22.64 to 22.69, 22.75 to 22.77
48	Removal to hospital of other prisoners	Paragraphs 20.2 to 20.4, 20.7 to 20.9	Paragraphs 22.64 to 22.69
49	Restriction on discharge of prisoners removed to hospital	Paragraphs 19.6 to 19.7, 20.5 to 20.6	Paragraphs 22.64 to 22.69
50	Further provisions as to prisoners under sentence	Paragraphs 16.15 to 16.22, 16.25, 19.14 to 19.21, 19.25, 21.15 to 21.16	
51	Further provisions as to detained persons	Paragraphs 17.8 to 17.12, 20.10, 20.22 to 20.27	
52	Further provisions as to persons remanded by magistrates' courts	Paragraph 20.10, 20.15 to 20.21	Paragraphs 22.39 to 22.41
53	Further provisions as to civil prisoners and persons detained under the Immigration Acts	Paragraphs 20.10, 20.28 to 20.31	Paragraphs 14.126 to 14.129
54	Requirements as to medical evidence	Paragraphs 15.45 to 15.47	Paragraphs 14.71 to 14.76
54A	Reduction of period for making hospital orders	Paragraph 15.47, 18.10	
55	Interpretation of Part III	Paragraphs 15.22 to 15.26, 15.42 to 15.44, 19.26 to 19.27, 21.19 to 21.24, 28.73 to 28.75	
56	Patients to whom Part 4 applies	Paragraphs 14.17 to 14.24, 15.22 to 15.26, 18.13 to 18.16, 2.32	Paragraphs 24.10 to 24.11
57	Treatment requiring consent and a second opinion	Paragraphs 23.7 to 23.8, 23.12 to 23.14, 23.17 to 23.24	Paragraphs, 19.79, 24.8 to 24.13, 25.7 to 25.10, 25.45 to 25.52, 25.53 to 25.71
58	Treatment requiring consent or a second opinion	Paragraphs 12.10 to 12.11, 23.7 to 23.8, 23.12 to 23.14, 23.25 to 23.62	Paragraphs 19.78 24.8 to 24.13 25.11 to 25.18 , 25.45 to 25.71

Section No.	Heading	See in particular	See in Code of Practice
58A	Electro-convulsive therapy, etc	Paragraphs 12.10 and 12.11 (and Figure 71)	Paragraphs 13.63 to 13.66, 19.80 to 19.84, 19.87, 24.8 to 24.13, 25.19 to 25.25,
59	Plans of treatment	Paragraph 23.22	Paragraphs 24.45 to 24.53
60	Withdrawal of consent	Paragraphs 23.23, 23.39, 23.54	
61	Review of treatment	Paragraphs 23.63 to 23.68, 24.49 to 24.51	Paragraphs 25.76 to 25.80
62	Urgent treatment	Paragraphs 23.25 to 23.40, 23.67 to 23.68, 24.33 to 24.44	Paragraphs 25.37 to 25.42
62A	Treatment on recall of community patient or revocation of order	Paragraphs 23.25 to 23.40, 23.62, 24.33 to 24.44	Paragraphs 24.10 to 24.13
63	Treatment not requiring consent	Paragraph 23.16	Paragraphs 24.40 to 24.44
64	Supplementary provisions for Part IV	Paragraphs 23.15, 24.3 to 24.32, 24.46 to 24.51	
64A	Meaning of 'relevant treatment'	Chapter 24	Chapters 24 and 25
64B	Adult community patients		
64C	Section 64B: supplemental		
64D	Adult community patients lacking capacity		
64E	Child community patients		
64F	Child community patients lacking capacity		
64G	Emergency treatment for patients lacking capacity or competence		
64H	Certificates: supplementary provisions		
64I	Liability for negligence		
64J	Factors to be considered in determining whether patient objects to treatment		
64K	Interpretation of Part 4A		

Section No.	Heading	See in particular	See in Code of Practice
66	Applications to tribunals	Paragraphs 6.24 to 6.30, 6.31 to 6.33, 10.29 to 10.33	Chapter 12, paragraphs 19.107 to 19.110
67	References to tribunals by Secretary of State concerning Part II patients	Paragraphs 6.55 to 6.58, 6.64 to 6.66	
68	Duty of managers of hospitals to refer cases to tribunal	Paragraphs 6.42 to 6.54, 6.63 to 6.66, 10.29 to 10.33	Paragraphs 12.10 and 37.39
68A	Power to reduce periods under section 68	Paragraph 6.63	
69	Applications to tribunals concerning patients subject to hospital and guardianship orders	Paragraphs 6.24 to 6.32	Chapter 12, paragraphs 4.52 and 30.16
70	Applications to tribunals concerning restricted patients	Paragraphs 6.24 to 6.30, 27.16 to 27.19	Paragraph 22.56
71	References by Secretary of State concerning restricted patients	Paragraphs 6.59 to 6.61, 6.63	
72	Powers of tribunals	Paragraphs 6.69 to 6.79	Paragraph 29.19
73	Power to discharge restricted patients	Paragraphs 6.80 to 6.88, 21.7 to 21.14, 27.2 to 27.10, 29.11 to 29.13	Paragraphs 22.78 to 22.80
74	Restricted patients subject to restriction directions	Paragraphs 6.89 to 6.97, 16.23 to 16.24, 19.22 to 19.24, 20.11 to 20.14	Paragraph 22.56
75	Applications and references concerning conditionally discharged restricted patients	Paragraphs 6.98 to 6.99, 21.11 to 21.14, 27.2 to 27.10, 27.16 to 27.26	Paragraphs 22.78
76	Visiting and examination of patients	Paragraphs 6.38 to 6.40	Paragraphs 11.7 to 11.10
77	General provisions concerning tribunal applications	Paragraphs 6.34 to 6.37, 6.62	Chapter 12
78	Procedure of the Mental Health Review Tribunal for Wales		
79	Interpretation of Part V	-	

Section No.	Heading	See in particular	See in Code of Practice
80	Removal of patients to Scotland	Paragraphs 34.24 to 34.30, 35.3 to 35.5, 35.12 to 35.14	
80ZA	Transfer of responsibility for community patients to Scotland	Paragraphs 35.20 to 35.26	
80A	Transfer of responsibility for conditionally discharged patients to Scotland	Paragraph 35.19	
80B	Removal of detained patients from Scotland	Chapter 34	
80C	Removal of patients subject to compulsion in the community from Scotland	Chapter 34	
80D	Transfer of conditionally discharged patients from Scotland	Chapter 34	
81	Removal of patients to Northern Ireland	Paragraphs 36.3 to 36.5, 36.10 to 36.11, 36.22 to 36.25	
81ZA	Removal of community patients to Northern Ireland	Paragraphs 36.19 to 36.21	
81A	Transfer of responsibility for patients to Northern Ireland	Paragraphs 36.16 to 36.18	
82	Removal to England and Wales of patients from Northern Ireland	Paragraphs 34.31 to 34.35	
82A	Transfer of responsibility for conditionally discharged patients to England and Wales from Northern Ireland	Chapter 34	
83	Removal of patients to Channel Islands or Isle of Man	Paragraphs 37.3 to 37.5, 37.11 to 37.12, 37.23 to 37.26	
83ZA	Removal or transfer of community patients to Channel Islands or Isle of Man	Paragraphs 37.16 to 37.22	

Section No.	Heading	See in particular	See in Code of Practice
83A	Transfer of responsibility for conditionally discharged patients to Channel Islands or Isle of Man	Paragraph 37.15	
84	Removal to England and Wales of offenders found insane in Channel Islands and Isle of Man	Paragraphs 34.40 to 34.41	
85	Patients removed from Channel Islands or Isle of Man	Paragraphs 34.24 to 34.25, 34.36 to 34.39	
85ZA	Responsibility for community patients transferred from Channel Islands or Isle of Man	Paragraphs 34.36 to 34.39	
85A	Responsibility for conditionally discharged patients transferred from Channel Islands or Isle of Man	Paragraphs 34.36 to 34.39	
86	Removal of alien patients	Paragraphs 41.3 to 41.9	
87	Patients absent from hospitals in Northern Ireland	Paragraphs 11.23 to 11.25	
88	Patients absent from hospitals in England and Wales	Paragraphs 11.14 to 11.15	
89	Patients absent from hospitals in the Channel Islands or Isle of Man	Paragraphs 11.23 to 11.25	
90	Regulations for purposes of Part VI	Chapters 34 to 38 (passim)	
91	General provisions as to patients removed from England and Wales	Paragraphs 35.15 to 35.18, 35.20 to 35.26, 36.12 to 36.15, 37.13 to 37.14, 41.10	
92	Interpretation of Part VI	Paragraphs 35.3 to 35.5, 35.19, 36.3 to 36.5, 36.16 to 36.18, 37.3 to 37.5, 37.15	

Section No.	Heading	See in particular	See in Code of Practice
114	Approval by local authority	Paragraphs 30.2, 30.8 to 30.31	
114A	Approval of courses etc for approved mental health professionals	Paragraphs 30.27 to 30.28	
115	Powers of entry and inspection	Paragraphs 7.2 to 7.5	
116	Welfare of certain hospital patients	Paragraphs 12.16 to 12.19, 28.156	
117	After-care	Paragraphs 29.2 to 29.13, 29.16 to 29.19	Paragraphs 19.111 to 112, 22.50, Chapter 33
117A	After-care: preference for particular accommodation	Paragraph 29.3	Paragraph 32.18
117B	After-care: exceptions for provision of nursing care		
118	Code of Practice	Paragraphs 3.2 to 3.9	
119	Practitioners approved under part IV and section 118	Paragraphs 3.22 to 3.23, 23.12 to 23.14	Paragraphs 25.45 to 25.52
120	General protection of detained patients	Paragraphs 3.14 to 3.21, 3.25	XXIV to XXVII
126	Forgery, false statements, etc	Paragraphs 33.2 to 33.4	
127	Ill-treatment of patients	Paragraphs 33.5 to 33.10	
128	Assisting patients to absent themselves without leave, etc	Paragraphs 33.11 to 33.12	
129	Obstruction	Paragraphs 33.13 to 33.14	
130	Prosecutions by local authorities	Paragraphs 4.2 to 4.22, 9.20, 33.16 to 33.17	
130A	Independent mental health advocates	Chapter 4	Chapter 6
130B	Arrangements under section 130A		
130C	Section 130A: supplemental		
130D	Duty to give information about independent mental health advocates	Paragraphs 26.30, 28.89	Paragraphs 6.15 to 6.16

Section No.	Heading	See in particular	See in Code of Practice
131	Informal admission of patients	Paragraphs 9.21 to 9.24,12.3 to 12.9, 13.2 to 13.4	Paragraphs 4.49 to 4.51, 14.11, 14.14 to 14.16, 19.57 to 19.70 26.46
131A	Accommodation, etc for children	Paragraphs 9.21 to 9.24	Paragraphs 19.90 to 19.104
132	Duty of managers of hospitals to give information to detained patients	Paragraphs 9.10 to 9.19, 10.26 to 10.28	Paragraphs 4.9 to 4.36, 4.48, 19.75 to 19.77
132A	Duty of managers of hospitals to give information to community patients	Paragraphs 26.28 to 26.29	Paragraphs 4.9 to 4.36, 29.34 to 29.35, 29.68,
133	Duty of managers of hospitals to inform nearest relatives of discharge	Paragraphs 25.89 to 25.91, 26.7, 26.112	Paragraph 4.33
134	Correspondence of patients	Paragraph 3.24, 5.2 to 5.19	
134A	Review of decisions to withhold correspondence		
135	Warrant to search for and remove patients	Paragraphs 7.6 to 7.16	Paragraphs 16.3 to 16.16, 28.9 to 28.10
136	Mentally disordered persons found in public places	Paragraphs 7.17 to 7.20	Paragraphs 16.17 to 16.29, 16.40, 19.105, 28.9 to 28.10
137	Provisions as to custody, conveyance and detention	Paragraphs 8.66 to 8.69, 10.16 to 10.19, 11.2 to 11.4, 11.21 to 11.22, 35.12 to 35.14, 36.10 to 36.11, 37.11 to 37.12	Paragraphs 22.32 to 22.38
138	Retaking of patients escaping from custody	Paragraphs 8.66 to 8.69, 10.16 to 10.19, 11.5 to 11.13, 11.21 to 11.22, 15.31 to 15.33, 16.10 to 16.11	
139	Protection for acts done in pursuance of this Act	Paragraphs 33.18 to 33.21	
140	Notification of hospitals having arrangements for special cases	Paragraphs 8.20, 12.5 to 12.9	Paragraphs 14.77 to 14.86
142A	Regulations as to approvals in relation to England and Wales	Paragraphs 30.44 to 30.50	

Section No.	Heading	See in particular	See in Code of Practice
142B	Delegation of powers of managers of NHS foundation trusts	Paragraphs , 26.7 to 26.8, 31.7 to 31.17	
143	General provisions as to regulations, orders and rules	-	
144	Power to amend local Acts	-	
145	Interpretation	Paragraphs 1.17 to 1.22, 1.29 to 1.31, 1.33 to 1.36, 2.33 to 2.36, 30.3 to 30.7, 30.38 to 30.43, 31.2 to 31.6	
146	Application to Scotland	-	
147	Application to Northern Ireland	-	
148	Consequential and transitional provisions and repeals	-	
149	Short title, commencement and application to Scilly Isles	-	

Note: Sections 16, 25A to 25J, 46, 93 to 113, 121,123 124, 125 and 141 have been repealed. In practice, sections 65 and 78 now apply only to the Mental Health Review Tribunal for Wales. Section 122 applies only to Wales.

Schedules

Schedule No.	Heading	See in particular	See in Code of Practice
1	Application of certain provisions to patients subject to hospital and guardianship	Paragraph 15.35	
	Part I – Patients not subject to special	Paragraph 4.35	
	Part II – Patients subject to special	Paragraphs 4.41, 21.3 to 21.6	

Note: In practice, Schedule 2 now applies only to the Mental Health Review Tribunal for Wales. Schedule 3 has been repealed. Schedule 4 (consequential amendments) and Schedule 6 (repeals) made amendments to other legislation, not the Act itself. Schedule 5 (transitional and saving provisions) dealt with transitional arrangements in connection with the implementation of the Act in 1983, some of those arrangements may still be relevant to a small number of patients, but these are not described in this Reference Guide.

Adapted and published by GRANGIS under the OGL Licence.
GRANGIS - UK PUBLISHING 2022.
Thank you for taking the time to leave us a review regarding this edition"

★★★★★

For further inquiries, please feel free to contact us at:
www.grangis.com / contact@grangis.com

www.ingramcontent.com/pod-product-compliance
Lightning Source LLC
LaVergne TN
LVHW060210210926
848481LV00008B/2686